MAR 1 5

The Truth About Big Medicine

The Truth About Big Medicine

Righting the Wrongs for Better Health Care

Cheryl L. Brown and John T. James

ROWMAN & LITTLEFIELD
Lanham • Boulder • New York • London

Published by Rowman & Littlefield
A wholly owned subsidiary of The Rowman & Littlefield Publishing Group, Inc.
4501 Forbes Boulevard, Suite 200, Lanham, Maryland 20706
www.rowman.com

Unit A, Whitacre Mews, 26-34 Stannary Street, London SE11 4AB, United Kingdom

British Library Cataloguing in Publication Information Available

Library of Congress Cataloging-in-Publication Data

Brown, Cheryl L., 1961-,
The truth about big medicine : righting the wrongs for better health care / by Cheryl L. Brown and John T. James.
p. cm.
Includes bibliographical references and index.
ISBN 978-1-4422-3160-3 (cloth : alk. paper) -- ISBN 978-1-4422-3161-0 (electronic)
1. Malpractice--United States. 2. Clinical competence--United States. 3. Licensure, medical--standards--United States. 4. Medical errors--prevention and control--United States. 5. Peer review, health care--United States. 6. Truth disclosure--United States. W 44 AA1. I. James, John T., author. II. Title.
RT50
344.0414--dc223
2014023249

Printed in the United States of America

To Alex, who often asked me, "Why Daddy?"
Why indeed!
Even now, after twelve years without you, I still have no answer.

And

To all who have been harmed or perished . . . we speak for you.

Contents

Foreword

For the first time in the history of modern Western medicine, a growing segment of the American public is acutely aware of and outspoken about the reality that medical treatment is a leading cause of preventable death and disability in the United States.

Propelling this activism is the sheer number of Americans affected by medical errors, hospital-acquired infections, unsafe drugs and devices, overuse of inappropriate medical treatment, and the failure of medical licensing and credentialing to protect the public.

While many dedicated physicians and nurses work diligently to keep patients safe, the health care sector has evolved into a self-sealing, impermeable system that is perfectly designed to foster unsafe practices. Too often, it exists for its own benefit rather than for those who are sick and in need of compassion and competent caring.

Health care is big business. Safety failures in medical care are accelerating as the guiding mantra is to maximize revenue.

The health care industry has uncanny similarities to the financial industry. Both sectors have price bubbles, toxic assets and products, a too-big-to-fail attitude, and privatized gains and socialized losses whereby the system benefits financially from the harm it causes and shifts the human and financial cost to individuals and society.

An informed and active citizenry is the only antidote to reset the health care system so that it serves the public interest, not private interests. The task is enormous. For decades the public has trusted that the system is working for them and has given generously to pay for a health care sector that consumes nearly 20 percent of the country's gross domestic product.

Now, many Americans are awakening to the reality of where their money has been going, who is getting it, and what they are really doing with it. They are demanding more transparency and accountability for how the money is spent. Public pressure is mounting on Medicare and other insurers to stop paying hospitals and doctors when patients are harmed.

The authors in this volume are among a growing cadre of national leaders advocating for safer, more accountable health care for all Americans. They hail from many walks of life and work experience and include a university-based oceanographer, a former chief toxicologist for NASA, a former senior federal government official, public interest advocates, former career army nurse officers, and physicians who have cared for patients and observed firsthand the challenges that ethical clinicians encounter.

They are united and courageous in a common cause. Most volunteer their time to acquire deep knowledge of the inner workings of the health care establishment, a knowledge that is on par with that of a full-time, well-compensated health care professional. Some have lobbied successfully for legislative and regulatory remedies that strengthen accountability for safer care.

As doctors to the system, they diagnose its ills and prescribe remedies. Their aim is open, honest, and accountable health care that serves the public interest, not the special interests. They speak truth to power and remind us of the purpose of health care, which is to heal always, harm never.

I hope that readers who are inspired will join the cause. It is a noble one.

Rosemary Gibson
  May 2014

Acknowledgments

I would like to thank the professionals who pulled together from every corner of the country to make this book happen. I also am grateful for the input on apology and disclosure from Lee Taft. Thank you to numerous family, friends, and supporters who kept saying "you go, girl." To my children, Greg, Wesley, and Savannah, for their daily support during a busy two years of watching mom write; I love you guys. (Dr. Cheryl Brown)

I am grateful for thoughtful reviews of one or more chapters by John Santa, MD, Kim Witczak, and Kevin Kavanagh, MD. (Dr. John James)

I would like to thank Alan Levine of Public Citizen for providing helpful documentation and Michele Moseratte Ramos and Rex Johnson for excellent suggestions and discussions to improve the chapter. (Dr. Yanling Yu)

I would like to acknowledge the help I received from Dr. Frank Sebat and Dr. Ian Grady to help write our report on the root cause of the Redding Medical Center disaster, and Gil Mileikowsky for helping me understand the problems with effective peer review. (Dr. Gerald Rogan)

Thanks to Kevin T. Kavanagh of Health Watch USA for offering his expertise on reducing health care–associated infections. Thanks also to John James and Cheryl Brown for taking the time to edit and share ideas on patient safety. (Dr. Daniel Saman)

Thanks to the thousands of people who shared their stories about medical harm with Consumers Union and the dedicated activists in the Safe Patient Project Network who work every day to create a safer health care system. (Lisa McGiffert)

Introduction

The Empowered Patient

John T. James, PhD, DABT,
and Cheryl L. Brown, DBA, RN

An empowered patient may function at three levels. At the personal level many Americans are awakening to the fact that health care in our country can be inordinately expensive, dangerous, and unnecessary. They ask challenging questions and seek other expert opinions before accepting the need for invasive medical care. At the activist level, many patient safety advocates are filling important roles in federal, state, and local boards, panels, and commissions that implement laws and policies indirectly affecting the spectrum of patient care. A few highly empowered patients are engaging at the third level, which is to promulgate new laws from state and federal governments that are in the best interest of patients—and not necessarily in the interest of an often callous, money-driven medical industry. The medical industry has well-paid lobbyists representing industrial interests to lawmakers, who in turn create laws that favor industry. This is never clearer than in the drug industry, where the patient-protective role of the Food and Drug Administration (FDA) has been compromised by the pharmaceutical industry.[1]

OUR AUTHORS

Many of our authors are patient safety activists that came to this cause because of a critical event in their lives when they were seriously harmed by medical errors or had a loved one harmed by medical errors. The authors have been and are engaged in correcting the wrongs while often attacking and exposing the root causes of the harm done to them or family members.

They are experts in facets of the medical industry that have been slow or unresponsive to the need for change. They battle with powerful, entrenched, and well-funded entities that often refuse to hear their messages that too much harm is done in the name of medical care. They have well-thought-out solutions to right the wrongs that continue to occur, and in their writings they show how patients can become activists for the cause of safer care. Physicians trying to mitigate patient harm were another type of writer we sought. These doctors have been on the front lines of identifying and trying to improve a facet of the medical industry that has caused unbridled harm to many patients or has left patients at risk of harm from inadequate quality control of medical procedures. Experts with experience in critical databases and legislation were also selected. These individuals have worked much of their careers trying to empower patients with control and insight into the medical industry's processes and information. One author is a retired official who once oversaw the "secret" National Practitioner Data Bank, which is a compilation of individual physician malpractice settlements and disciplinary actions. Another worked tirelessly in many states to pass laws that gave patients more control and insight into their care. Their experience and insight provide foci for action and a roadmap for how to make or change laws that work for improved patient safety.

TOO MUCH HARM

Many caregivers are burned out by the present systems within which they work. Ninety percent of practicing physicians would not encourage others to join the profession. The number of suicides among doctors has reached about three hundred each year, and the pressure to see more patients to make ends meet has reduced the average primary-care visit to only twelve minutes.[2] Obviously, it is not in the patients' best interest to visit a physician who is nearly burned out. Patient safety activists have a strong interest in helping physicians enjoy their professional work and avoid burnout. Far too many Americans are harmed when they seek only to be healed from a disease.

Medicine is remarkably complex and undergoes constant updating of best-practices information. In many specialties and in the general practice of medicine, it would be a full-time job just to keep up with new findings and guidelines. One should not be surprised that medical errors occur with disturbing frequency. Based on recent data, the pre-2000 estimates of harm while hospitalized seem to be worse underestimates than had been thought. One review using four limited studies of adverse events in US hospitals estimated that in 2007 approximately 440,000 Americans had their lives significantly shortened by preventable adverse events in hospitals.[3] The investigation included estimates of five types of errors: commission, omission, communication, context, and diagnostic. Previous studies had not considered such a broad spectrum of ways in which medical errors could occur and they also did not consider the limitation of finding evidence of errors in medical records.

VARIETY IN ACCESSING CARE

There are several avenues whereby we enter into the medical system. We enter through doctor's offices, screening clinics, ambulatory surgical centers, convenient neighborhood walk-in stores, emergency rooms, and prescheduled appointments. Urgent care facilities and retail clinics in drug and grocery stores are springing up almost daily. These facilities have a different business model than retail clinics. The business model for urgent care facilities centers on readily available, high-cost, low-volume care. Some facilities charge up to $1,000 to walk in the door and seek medical attention. These are typically manned by a licensed physician. On the other hand, retail clinics are typically manned by a nurse practitioner or physician assistant, and the business model is one of low-cost, high-volume care available well into the evening. The cost of those visits typically ranges from $59 to $99, and they often substitute for more traditional visits with pediatricians.[4]

Accountable care organizations (ACOs) are groups of doctors, hospitals, or other health care providers who join together to deliver coordinated, high-quality health care to Medicare patients.[5] In principle at least, ACOs could contribute substantially to solving some of the problems highlighted in this book. The goal of ACOs is to ensure that patients receive the right care at the right time and do not receive unnecessary or duplicated care. When the Medicare program observes that an ACO is saving money for the program, then the ACO will share in the money saved. A pioneering ACO has been formed in Texas by the Kelsey-Seybold Clinic.[6] This ACO intends to achieve the goals of Medicare by coordinating care based on best evidence and through use of information technology. The quality measures include outcomes, accountability for proper care, and patient satisfaction. Emphasis will be placed on proactive and prevention services.

PROFIT VERSUS NONPROFIT HOSPITALS

Hospitals of various kinds, numbering roughly 7,500, exist throughout the country. Some of these operate for profit and others are operated as nonprofit entities.[7] In the name of profit, hospitals can be far too aggressive. For example, Marty Makary, MD, noted in his book *Unaccountable* that a surgeon colleague was urged through an e-mail from his department head to do more operations at the end of the year as bonus-giving time was approaching.

The surgeon replied, asking if his boss would like him to start removing normal gallbladders.[8] The idea that many nonprofit hospitals operate in a nonprofit manner has been challenged recently by a series of exposés by Rita Healy. Her latest report revealed that nonprofit hospitals threw lavish parties such as the Cedars-Sinai Medical Center's Board of Governors Gala in which a $125,000 Lexus was given away. In California alone, more than 100 hospital executives earn more than $1 million per year.[9] One must ask, "Where is the charity in all this, and why do such nonprofit enterprises benefit from a tax-exempt status?"

CRITICAL ACCESS HOSPITALS

Hospitals come in various sizes ranging from large tertiary-care institutions (often with formal teaching functions) to moderately sized suburban/community institutions to small rural hospitals called critical access hospitals (CAH). CAHs number nearly 1,300, with typically twenty-five or fewer beds, and are located approximately thirty-five miles from alternative facilities with acute care capability. The CAH designation was created in 1997 by Congress to stem the tide of closing hospitals that serve rural populations. However, it seems that CAHs have struggled to improve over the past decade compared to their larger counterparts. Based on outcomes in patients with heart attacks, congestive heart failure, or pneumonia in 2010, CAHs had mortality rates approximately 2 percent higher than their larger counterparts (13.3 percent versus 11.4 percent).[10]

SAFETY NET HOSPITALS

"Safety net" hospitals offer another distinctive health care setting. They serve an underprivileged population that often cannot pay for their care. These hospitals tend to be large and located in urban areas. Otis Brawley, MD, in his book *How We Do Harm* describes the culture at what he says is the largest hospital in the United States (950 beds)—Grady Memorial Hospital in Atlanta, which serves the indigent. He describes appalling conditions and notes that historical-racial segregation has given way to economic segregation—the rich do not want to come to Grady Memorial; it is for the poor.[11]

NURSING HOMES

Nursing homes offer various intensities of patient care. Patients that are too ill to return home after staying in an acute care hospital may require admission to a skilled nursing facility (SNF). The Office of Inspector General of the Department of Health and Human Services recently published a study of a nationally representative sample of medical records from SNFs to determine how often patients are harmed in these facilities. The investigators found that one-third of patients, having stayed thirty-five days or less, experienced harm or an adverse event while in an SNF. The preventability of such events was determined to be 59 percent, and many of the victims had to be returned to an acute care hospital for additional critical treatment after the harm or adverse event.[12] These hospital readmissions cost Medicare an estimated $2.8 billion in 2011. Advocacy for high-quality patient care in SNFs is clearly as important as advocacy in acute care hospitals. Many of us and our loved ones will spend our latter days in a nursing home receiving assisted living and medical care as our abilities and health conditions gradually deteriorate. Although many nursing homes offer skilled and compassionate care, recent studies found widespread overuse of antibiotic[13] and antipsychotic[14] prescriptions in this vulnerable population. This is to say nothing of the challenges of advocating for a seriously ill loved one in a for-profit nursing home that has cut nursing staff to the bone.[15]

MEDICAL DEVICES

Medical device manufacturers and their advertising networks are quickly becoming a political and economic force in America. Chapter 4 shares how device creators, through political influence, have been successful in limiting new regulations that would better protect patients from poorly designed or improperly manufactured devices. The FDA regulations on devices are weak because of beliefs that regulations stifle innovation. In March 2014 at least two device manufacturers created TV commercials, joining the drug manufacturers in advertising through this type of programming. One of the more egregious stories is that of the harm caused to women by transvaginal mesh implants manufactured by Johnson & Johnson. Harmed women are using social media to vent their frustrations over the lack of justice for the harm these devices caused. The harm includes erosion of tissue and perforation of bodily organs.[16] Tragically, multiple surgeries may be required to repair the damage.

HEALTH INSURANCE AND MEDICAL BILLS

Health insurance companies represent a process that expects money from us with fear as the underpinning driver. We buy health insurance because we fear that if we become seriously ill and need prolonged treatment, we will be left with serious harm to our net worth. Most bankruptcies result from patients' inability to pay their medical bills, and those who file for bankruptcy in the face of high medical bills often have some type of medical insurance.

Based on a national survey before the recent recession, medical bills were responsible for more than 60 percent of bankruptcies, and three-fourths of these people claimed to have health insurance.[17] A study from the Centers for Disease Control and Prevention noted that an average of 20 percent of Americans under sixty-five are living in households with difficulty paying medical bills. For those without insurance the portion was 36 percent, and for those with health insurance the portion was 14 percent.[18] Health insurance is not a guarantee that you will be able to pay your medical bills without serious injury to your net worth.

MEDICAL IMAGING

Technology developers and their marketing staffs play a growing role in American medicine. Large and complex machines have been built for screening and treating injuries and disease. Improper use and poor image interpretation skills are a setup for harmful events. Chapter 11 deals with overuse and misuse of imaging. Technology has also been developed to assist surgeons during operations. However, it is sometimes used well before improved outcomes have been demonstrated for that technology. Furthermore, as the technology is employed in patient care, physicians may find that the new technology may be more harmful than the older approach it was meant to replace. One example of this is the da Vinci robot used for robotic surgery. The Advisory Board Company summarized the issues with the robot and why the manufacturer recalled almost 1,400 of the devices; the FDA is investigating this device with an eye to vast underreporting of complications.[19]

CLINICAL TRIALS, APPLIED RESEARCH, AND PATIENT-CENTERED OUTCOMES

One author had the privilege of doing *basic* medical research in laboratories on the Bethesda Campus of the National Institutes of Health. This was during the days of President Nixon, whose plan was to win the war on cancer in a decade or less. Since that didn't happen, basic research still holds the promise of reducing harm from this dreaded disease. Clinical trials are also an important applied research effort that can lead directly to improvements in patient care. Typically, these involve a comparison of outcomes of a promising new treatment to outcomes elicited by the standard of care. One highly successful clinical trial in 1982 involved a comparison of the value of a β-blocker with the prevailing standard of care for patients with heart failure. The β-blocker was so successful that the trial was stopped early because those not receiving the β-blocker were dying much earlier than those who received it.[20] Unfortunately, the medical care industry's inability to transition this finding to clinical practice meant another twenty-five years before full use of β-blockers for patients with heart failure happened.[21] A small part of the national expenditure on health care is devoted to basic and applied research, and recently more attention is being given to transitioning the results of applied research to clinical use. A relatively new institute called the Patient Centered Outcomes Research Institute (PCORI) intentionally engages patient advocates in deciding which proposed research will be of most value to patients. An empowered patient can consider contributing to one of the PCORI decision groups.[22]

MEDICAL SCHOOLS: FOREIGN OR DOMESTIC?

The number of first-year enrollees in US medical schools reached an all-time high of 20,055 in 2013, partially in response to a prediction of a shortage of doctors.[23] In the past there has been concern that graduates of foreign medical schools may be less capable than their US-educated counterparts.

One study of in-hospital deaths from heart attack or congestive heart failure in Pennsylvania hospitals found that non-US citizens who graduated from foreign medical schools actually had better outcomes than their US-citizen counterparts that graduated from US medical schools. US-citizen graduates of foreign medical schools seemed to perform a bit worse than the other two groups.[24]

MEDICAL CARE COSTS

Health care in the United States costs far more per person than in any other developed country. In constant 2009 dollars the cost per capita in the United States has grown from $500 in 1950 to $8,200 per year in 2009. In the same constant dollars, the average new car cost increased from $13,000 to $20,000 per year. One could argue that medical care has developed marvelous new technology in the intervening years, and that is true. But car makers have also developed and adapted marvelous new technology to improve reliability and safety of their products. At present the medical industry consumes 17 percent of our gross domestic product, whereas in other developed countries it is no more than 10 percent.[25] Most health care economists agree that we cannot go on like this, yet solutions to the high cost of medical care seem to be elusive. A common estimate of the waste in medical care spending now is about $750 billion per year.[26] Two causes of this waste are, first, that our system is underloaded with less-expensive primary care physicians compared to other countries and we, as a consequence, lack an emphasis on preventive care.[27] Second, costs for procedures are often not known by hospital personnel and physicians, so knowing costs ahead of time for a scheduled procedure may be challenging. If one is in an emergency situation, say because of a possible ruptured appendix, the cost of removing it has been shown to vary more than a hundredfold in the State of California.[28] There is no rational explanation for such variation in cost except for a free-enterprise medical system run amok. This must change.

MEDICAL RECORDS

Our nonstandardized national system of medical record keeping is nothing short of a profound tragedy. A recent president's administration decided that formatting and provision of electronic medical records throughout the country should follow the capitalist model and be subject to competition. That competition persists today and leaves patients at increased risk, because medical records have become a patchwork of disorganized information. For example, if you have a heart attack at 2 a.m. on a Sunday away from home and nowhere near your medical care community, would you have access to your medical records? You certainly would if you lived in other countries such as France or Taiwan. There each and every citizen is issued an electronic card with their medical record and billing information.[29]

CHOOSING A DOCTOR

Consumers have few resources to help select quality, cost-effective care in the United States. The US medical industry operates more or less on a free-enterprise model. That model depends on consumers of the product in question being able to make wise choices about where to obtain the product—in the present case, safe and cost-effective health care. How do you choose the best hospital in your area for the kind of care you need? Some websites offer limited ratings of hospitals, but these are typically for selected procedures; some involve a most important element—customer/patient feedback. Choosing a physician wisely is more difficult than selecting a hospital. Although there are websites that purport to rate physicians based on perceived quality of care received by patients, these would not withstand a test of statistical validity.

SELF-REGULATE?

Doctors and hospitals want autonomy to engage the patient as they see fit, and patients naively expect someone to be in charge of ensuring quality care. That's not the way it is. Much of the medical industry self-regulates. Medical boards that are expected by the public to discipline physicians are run by physicians. Organizations that accredit hospitals are funded by hospitals, and drug and device regulation is heavily constrained by powerful special-interest lobbies.

PATIENT BILL OF RIGHTS

The best way forward for attaining a national patient bill of rights is to get a bill passed in one or more key states. After some experience with such a law in a few states, a polished model of the law should be brought forward at the national level. We would note that the bill of rights we envision is much more far-reaching than previous versions developed by political entities such as President Clinton. Clearly he did recognize the value of a national, enforced patient bill of rights.[30]

WHAT WE HOPE TO ACCOMPLISH

Our readers will learn about regulatory gaps that facilitate patient harm; medical boards that don't completely regulate a doctor's quality of care; failed peer review allowing physicians to practice outside any effective oversight by their colleagues; and weaknesses in the FDA's ability to regulate drugs and devices that brought harm and early death to patients. Our readers will get answers to questions such as who regulates the quality of those who read images that guide so much of modern medical care; who has oversight of safe practices in doctor's offices; who has access to information on doctors that have malpractice judgments against them; and who ensures that you receive enough information to give your informed consent for invasive procedures. Readers will also benefit from learning the legalities behind physician apology and disclosure after a harm event, plus who writes the laws passed by legislatures.

Our writers inform the reader on ways they can protect themselves from harm by gaps left in place from weak oversight and regulatory structures. The empowered patient will understand as much as they can about their health care needs and ask questions until they have enough information to make an informed decision. Powerful, confident patients will investigate the quality of hospitals and doctors that will be responsible for their care and will render feedback if that care is suboptimal or poor. Knowing that FDA approval does not necessarily mean a drug is safe and effective for you, powerful, well-informed patients will not take a drug until they understand whether it is effective and reasonably safe.

In the pages of this book we propose legislative/regulatory ways to make patient care safer. We have no interest in creating a climate in which all bow before onerous overregulation. However, we do seek to level the playing field between the consumer and the provider of medical care. In the past our nation passed laws to protect groups of Americans from exploitation by more powerful groups. Patients must have rights based on national legislation with enforcement outside the Department of Health and Human Services. These laws should originate with patient advocates and especially should not come from politicians beholden to the medical industry for reelection funds. One such bill of rights has been proposed by a patient activist. [31]

This book profiles successful efforts leading to improvements in laws, or new laws, that protect patients from harm. Together we must provide better ways for the provider community to respond when they have caused harm. Human beings make mistakes, and there must be a better way to capture mistakes, find their root causes, and then correct the system to prevent further harm. Secrecy should have no place in our vision of a patient-centered health care system. No one wants to admit that they hurt or caused the early death of another human being, yet mistakes must be acknowledged, disclosed, investigated, and shared with others so that we all learn in the interest of not repeating them.

Chapter One

The Failure of State Medical Boards to Protect the Public

Yanling Yu, PhD

For my father.

AN AWAKENING JOURNEY

Who wants to learn about state medical boards by losing a loved one to negligence? I do not know anyone who would want this experience with the agencies that are supposedly responsible for disciplining negligent or incompetent doctors to protect the public.

In March 2008 my father was hospitalized for acute bronchitis. To improve breathing, he was put on a noninvasive ventilator called bilevel positive airway pressure (BiPAP), a device commonly used at home for people with sleep apnea. After a course of antibiotics, my father's infection was gone, but he still needed periodic assistance with BiPAP, so he was referred to a regional hospital that specializes in weaning people off ventilators.

My father spoke no English, so I was his medical power of attorney and had been his advocate for years; I went with him to every doctor visit and was with him 24/7 during his hospital stays. This time was no exception. On the way to the special facility, my father asked me how long he had to stay there and when he could go home, where he would rather be. I told him he was one step closer to coming home because he was going to get good help. However, none of us knew this would be a fatal trip.

Arriving at the facility around noon, my father was still wearing a red allergy band that was put on him at the original hospital for his well-documented sulfa-drug allergy. In 2004 he was twice given a sulfa antibiotic called Bactrim. Both times, he suffered life-threatening reactions with severe

1

gastrological distress, mild renal failure, and abnormal electrolytes. Because of this well-documented allergy, the admitting nurse put an additional red allergy band on his wrist and noted the sulfa allergy on the medication reconciliation forms.

On the second day after admission, the attending physician, who was the medical director and the only regular doctor at the facility, prescribed a drug called Diamox, claiming it would reduce my father's elevated CO_2. Since this was a new medication for him, we asked questions about the drug, in particular the risks. Dr. X said Diamox would reduce blood pH but had no risks for my father. The doctor mentioned nothing about it containing sulfa. I was uncomfortable about lowering the blood pH when it was normal at admission, so I expressed concerns. The doctor became irritated and lectured us: "I have been a pulmonologist for over twenty-five years and have treated many COPD patients with Diamox. You people need to stand back and let me do my job." Intimidated by his abrupt manner, we did not ask any further questions. We assumed the doctor knew what he was doing, but this was a deadly mistake.

On his second day on Diamox, my father started a cascade of complications. He first developed ten episodes of diarrhea, followed by a noticeable decrease in his blood pH that required him to be kept on BiPAP longer. But these were just the tip of the iceberg. Shortly after the fourth dose, my father complained of dizziness and a headache as his blood pressure plummeted. To address his life-threatening hypotension, the hospital stopped further Diamox and administered emergently large amounts of IV fluids, which severely compromised his heart condition. His body was swollen up and his skin started to break down with large blisters and open bedsores. Devastated, we watched helplessly as my father spiraled downward, not knowing what had caused his sudden hypotension and rapid deterioration.

My father had been doing well on admission at the weaning facility. He was documented in the medical records as "stable," "alert," "smiling," "chatting with family," and finishing 100 percent of hospital meals. He was looking forward to having lunch and made jokes with my mother, who was also at the hospital. Now, only a week after Diamox, my father was suffering from acute respiratory failure, acute heart failure, and acute renal injury. Dr. X neither informed us nor documented the latter critical condition in the medical records; he never treated it either.

Crying out loud for help, I raised concerns to the doctor and hospital staff that my father might be having a drug reaction. But no one addressed my concerns. Dr. X blamed my father's health for his sudden deterioration.

On April 18, Dr. X told us he could do nothing further to help my father except a tracheotomy. It was against my father's physician directive signed by this doctor at admission. On April 20, we took my father home.

At the time of discharge, he could no longer eat, drink, talk, or breathe without BiPAP. The skin inside his mouth was peeling off due to the prolonged hours on BiPAP, and he suffered from two large, open bedsores. I rode home with my father in the ambulance. Sitting next to him and holding his hand, I wanted to tell him we were finally going home. But I could not say a word, and only had tears running down my face. His eyes were wide open, looking out of the small back window of the ambulance; I saw white, puffy clouds in the sky.

Three days later, my father lost his fight to the negligent use of Diamox only two weeks after being admitted for a simple weaning. After he passed away, we learned that Dr. X used Diamox as a respiratory stimulant that is noted in drug monograph as off-label and investigational. We also found numerous drug warnings in medical literature: (1) Diamox is contraindicative for my father's severe sulfa allergy and COPD;[1,2] (2) diarrhea, dizziness, headache, and lowering blood pH (a result of drug-induced metabolic acidosis) are among the significant side effects of Diamox, and the drug label has special warnings for the elderly and for patients with respiratory acidosis like my father;[3] (3) the latter side effect can be detrimental, and therefore the drug is rarely indicated for COPD patients;[4] (4) no quality clinical data have shown Diamox to be effective and safe when used as a respiratory stimulant on COPD patients;[5] (5) contrary to what Dr. X told us, Diamox can increase CO_2 for patients with severe COPD, so that they may develop severe acidosis and acute respiratory failure while on Diamox;[6,7] and (6) the risks of Diamox for these patients have been amply documented in medical literature since the 1990s and outweigh any benefit.[8]

We were shocked by our findings. Had we been informed about these significant risks and contraindications, we would never have allowed the administration of Diamox, because any one of these risks could have harmed my father.

Having lost our trust in this doctor and the hospital, we sought legal advice. After reviewing hospital records, nine out of ten attorneys believed there was malpractice but told us that a lawsuit was not economically feasible for my elderly father. One attorney suggested that we file a complaint with Washington State Medical Quality Assurance Commission (MQAC), our state medical board that supposedly investigates poor quality of care. Before dismissing us, the attorney warned us that MQAC rarely took actions against doctors.

Like most Americans, we had never heard of a state medical board before. We went to the commission's website and read: "It is the purpose and responsibility of the Medical Quality Assurance Commission (MQAC) to protect the public by assuring quality health care is provided by physicians and physician assistants."

Gathering all of the hospital records and medical references, we wrote MQAC a long, detailed letter, hoping this state agency would investigate what went wrong. However, six months after my father's death and the day before Thanksgiving, we received a brief letter from MQAC, stating that the commission was unable to present sufficient evidence to support disciplinary action. The letter offered no explanation for this decision.

On the same day that MQAC's letter arrived, we received in the mail a copy of an internal pharmacy note from the hospital. It documented that, before my father was given the first dose of Diamox, the hospital pharmacist warned Dr. X and the attending nurse of the risks of a drug reaction and anaphylaxis. Despite this warning, they went ahead with the drug treatment and told the nurse to monitor my father for anaphylaxis.

We were appalled. Why would anyone want to expose my vulnerable, elderly father to the risk of anaphylaxis when he had no medical emergency and was stable and improving? Why did this doctor not inform us about this significant drug warning and monitoring, when I was at his bedside 24/7? Why did no one ask my father if he felt any symptoms during the supposed monitoring, and why did no one address our concerns about a potential drug reaction after his blood pressure suddenly plummeted? According to the pharmacist's note, the drug warning was communicated to Dr. X three hours before we asked about the drug risks, yet he told us there were no risks and we should stand back and let him do his job.

To find out what the board investigated, we filed a Public Record Act request and discovered that MQAC never investigated the patient rights violation and was never aware of the pharmacist's warning. The doctor was also dishonest, falsely claiming a medical emergency at the time he prescribed the drug and using a single BiPAP-altered pH to fabricate a disorder of metabolic alkalosis that he never documented in medical records. When asked why he did not inform and treat my father for his acute renal failure, the doctor denied the condition and falsely quoted a lab test before the acute event.

MQAC never investigated and verified any of the false, self-serving statements with medical records. In the case summary, the MQAC reviewing member documented only "what the daughter said" and "what the respondent said." All statements from the doctor were accepted without question, even though many were contradictory to the medical records and could be easily verified even by a layperson. We were never given an opportunity to respond to Dr. X's false statements before MQAC made its decision.

Based on Washington State Uniform Disciplinary Act, RCW 18.130.180, we believe there was substantial evidence that Dr. X committed unprofessional conduct. He was incompetent, negligent, and dishonest, and he violated both federal and state patient rights and informed consent statutes.

In the following months, we contacted MQAC several times, asking for explanation of their decision. Finally, ten months after my father's death and four months after the board closed the case, they arranged a conference for us to meet with their chief investigator, whom I'll call John Marks, and a staff attorney I'll call Kathy Embry. However, only a few minutes into the discussion, we realized that these staff members had no intention to listen to us.

At the beginning of the meeting, John Marks made a rule that no medical issues would be discussed because we were not medical doctors. Following his "rule," he refused to look at the pharmacist's note and medical literature that warns against the use of Diamox in patients with severe COPD. Then, when we asked why MQAC did not investigate the patient rights violation, Marks claimed it was a legal issue and he could not discuss this with us either because we were not lawyers. He claimed that if we believed the doctor killed my father, we needed to go to an attorney; the state could not help us. When we pointed out that the doctor's statements were contradictory to the medical records, the investigator insisted that MQAC does not make mistakes. During the entire meeting, the two MQAC staff members repeatedly reminded us that it was serious to take a doctor's license away. Finally, they ended the meeting abruptly and walked out of the room. This meeting was the most disrespectful, abusive experience that we'd ever had in our lives; we were treated as if we were criminals.

I will never forget that day, when we were finally awakened to the reality that our state medical board does not exist to help patients find the facts, and there is no recourse and accountability. MQAC is more interested in defending their fellow physicians' reputations and licenses than in protecting patients. Such self-serving interests are in serious conflict with the public safety.

A BRIEF HISTORY OF STATE MEDICAL BOARDS

> Safeguarding the public's health and safety is the paramount responsibility of every disciplining authority and in determining what action is appropriate, the disciplining authority must first consider what sanctions are necessary to protect or compensate the public. —Washington RCW 18.130.160(12)

Each state has laws and regulations to define competent medical practice and to delegate exclusively the sole regulatory powers to a state medical board. As spelled out by statutes, the primary responsibility of state medical boards is to protect public health and safety by ensuring that all physicians in the state are properly licensed and comply with various federal and state laws and regulations governing the practice of medicine. Thus, medical boards are expected to protect the public against unethical, negligent, or incompetent doctors. Most Americans assume today that this state regulatory system exists to ensure patient safety. Unfortunately, state medical boards have a track record of paying less attention to patient safety than physicians' welfare. This lack of interest can be traced to the creation of medical boards during the years of their inception.

State medical boards were created by organized medicine pushing for laws to regulate the practice of medicine in the late 1800s. Arguably, the regulations were established to defend their own professional territory and to curb competition from "unorthodox" practitioners, rather than to protect the public.[9] Despite that, state legislatures clearly designate public protection as the boards' primary duty. Backed by state government, boards regulate medical professions primarily through licensure and discipline.

Practicing medicine requires a license in the United States.[10] As "gatekeepers," medical boards are supposed to ensure that those entering the practice meet minimum requirements, including graduation from a recognized medical school, postgraduate training, and passing the national medical licensing examination.[11] After physicians are licensed, medical boards periodically reregister licensees to continue their active status, which is contingent on their completion of continued medical education (CME). However, few boards assess physicians' performance and ensure care quality, such as checking the appropriateness of CMEs, verifying recertification, or conducting random practice audit.[12] Thus, to ensure medical quality, state medical boards focus their responsibility largely on disciplining professional licensees.[13]

Medical boards' discipline is mostly a passive process in response to complaints. According to a case study by the US Department of Health and Human Services,[14] 60 to 90 percent of complaints come from the general public and are predominantly concerned with poor quality of care. On average, 75 percent of cases are closed on the grounds of insufficient evidence, and boards are given a broad discretion to determine what to investigate. If the board does decide to take action, the form of discipline ranges from a stipulation to informal disposition (STID) to license revocation. Under a STID, a physician admits no wrongdoing but agrees to take some form of education class or rehabilitation. While varying among states, unprofessional conduct is usually defined as abuse of a patient; inadequate record keeping; failure to meet the standard of care; illegally prescribing drugs; failure to meet continuing medical education requirements; dishonesty; conviction of a felony; or delegating the practice to an unlicensed individual.[15]

Throughout the 1960s to the early 1990s, medical boards took few disciplinary actions on the basis of medical malpractice or incompetence, focusing almost entirely on criminal activity and substance abuse. Few people called attention to the inadequate disciplinary actions taken by medical boards.[16] This situation did not change significantly over the next twenty years. As noted by Dr. Robert Derbyshire, a former president of the Federation of State Medical Boards (FSMB), the disciplinary statistics rose insignificantly from 0.06 percent of all licensed physicians to 0.14 percent between 1963 and 1981.[17]

Consumers have long been a strong voice in criticizing the state medical boards for their conflicts of interest. As early as the 1980s, several prominent newspapers around the country published a series of articles reporting the lack of actions against incompetent doctors and questioning the effectiveness of the boards in protecting patients from medical harm.[18] For example, in 1986, Andrew Stein, the president of the New York City Council, wrote in the *New York Times*: "American doctors are killing and maiming thousands of patients every year—and, for the most part, they are getting away with it. It is time that we in government, and the medical profession, came up with some remedies for this national tragedy." He called for accountability, and at the same time Public Citizen estimated that as many as 200,000 Americans were injured or killed in hospitals each year as a result of negligent care.[19] To hold state medical boards accountable for protecting patients from bad doctors, Public Citizen has continued to publish its reports on questionable doctors and boards' disciplinary actions over the years.[20]

As skepticism and distrust grew, the public demanded more accountability and transparency. Gradually, nonphysician members, so-called "public members," were included in most medical boards to help balance the interests of physicians and the public, although boards were still dominated by physicians. Some states also enacted a sunset review policy to evaluate an agency's existence based on its effectiveness and performance.[21] All these changes signaled a greater government oversight and public accountability.

In response to public concerns, the federal government took a great interest in state medical boards between 1986 and 1993. During this period, the Office of Inspector General (OIG) of the Department of Health and Human Services (HHS) published eight reports based on their reviews of state medical boards' quality assurance activities, licensure and disciplinary functions, and performance. The OIG found that "in most states, violations involving drugs or alcohol seem to account for three-fourths or more of all disciplinary actions." And most disciplinary actions "involved reprimands or voluntary stipulations, which are often agreed to in informal proceedings." There were strikingly few disciplinary actions on the basis of medical malpractice or incompetence.[22]

Four years later, the OIG evaluated thirty-six state medical boards and found that they rarely documented complaint sources and types in their annual reports and provided minimal data for the public to evaluate these boards' performance.[23] In a 1993 report, the OIG further examined nine state medical boards, aiming to help improve state licensure, discipline, and other quality assurance efforts. The OIG listed a critical issue that the federal initiative intended to address: "States have much difficulty pursuing quality-of-care cases. These cases are time-consuming and complex and require legal and medical expertise. States often have problems identifying significant cases and investigating them. Some States have medical practice acts that make pursuing these cases even more difficult."[24]

Despite the federal oversight efforts in the past, however, state medical boards are still facing the same problems today.

THE SAME ELEPHANT IN THE ROOM

Twenty-eight years have passed since Andrew Stein called on the state medical board to stop the killing of thousands of patients each year by dangerous doctors. While medicine has become more technology laden and new drugs are pushed onto the market every year, US health care has not become any safer, and leniency is still too common among state boards. At the same time, the media around the United States continues to highlight public concern on preventable medical harm resulting directly from inactions of state medical boards.

Déjà Vu, Again?

In 2006, the *Seattle Times* published a series of articles, License to Harm. The *Times* investigation found that a large number of Washington health care professionals, including physicians, sexually abused hundreds of patients for years. Yet the Washington state regulatory boards, including MQAC, made it easy for the abusers to get away with it again and again. As a result, hundreds of doctors, counselors, and others kept practicing despite their sexual misconduct.[25]

In 2009, investigative reporter William Heisel and his team investigated 128 disciplinary actions of more than 100 physicians in every state and the District of Columbia. Nearly half of them were responsible for injuring or killing 290 patients. Yet 82 percent of them were still licensed to practice medicine.[26]

In 2010, the *Chicago Tribune* uncovered sixteen convicted sex offenders who held Illinois medical licenses within the past fifteen years. None of them had their license permanently revoked. In many cases, physicians were allowed to continue practicing in spite of allegations of serious misconduct and even convictions. The Illinois medical board believed that by law they could not permanently revoke a physician's license unless there had been two felony convictions.[27]

In 2010, the *St. Louis Post-Dispatch* found that Missouri doctors who provide substandard care often continue to practice without worry of any disciplinary action or their names appearing in public records. Sending confidential "letters of concern" is the most frequent action by the board, carrying no repercussions. Doctors can get more than one such letter without informing the public. The Missouri board hasn't used its emergency power to suspend a doctor's license in at least twenty-five years and often doesn't seek action against a doctor until police, drug enforcement agents, or other states' medical boards have taken actions.[28]

In 2012, the Albany *Times Union* reported that the number of doctors who received serious disciplinary actions from the New York state medical board had declined significantly since the mid-1990s. Even though the number of practicing doctors increased by 1.4 times and patient complaints had risen 38 percent, revocation and surrenders of medical licenses, the most severe actions, plummeted from 184 in 1996 to 96 in 2011. License revocations fell 46 percent and license surrenders dropped 22 percent. At the same time, slap-on-the-wrist punishments called "censure and reprimands" increased by 67 percent.[29]

In 2012, the Minneapolis *Star Tribune* reported that in Minnesota, a doctor only needs to meet the minimum standard to avoid state discipline, as in the case of Dr. James Wasemiller. Over thirty-five years, he has defended a dozen malpractice claims against him in two states, injured a number of patients, lost his malpractice insurance because he was considered to be too much of a risk, and forfeited his surgical privileges at a Minnesota hospital. He also failed parts of a clinical skills test requested by the state medical board. Despite his record, the Minnesota board didn't suspend him until 2011, as the board favors correcting problems over punishing misconduct or mistakes.[30]

In 2013, Madison's *Wisconsin State Journal* reviewed 218 cases leading to discipline from 2010 to 2012. More than half of the disciplined doctors received reprimands, warnings that go on their records but don't limit their practices. In at least fifty of the cases involving reprimands, patients were harmed or died. The reprimands were used for a wide range of problems, from poor record keeping and improper drug prescribing to missed cancer diagnoses and fatal mistakes. The medical board defended their actions, as they preferred rehabilitation to punishment.[31]

In 2013, the *Texas Observer* reported a number of patient harms and deaths associated with care given by Dr. Christopher Duntsch. Between 2012 and 2013, he was the subject of repeated complaints from a half dozen doctors and lawyers begging the medical board and the hospital where Dr. Duntsch worked to take actions. Dr. Duntsch continued to practice, despite his well-documented mistakes. It took the Texas medical board more than a year to stop this doctor, while he kept operating on patients who ended up seriously injured or dead.[32]

Though public outcries continue, they are often forgotten due to the short memory of society as a whole. Every day patients continue to put their lives and trust in the hands of physicians without knowing whether they are competent or if they follow the standard of care until a harm occurs. The role of medical boards in allowing negligent doctors to continue to practice cannot be ignored any longer, given the slow progress in patient safety and the alarming number of patient deaths due to preventable medical errors.

Epidemic Harm by the Same System That Is Supposed to Heal

In its 2000 report "To Err Is Human," the Institute of Medicine (IOM) estimated that up to 98,000 people are killed each year because of preventable medical harm. The IOM declared that "it is simply not acceptable for patients to be harmed by the same health care system that is supposed to offer healing and comfort," thereby setting a goal to reduce medical errors by 50 percent over five years.[33]

In the same year as the IOM report, Dr. Barbara Starfield showed grim statistics of US health care: 12,000 deaths from unnecessary surgeries; 7,000 deaths from medication errors in hospitals; 20,000 deaths from other errors in hospitals; 80,000 deaths from hospital-acquired infections; 106,000 deaths from prescribed medicines.[34] This brings the total annual deaths to 225,000, making medical care the third leading cause of death, right after heart disease (597,689) and cancer (574,743).

A more recent study found that the number of preventable deaths may have doubled, according to Dr. John James, a former NASA medical scientist and a patient safety advocate. When taking into account hidden adverse events that are not documented in medical records, errors of omission, and diagnostic errors, Dr. James estimated that the number of deaths associated with preventable medical errors may be 440,000 annually.[35] This number is roughly one-sixth of all deaths in the United States each year.

It is extremely disturbing that patient deaths due to preventable medical harm are not being reduced. Instead this harm has reached both epidemic and pandemic levels. How did we get here, since Andrew Stein called for tough sanctions on bad doctors in the 1980s and since the IOM called for a 50 percent reduction in medical harm in 2000? As Dr. Philip Levitt argued, the silent casualties will continue so long as the inept doctors remain untouched.[36]

Continuing to Practice Despite Negligence and Misconduct

Despite 440,000 patient deaths each year from preventable harm, state medical boards continue to allow many physicians to keep practicing even after findings of serious misconduct that puts patients at risk. Based on the data from the National Practitioner Data Bank, Public Citizen reported that just 5.1 percent of doctors account for 54.2 percent of the medical malpractice payouts. Of the 35,000 doctors who have had two or more malpractice payouts since 1990, only 7.6 percent have ever been disciplined. Public Citizen also found that 5,887 physicians who had one or more hospital clinical privilege restrictions had never been disciplined by any state medical board.[37] When a hospital has restricted a physician's practice, the problem is normally very serious, yet the state medical boards fail to act.

Also, according to a 2013 investigation, *USA Today*[38] reported that:

- From 2001 to 2011, nearly 6,000 doctors had their clinical privileges restricted or taken away by hospitals and other medical institutions for misconduct involving patient care. Yet 52 percent of them were never fined or imposed with a license restriction, suspension, or revocation by medical boards.
- Nearly 250 of the doctors sanctioned by health care institutions were cited as an "immediate threat to health and safety." Yet their licenses were not restricted or taken away. About 900 were cited for substandard care, negligence, incompetence, or malpractice, yet they kept practicing with no licensure action. Even the most severe misconduct goes unpunished.
- Among the 100,000 doctors who had malpractice claims from 2001 to 2011, roughly 800 were responsible for 10 percent of all the dollars paid, and their total payouts averaged about $5.2 million per doctor. But fewer than one in five faced any form of licensure action by their state medical boards.

I also learned about Washington State medical board's leniency firsthand. After MQAC's failed investigation, the Center for Medicare and Medicaid Services (CMS) investigated our complaint of patient rights violation at a regional hospital. When questioned by the federal investigators why he did not inform us about the drug risks and warnings, Dr. X responded, "It never crossed the synapse that day." Two years after my father's death, the federal agency confirmed the violations of his rights and informed consent. CMS also cited a violation of medical records because the pharmacist's warning was never documented or included in my father's medical records. Despite the federal findings, MQAC refused to consider the evidence, claiming they had no jurisdiction over the federal findings.

To raise awareness of the unsafe use of Diamox, Dr. M, a university professor and physician and a well-respected, world-leading expert and researcher on Diamox and its impacts on pulmonary functions, offered to evaluate the use of Diamox on my father. After reviewing his medical records, Dr. M opined that my father did not need Diamox and he was at a very serious disadvantage and at extreme high risk for all the known adverse effects of the drug. Given his advanced age and medical condition as well as so little chance of the drug working, Dr. M stated that the administration of Diamox was below the standard of care and negligent, causing irreversible harm to my father. When we submitted Dr. M's review to MQAC's executive director and the then-commission chair, they insisted that Dr. X's care met the standard and kept mute about the risks and harm that were raised by Dr. M.

What happened to my father is unfortunately the norm in many states. Because of boards' failure to sanction their colleagues, inept physicians continue to practice while harming more unsuspecting patients. For many bad doctors, the system works exactly as designed.

As Dr. Robert Derbyshire wrote in 1983, "While physicians have always insisted upon policing their own ranks, many people now question the effectiveness of self-regulation in protecting the public against unscrupulous, unethical, and incompetent physicians."[39] He asked, "How effective is medical self-regulation?" Sadly, the public is still vexed with the same question that Dr. Derbyshire asked thirty years ago.

Why have state medical boards consistently failed the public? To examine the root cause of the problem, we must look into the premises for self-regulation, a topic that has been visited by many over the years.

THE ANATOMY OF MEDICAL SELF-REGULATION

The cornerstone of self-regulation is the medical profession's autonomy, which grants physicians the freedom to exercise their professional judgment to practice medicine. The public believes that, as trained professionals with specialized expertise, physicians have absolute authority on medical knowledge. The public expects that physicians undergo a rigorous, periodic examination of knowledge;[40] that they are able to self-assess and maintain professional competence; and that they will practice in the best interest of patients. In return, the public's beliefs and expectations enable physicians to regulate themselves because they have the knowledge and expertise to evaluate the quality of care.

However, as argued by Mehlman,[41] the medical profession has far less knowledge and expertise than the public believes. According to IOM, only 15 percent of medical practices are based on solid clinical trials, which are the gold standard for validating medical practices.[42] When examining the 431 "evidence-based practice guidelines" produced by specialty organizations, Dr. Brawley noted that "67 percent of those guidelines didn't describe the participants in the guideline making, 88 percent didn't provide information on how relevant literature was identified, and 82 percent didn't grade the strength of the evidence. Only 5 percent met these three criteria."[43] As Dr. Brawley argued, some guidelines are reasonable, but others are commercial documents based on self-interest and are harmful.

Still, even when solid clinical studies and evidence-based guidelines suggest the proper treatment, doctors often fail to follow the evidence. The problem is "no one rates them, no one regulates them."[44] A good example is a national random survey of 599 physicians who prescribe medications. About 41 percent of them prescribed drugs for off-label indications with the erroneous belief that these off-label indications are approved by FDA, despite uncertain drug efficacy or no supporting evidence.[45]

When medical practice is very much guesswork,[46] lacking evidence-based guidelines on standard of care and lacking public transparency on what is known and what is not known, the premise for self-regulation is placed in serious doubt. In the following, I will dissect the anatomy of medicine self-regulation, arguing that its premise of self-assured competency is mostly a fairy tale and thus self-regulation is no more than a broken contract with the public. These factors will explain why medical boards, heavily populated with physicians, have consistently failed to effectively regulate medical professionals and why a lack of transparency remains a hallmark of medical self-regulation.

A Flawed Premise for Self-Assured Competency

To ensure quality of care, the medical profession largely depends on individual practitioners' self-maintenance for competency. However, evidence suggests that physicians have limited ability to accurately self-assess their competency[47] and fewer than 30 percent of physicians examine their own performance, demonstrating a poor ability to independently self-assess and self-evaluate their quality of care.[48] Most education programs like CMEs aim at maintaining minimum professional standards and rely heavily on self-reporting of individual physicians. Furthermore, studies show that physicians lean toward continuing education that reinforces what they already know rather than focusing on areas where they are weak.[49] This puts the assumption in doubt that self-regulating physicians will be able to recognize and acknowledge their own knowledge gaps.

In discussing "faith-based medicine" versus "evidence-based medicine," Dr. Brawley described apathy among his physician colleagues:

> Why do my colleagues ignore science? Some do it out of ignorance. Some do it out of greed, some do it out of a weird apathy. This last group is composed of people who are satisfied with not knowing, with not being informed. They are not technically ignorant. They know what they do not know. They know there is something to learn. They just don't want to learn it.[50]

The lack of drive to learn and inability to identify knowledge gaps offer little assurance to the public about medical professionals' competency and quality of care. Equally disturbing is the lack of correspondence between self-rated performance and actual performance.[51] According to Kruger and Dunning,[52] overestimation by the poorest performers is unfortunately the

natural consequence of being a poor performer. Since to perform well requires the skills to know what a good performance is, people with incompetence tend to believe they are above average, thus lacking the ability to
realize how poorly they are performing.[53] As a result, the claim to self-
regulating based on individuals' self-assurance of competency is overly opti-
mistic.

Since it is questionable that physicians will be able to maintain their
professional competency through self-assessment, it is extremely critical for
state medical boards to ensure that physicians maintain adequate clinical
skills through CME and keep up with medical science, so that they will not
place their patients at risk of harm.

Despite the public expectation that physicians keep up medical knowledge[54] in return for the privilege of self-regulation and despite the increasing
pressure from the public demanding accountability for the medical profession to deliver quality of care, state medical boards have been slow in their
progress to assure physicians' competency. There is little effort by medical
boards to determine whether the learning is successful or whether it addresses the right areas of individual competence. For instance, in Washington
State, physicians are required to complete 200 hours of CMEs every four
years to maintain their licenses. Because the courses are not specified, there
is no requirement for physicians to take CME in the fields that they are
practicing, and there are no checks on the results of their learning. The board
also does not measure whether the physicians' competency has been improved through these CME classes. Physicians are only required to report to
MQAC by a signature stating that they have met the CME requirements,
without demonstrating they are keeping up with the science and advances in
medicine.

As a self-claimed pulmonologist, Dr. X obtained his MD in 1981 from the
American University of the Caribbean, which was first opened in August
1978 and had a questionable teaching quality in the early 1980s.[55] Later, Dr.
X took board examinations in pulmonary medicine twice but flunked both
times, so he has never been board certified in pulmonology. He learned to
use Diamox to stimulate COPD patients' breathing during his residency in
the 1980s. Since then he has used it off-label as his "routine practice" to
wean people off ventilators despite numerous warnings in medical literature.
He admitted that he was "not a follower of Diamox research" and not aware
of any drug warnings in medical literature. He took no courses to stay current
with evidence-based practice on Diamox. Astonishingly, MQAC is not concerned about this doctor's apathy and incompetence as well as the potential
harm to many other COPD patients; they told me to contact the Food and
Drug Administration if I was concerned about this doctor prescribing Diamox improperly.

Medical boards also lack assurance of physicians' competency in many other states. For example, after his teenage son Alex was killed due to the incompetence of the treating cardiologist, Dr. John James discovered that in Texas only 1 percent of physicians' CMEs are verified each year by the Texas medical board.[56] The situation is worse in Colorado, Indiana, Montana, New York, and South Dakota, where physicians have no requirements to take basic CMEs as a condition of license renewal.[57]

In addition, not all CME courses are aimed at improving quality of care. Many CMEs are financed and accredited by pharmaceutical and medical device companies as marketing strategies to promote the sale of drugs or devices.[58,59] As a study shows, industryfunding for accredited CMEs increased by more than 300 percent in recent years.[60] Not surprisingly, some physicians' prescribing patterns are guided not by evidence but by the interests of industrial sponsors.[61] Then other CMEs are offered so casually that doctors can earn their credits by taking audio-digest courses "anywhere and anytime" while on vacations; these credits are fully accredited by the California Medical Association.[62]

Therefore, a license renewal or a CME course does not guarantee a doctor's competency. Unfortunately, a physician's shortcomings often will not come to light until a patient is harmed or dies.

Self-Regulation—A Broken Contract with the Public

To spot physicians' incompetence and the resulting harm to patients, the medical profession has traditionally relied on physicians to report these incidents and their impaired colleagues. This tradition is founded in the specialized knowledge and skills that physicians possess and therefore their ability to evaluate the clinical performance of their colleagues.

For nearly 200 years, the ethical standards of the medical profession have required physicians to report potentially injurious conduct by colleagues. The ethics code states that physicians have an ethical obligation to report impaired, incompetent, and unethical colleagues in accordance with the legal requirements in each state.[63] In recent years, some states have adopted mandatory reporting. Under the law, physicians are obligated to report to the licensing board the conduct of any colleague who may be impaired, incompetent, or unethical. Failure to report can be grounds for disciplinary action. In reality, however, only a small percentage of complaints received by medical boards originate from physicians. This suggests that most physicians' attitudes have changed little when it comes to reporting their impaired or incompetent colleagues, despite the Code of Medical Ethics.

As in a story told by Dr. Makary,[64] a group of approximately 3,000 surgeons at a national conference were asked to raise their hands if they knew a colleague who should not be practicing because he or she was dangerous. Every hand went up. By statistics, however, few of these surgeons may have reported their dangerous colleagues. According to a survey of 1,891 US physicians, more than one in three said that they do not always feel responsible to report their impaired or incompetent colleagues. About 17 percent said they knew of physicians who were practicing despite impairment or incompetence in the previous three years, yet only two-thirds of them reported the incidents.[65]

Aside from inadequate individual responsibility, the system does not help identify impaired physicians either. Many continue to practice and put their patients at risk of harm because most states allow the reporting of such impaired physicians to the state's confidential physician health program (PHP) instead of the state boards. As a result, the problem of impaired physicians has largely escaped the public's attention.[66]

The code of silence and unaccountability indeed characterizes American medicine today. Failure to maintain ethics overshadows their medical professionalism, which has failed to place the interests of patients above those of the physicians and to maintain professional standards of competence and integrity. This misplaced self-interest has turned self-regulation into self-protection, at the expense of patient safety.

Self-Regulation or Self-Protection

If the expectation that medical professionals will report their incompetent colleagues is a bit of fantasy, the assumption that their chief watchdogs, state medical boards, can be trusted to protect the public is even farther from the truth. To argue, one only needs to look into the strong ties between medical boards and medical professionals. In most states, physician board members are nominated by medical societies and appointed by the governor. In Washington State, one current MQAC member is also a trustee of the state medical association. Seldom meeting with patients and the general public, the MQAC chairs meet members of the medical association annually to brief on board functions, rules, licensure procedures, and disciplinary policies.

As extended arms of medical associations dressed in state agency clothing, the boards are more interested in protecting their fellow physicians than the public, which invariably leads to hostile attitudes toward members of the public who file complaints. At a recent public meeting, two MQAC physician members and one public member complained that the public just wants to chop doctors' heads off and take their licenses away. They suggested using a mock video to educate the public on what it is like to sanction a doctor. These comments echo a shared common belief among medical professionals that the public does not have the ability to understand complex medicine and recognize medical errors; therefore, it is incapable of judging a physician's care. The comments also show how far these board members are out of touch with reality and the public, who just want accountability and to be treated with respect and honesty. This is the minimum they should expect when they have been harmed or lost loved ones to preventable medical errors.

With such biased attitudes and conflicts of interest, boards rarely take patients' perspectives seriously and often view their testimonies about medical harm as "subjective and emotionally overwrought." To brush patients' stories aside, "a doctor's credentials as a fine human being may take precedence" and board physician members often look for "an alternative explanation and use what they know from the community."[67] Not surprisingly, state boards dismiss most of the patients' complaints each year on the basis of "insufficient evidence" and take few serious disciplinary actions.

Using the FSMB physician sanction records between 1992 and 2004, Grant and Alfred found that the number of mild sanctions (reprimands or license modifications) increased by about 10 percent, whereas severe (revocation, suspension, and surrender) and medium (probation, limitation, or restriction) sanctions all decreased in later years. When examining the basis for sanctions, the authors noted that 66 percent of the total sanctions were categorized as "not applicable."[68] This category is for informal board actions such as STIDs in Washington State, when physicians enter an agreement with the board to some form of corrective action such as additional training. The agreement allows physicians to continue to practice without admitting any unprofessional conduct.

According to records from the Data Bank's Public Use Data File, STID is the most common action from MQAC to resolve public complaints even in cases involving patient harm or death. In an example recently reported by Bill Heisel,[69] Dr. John Perry, a board-certified obstetrician and gynecologist, injured five patients from 2004 to 2005, including one patient who almost died. In later years this same doctor also committed sexual misconduct and mistreated a cancer patient. It took MQAC nine years before they revoked this physician's license, only after he had injured multiple patients and hidden a malpractice payout.

Why does the medical board only ask a doctor to pay a small fine or take a class when more severe sanctions should have been given from the very beginning? Some recent comments by MQAC members offer a glimpse into their mind-set. Last year, an MQAC physician member told us that he would not take a doctor's license away just because of "one event"; he justified that it would put the doctor's other patients at risk. In the MQAC winter 2013 newsletter, Dr. Bruce Cullen, another physician member, wrote about a medical error that exemplified what MQAC believes to be reckless behavior: "When an otherwise competent physician makes an error, the Commission would prefer that the physician be educated and rehabilitated, rather than severely penalized and removed from practice."[70] However, MQAC is more than willing to assume "an otherwise competent physician" and to avoid any penalty, even when incompetence is evident. Besides his four malpractice lawsuits over the years, Dr. X has had seven complaints against him, five of them since 2008, for allegations ranging from patient rights violations and performing unnecessary procedures to poor quality of care that resulted in serious patient harm or death. MQAC never issued him even one STID. MQAC appears to be more interested in protecting physicians or rehabilitating them than safeguarding patients' welfare, thus allowing some incompetent and negligent doctors to continue to harm other patients, event after event.

To further illustrate Washington State's discipline pattern, figure 1 shows the total number of serious violations by Washington State physicians who were sanctioned between 2002 and 2012. The number of STIDs counts for 83 percent of the total under the category of "violation not classified" and has almost doubled in recent years. This suggests that the Washington medical board is getting more lax on incompetent doctors, and slapping the wrist has become increasingly common in the board's discipline history. It is also striking that, during this eleven-year period, MQAC made only nine emergency license suspensions for immediate threat to the public (none since 2008) and merely eleven sanctions on the basis of substandard care. Even though the population of practicing physicians has increased each year in this state, the number of licensure actions resulting from negligence and incompetence has been decreasing since 2009, in comparison to sanctions based on

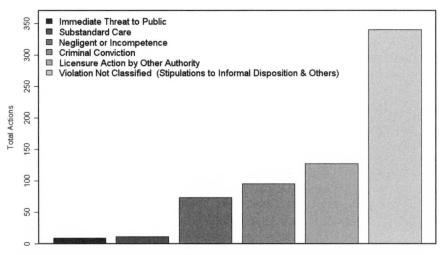

Figure 1.1. Serious Violations Resulting in Licensure Actions by Washington Medical Board (2002–2012)

criminal convictions (figure not shown). This pattern indicates that MQAC is less likely to sanction doctors for incompetence involving clinical judgment than those easy ones involving moral character, crimes, or actions already taken by other disciplinary authorities.

The sanction pattern in Washington State is not atypical. For example, in both Texas and Kansas, the bases for sanctions are dominated by drug- and alcohol-related misconducts or criminal convictions (figures 1.2 and 1.3), as opposed to other sanctions.

Misconduct and criminal convictions comprise 44 percent of all serious sanctions for Texas and 55 percent for Kansas. The few sanctions based on medical quality were criticized in a 1990 study by the Office of Inspector General[71] and also noted recently by Sawicki,[72] who examined nationwide action records reported by state medical boards. The sanction records shown in figures 1.1 and 1.2 suggest that for some medical boards, disciplinary priorities have changed little in the past three decades.

The consistent lack of substantial sanctions involving incompetency in clinical practice is extremely troublesome, when misdiagnoses contribute a significant number of preventable medical errors and harm.[73, 74] Based on a survey of more than 6,000 physicians, 47 percent said they encounter diagnostic errors at least monthly; 64 percent said that up to 10 percent of misdiagnoses they experienced directly resulted in patient harm; and 96 percent believe diagnostic errors are preventable at least some of the time.[75] According to a recent study published by *BMJ Quality and Safety*,[76] diagnostic

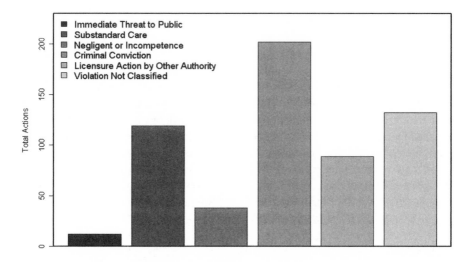

Figure 1.2.   Serious Violations Resulting in Licensure Actions by Texas Medical Board (2002–2012)

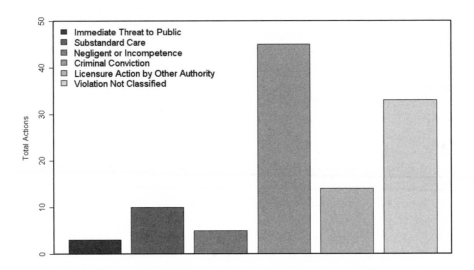

Figure 1.3.   Serious Violations Resulting in Licensure Actions by Kansas Medical Board (2002–2012)

errors affect at least one in every twenty adults in the United States who seek outpatient care, or approximately twelve million Americans every year. About half of these errors could potentially be harmful.

Diagnosis is the most critical skill that measures a physician's competency and abilities. Research shows that diagnostic errors occur because of cognitive biases in clinical decision making, sometimes coupled with negligence, not because a disease is rare or exotic.[77] For example, diagnostic errors (44 percent) occurred most frequently due to failure to order, report, and follow up laboratory results, followed by failure to consider competing diagnoses (32 percent), history taking (10 percent), physical examination (10 percent), and referral or consultation errors and delays (3 percent).[78] Another frequent but less noted source of diagnostic errors is the failure to recognize and listen to patients and their families about patients' medical histories, symptoms, and related complications. To reduce diagnostic errors, physicians need to practice based on science instead of personal "intuition" or what they believe, stay current with advances in medicine, respect values and perspectives of patients and their families, improve diagnostic skills by getting feedback, and overcome inflated confidence and other innate cognitive biases that detract from optimal reasoning and learning.[79, 80]

There are, however, abundant obstacles along the way. "Ego, arrogance, and excessive self-confidence lead doctors to confuse what they know with what they believe."[81] Compounding this problem are the medical boards' failure to rigorously review physicians' clinical practices that are not evidence based. This failure can create serious risks of patient harm. As John Banja[82] pointed out, "Many serious medical errors result from violations of recognized standards of practice. Over time, even egregious violations of standards of practice may become 'normalized' in health care delivery systems." This normalization "explains why flagrant practice deviations can persist for years, despite the importance of the standards at issue." By failing to recognize unsafe practice deviations and to take necessary actions, state medical boards are in essence normalizing poor quality of care and have turned the medical regulatory system into self-protection, a system that needs secrecy to survive.

The Veil of Secrecy: A Survival Instinct for Self-Regulation

Medical boards have a long history of secrecy in the licensing and regulation of physicians in the United States.[83] Often the boards do not inform complainants about their investigation results or the rationale behind a board's decision, in particular when cases are closed without investigation. Medical boards also rarely document their decisions behind closed doors, such as in Washington State. When MQAC refused to reopen my father's case despite the clear and convincing evidence, they told us that their decision was based on two additional internal reviews and one external review. However, they denied our access to these reviews except for a copy of the heavily redacted external review by an "independent reviewer," Dr. C. After having to hire an attorney to get a complete record, we discovered that MQAC did not seek Dr. C's review to investigate my father's care until one month after they had closed my father's case, and it was necessary in MQAC's mind to defend their decision before a state legislator we had asked to intervene. To meet MQAC's tight meeting schedule, Dr. C reviewed my father's records and our complaints to MQAC in less than three ways, and he justified the use of Diamox based on "*its occasional efficacy.*" As for the other two internal reviews, one of which was also for the sole purpose of meeting with the legislator, MQAC claimed they had no written records. Not documenting boards' reviews and decisions has become an effective way to avoid transparency and public accountability.

Besides the lack of documentation on boards' decisions, a number of states also have a variety of secretive, remedial programs under which a board would send a physician a confidential letter or request an informal meeting to express the board's concerns. These informal communications are excluded from the public eye. In Oregon, for example, if the medical board decides to close a case due to insufficient evidence but nonetheless has concerns, a confidential "letter of concern" will be sent to the licensee for practice improvement. These cases will not be revealed to complainants and the general public.[84] Other states also have similar confidential, nondisciplinary resolution, such as Kansas and Colorado.[85, 86] Complainants will not be informed if medical boards had concerns, and the public will never know how many legitimate complaints were rejected but resolved secretly through this type of confidential resolution.

In other states such as Texas, the remedial plan has some restrictions so that it may not be used to resolve complaints concerning a patient death, felony, sexual misconduct, or fraud. Such remedial plan agreement is said to be public information.[87]

Under increasing public pressure in recent years, medical boards have taken steps to increase transparency of physician profiles. Over 90 percent of medical boards post information about physicians' license status and in-state board sanction histories on public websites. But only 64 percent of the boards post board certification, 42 percent post criminal convictions or medical malpractice, one-third post disciplinary actions in other states or by hospitals, and only 18 percent post informal board actions. Washington State is among less than a handful of states that post minimal information on physician profiles, including only license status and in-state board actions on their public website.[88, 89]

In many states, medical boards rely on self-reported information from physicians, such as board certification, clinical privilege actions, and malpractice payments. However, according to Dr. Robert Oshel, the former associate director for research and disputes of the Data Bank, the self-reported information may not be complete and reliable because physicians tend to "forget" to report negative actions or malpractice payments. Often medical boards do not use Data Bank records to verify the accuracy and completeness of physicians' self-reports (Robert Oshel, personal communication, 2014).

While various improvements have been made so the public can easily access physician profiles, the public expectation for a more transparent disciplinary process often clashes with the veil of secrecy, making the progress extremely slow. After MQAC closed my father's case in 2008, we called the MQAC executive director and asked for an explanation. She refused to give one, stating that "the law does not require me to tell you anything, so I will not."

To address the lack of transparency in the board's investigational process and the lack of responsiveness to patients and their families who filed complaints about poor quality of care, we worked with a state legislator to pass a medical board transparency bill, "an act relating to providing greater transparency to the health professions disciplinary process" in 2011.[90] Under this law, a patient filing a complaint is guaranteed the right to request case reconsideration based on new information within thirty days of case closure. Also, by law, the disciplining authority shall notify the complainants in writing of its final decision on the request for reconsideration, including an explanation of the reasoning behind the decision.

Despite this new law requiring greater transparency, recent experiences from a number of Washington patients and their families say otherwise. A number of legitimate requests for case reconsiderations were denied on the same arbitrary basis of "no new information," even though much of the evidence was never brought before the board. Since there is no third-party review to listen to patients' sides of the stories, there is no mechanism for them to appeal a board's decisions or simply get their concerns heard. Transparency has become totally disposable at the board's biased discretion.

I recently surveyed a group of patients and patient family members from the ProPublica Patient Harm Community about their experiences with state medical boards. Of the thirty-six people who responded from sixteen states, 94 percent filed complaints with state medical boards because of personal experiences of preventable medical errors and harm. When asked if they were satisfied with the outcome of their complaints, 91 percent said no and only 17 percent said the board took some form of disciplinary action. When asked what improvements are necessary for medical boards to protect the public, transparency was the number one response with an overwhelming 89 percent, followed by 77 percent for allowing a third-party review and proactive investigations, 75 percent wanting tougher sanctions, and 72 percent for more public members on state medical boards. While the sample size is small, the survey results show a profound public distrust of state medical boards over their secretive investigations and ineffective discipline actions.

Given the great dissatisfaction with the state medical profession's self-regulation and the overall poor performance of medical boards, should they ever be trusted to protect the public against impaired, incompetent, or negligent doctors?

CAN THE PUBLIC EVER TRUST STATE MEDICAL BOARDS?

The following recommendations are needed to address the public distrust and to maximize public protection under the current, inept medical regulatory system.

(a) **Greater transparency and accountability.** To win public trust, state medical boards must take steps to ensure a more transparent process in handling public complaints and investigation. Copies of physicians' replies and medical consultants' reports should be provided to complainants so that they will have an opportunity to respond before the board makes its final decision. The boards should address every complaint from the public when cases involve serious harm or patient death. The boards should also provide complainants with information on laws and regulations, based on which decisions are made.

All information involving informal remedial resolutions should be available to the public on the state physician profile websites and submitted to the Data Bank. Today many physicians are licensed in a number of states, making it easier for them to move around and hide their history from unsuspecting patients. The Data Bank is a critical national resource for medical boards and others (but not for the public) to check on disciplinary actions and other issues in a physician's record from all of the states. To increase health care transparency, the Data Bank should be open to the public. This transparency includes allowing the public to use state websites and the federal Data Bank site to check the records of doctors from whom they seek treatment. The patient has a right to know if a doctor has been disciplined, has any malpractice payout, is subject to any kind of board action including remedial education, or is impaired due to substance dependence.

(b) **Third-party review.** Complainants from the public should be guaranteed the right to file for an appeal of a board's decision by requesting a third-party review outside the medical board. In theory, this review could help reduce the abuse of power by medical boards and minimize conflict of interest by medical professionals. The third-party review and appeal should be handled by an administrative judge or an agency that is independent from any medical industry or medical boards.

(c) **Proactive investigation.** Upon receiving complaints from the public, medical boards should conduct thorough investigations by verifying complainants' and providers' responses with medical records. The board investigators should provide opportunities via either phone conversations or personal interviews with complainants before the case is closed, giving complainants an opportunity to respond to the comments from physicians and medical consultants. The public should be allowed to ask for case reconsideration by providing new information relevant to the case without time limit, when a case involves serious patient harm or death. Medical boards should also verify physician profiles through regular querying of the Data Bank and other state boards' sanction records.

(d) **Balance of interests.** Under the current medical regulatory system, boards' actions will inevitably continue to be heavily influenced by the professional interests of practitioners that they license. Therefore, the self-serving interest of the medical profession must be balanced with that of the public. Progress has been made in many states by increasing the number of public members on state medical boards; however, having more public members does not necessarily represent patients' perspectives and ensure proactive, tougher sanctions.[91] So to best serve public interest, medical boards should include people with experiences of preventable medical errors or harm, patient safety advocates, and people with scientific backgrounds who are qualified to challenge the shallow investigations and biased reviews conducted by the medical boards.

(e) **Strengthen oversight and public accountability.** At present, only twenty states have sunset provision with the review frequency varying from four years to fifteen years and some with the frequency "unspecified."[92] To ensure boards' responsiveness to the public and accountability, states should adopt regular performance auditing and sunset reviews on medical boards with inputs from the public, which is a critical mechanism to reduce the boards' abuse of power and conflicts of interest. There should also be regular federal reviews of state medical boards. Because of OIG's significant historical oversight role involving state medical boards' performance and because of medical boards' important role in protecting Medicare and Medicaid patients from questionable doctors, Dr. Sidney Wolfe of Public Citizen has called upon the US Department of Health and Human Services to reinitiate OIG investigations of medical boards.[93] The OIG has not issued a comprehensive evaluation on state medical boards since 1993. The OIG should renew this federal initiative; it is long overdue.

(f) **Standardize sanction guidelines across states.** Doctors are moving around more nowadays among states. It is thus important to standardize the state sanction policies and guidelines. Of all medical boards, 75 percent use "preponderance of evidence" as the standard of proof required, whereas 21 percent use "clear and convincing evidence."[94] Because of different state laws and disciplinary guidelines, inconsistent sanctions widely exist. The same offense can lead to revocation of license by one state's board, whereas another state may only send a letter of concern or order the doctor to take a class. Therefore, the standard of proof of "preponderance of evidence" and sanction policies should be unified among all states. The inconsistency also exists even within states due to the board's arbitrary decisions and lack of defined standards of care.

(g) **Apply standard of care guidelines in boards' investigations.** Evidence-based guidelines should be used in board investigations involving standard of care. These guidelines must be discussed by the so-called experts hired by the medical boards. An anonymous expert should not be allowed to blithely declare that the standard of care has been met without thorough documentation. In recognizing personalized medical care, patient references must be respected, communicated, and documented when making evidence-based medical treatment decisions. Principles of patient-centered care, informed consent, and "first, do no harm" must be built into the standard of care and sanction guidelines.

(h) **Increase transparency on physician profiles.** To help patients make informed decisions when choosing health care providers, physician profiles should be more transparent and posted on publicly accessible websites. The physician profiles should include all important information on the quality and experience of the physicians, with all criminal and sanction histories. Boards should not be dropping records from their websites every so often. They should include all in-state and out-of-state disciplinary history records for a physician. Medical boards should also be proactive and use various data sources such as the Data Bank to verify the completeness and accuracy of any self-reported information from their licensees before posting the information on their websites.

Physician profiles on medical board websites must be easily accessible, allowing consumers to search by city and discipline. In most cases, one has to know the physician's name in order to search a record. This is not true public information. Allowing more general searches will give consumers more information on all physicians in their region.

(i) **Ensure physicians' competency.** Medical boards should set their regulatory priority on clinical quality and safety and impose proper sanctions when care falls below the professional standard. At the same time, boards should annually ensure physicians' competency through relevant CME and other education programs, by establishing a mechanism to determine whether an individual physician's learning is successful and addresses the right areas of competence. Since overdose, overtreatment, and overdiagnosing have caused significant patient harm and drive up medical costs, state medical boards must take discipline actions on unnecessary treatments to protect the safety of unsuspecting patients.[95]

(j) **Get tough on falsification of medical records.** A study[96] revealed that patients, six to twelve months after their hospitalization, could recall three times as many serious errors as were evident in their medical records. These errors reported by the patients were legitimate as verified by the investigating medical team. Thus, legislatures must institute laws requiring medical boards to determine if medical records were falsified, if information was intentionally or accidentally omitted from medical records, or if information was deleted from medical records when a harmful event occurred. Tampering with evidence in medical records should be treated as a criminal act.

(k) **Ensure adequate funding.** The changes recommended above will require additional funding by the state legislatures. The public must persuade their legislators to provide sufficient funding for the medical board to actually protect patients from dangerous physicians.

Public trust of medical boards has been nearly eroded after several decades of failure to protect the public from dangerous doctors and preventable medical harm. It will be a tremendous uphill battle for medical boards to rebuild this lost trust. The public must prod the boards up that hill and demand the change.

Chapter Two

Secrets of the National Practitioner Data Bank and the Failure of Medical Licensing Boards, Hospitals, and the Legal System to Protect the Public from Dangerous Physicians

Robert E. Oshel, PhD

Want to find out if your doctor, or one to whom you have been referred, has a record of malpractice or medical disciplinary issues such as having a license or clinical privileges suspended or revoked? Good luck. It is easier to find out if your toaster has been recalled than to find out if a doctor has been "recalled"—disciplined by a hospital, managed care organization (MCO), state licensing board, or professional society—or paid malpractice claims.

But even if you could get that information, could you be confident that the licensing boards, hospitals, and MCOs responsible for protecting the public from dangerous physicians have always acted when they should have to protect the public? Could you be confident that most harmed patients or their survivors had been compensated by malpractice payments?

This chapter examines these two questions: can you find out the information you need to protect yourself from potentially dangerous physicians and is it likely that those charged with protecting the public or at least compensating those harmed by medical malpractice have actually done so?

THE DATA BANK: A SOURCE OF INFORMATION ON
POTENTIALLY DANGEROUS PHYSICIANS

You can readily find out the safety status of consumer products like your toaster at a federal government website: https://www.cpsc.gov/cpscpub/prerel/prerel.html. That's important information, but most people would say it is even more important to be able to find out about the competency of their physician. Unfortunately, in contrast to the easy availability of safety information on toasters and other consumer products, it is impossible for you to find comprehensive information about your physician's competence and conduct from a federal government website or anywhere else.

The National Practitioner Data Bank (herein called the Data Bank; sometimes referred to as the NPDB) was established by the Health Care Quality Improvement Act of 1986 (the HCQIA) to collect and disseminate such comprehensive information on medical practitioner competence and conduct. After four years of preparation by the US Department of Health and Human Services (HHS), the Data Bank began doing so in 1990.[1]

The signing of the act by President Ronald Reagan marked the first time the federal government assumed any role in protecting the public from dangerous and miscreant physicians and other health care practitioners. President Reagan, who generally opposed expanding the role of the federal government, was himself a victim of medical error during treatment after he was shot by John Hinckley; he suffered complications resulting from an improperly placed central line.[2]

A federal data bank was needed because physicians and other practitioners were getting into trouble in one state and then moving to another state to practice without any notice of their dangerous or miscreant past to the new state's licensing board or to hospitals or MCOs which granted them clinical privileges. In many cases only after more patients were harmed would a physician's past problems in another state come to light.[3]

Besides establishing a federal repository for malpractice payment and medical disciplinary information, the HCQIA provided legal protection for hospitals and other institutions with peer review activities and for the members of peer review panels. (See chapter 3 for more on hospital peer review.) The intent was to encourage physicians to review their colleagues' care by removing the possibility that either institutions with fair peer review processes or physicians who acted in good faith could be found liable for money damages for participating in peer review. Similarly, no individual could be found liable for money damages for providing truthful information for use in peer review. These protections were necessary because of the chilling effects of large damage awards against apparently good faith hospital peer reviewers. Peer review was seen as a crucial component of hospital efforts to protect their patients from injury, and it was feared that in the absence of legal protection peer review would collapse. No one would participate if they could be sued and made to pay damages.

WHY YOU NEED—BUT CANNOT GET—INFORMATION TO PROTECT YOURSELF FROM QUESTIONABLE PHYSICIANS FROM THE DATA BANK

The Data Bank began operating in September 1990, and since that time it has become the most comprehensive source of information anywhere about a doctor's malpractice and medical discipline record. But you cannot get its information. As the Data Bank's website says:

> The general public is not permitted to access the Data Bank. You may view limited public information that does not identify organizations or practitioners. Only health care organizations and practitioners may access the Data Bank. [4]

A provision in the HCQIA, included at the insistence of the American Medical Association (AMA) when the law was being drafted, keeps the information secret. The Data Bank's reports are specifically exempted from disclosure under the Freedom of Information Act, and there are severe penalties for their unauthorized disclosure or misuse by those who are authorized to see them.

Only licensing boards, hospital or other peer reviewers, and certain others authorized by the HCQIA and subsequent legislation are permitted to see the Data Bank's information. [5] Even malpractice insurers cannot access the data to help them determine whom to insure.

Hospitals routinely get and use the information, but as will be discussed later, they do not necessarily act on it to protect the public, especially in the case of physicians already on their staffs. Hospitals are required by law to query the Data Bank for any reports it may have on all new applicants for their medical staffs. In addition, hospitals must query the Data Bank concerning all members of their medical staffs every two years [6] to be sure they have relatively up-to-date information on the malpractice and medical disciplinary action records of anyone holding clinical privileges.

Other authorized users (health maintenance organizations, MCOs, other providers with peer review activities, professional associations, licensing boards, and certain other agencies) are not required to obtain or use the data, but they often do so. Indeed these voluntary users find the information so useful that about 72 percent of the Data Bank's total of more than 4,250,000 queries each year are submitted voluntarily (mostly by health maintenance organizations and similar providers); required hospital queries account for only about 28 percent of queries. [7]

The high percentage of queries to the Data Bank which are submitted voluntarily is an indicator of the value users place on the information, since they must pay $3.00 per name when they query.[8] The fact that the Data Bank's voluntary users find the information on physicians' records useful enough to spend over $14.5 million each year to get it strongly suggests that the information also would be valuable to individual health care consumers.

One reason authorized users find querying the Data Bank valuable is because they are getting information from the Data Bank they do not get from any other source—including physicians' own applications. Apparently physicians with something to hide in their past often try to hide it.

A survey of Data Bank users found that 9 percent of the time when users received a response from the Data Bank that included one or more reports of malpractice payments or medical disciplinary actions concerning a practitioner, they learned new information—information they had not found in any other source, including the physician's application—that led them to make a different decision on licensing or granting privileges to the practitioner than they would have made if they had not received the Data Bank's information. This means that the Data Bank's information changes about 40,000 credentialing and licensing decisions each year.[9] Since the Data Bank's information is largely negative, it means that each year about 40,000 licenses or medical staff memberships weren't granted or were limited because of the malpractice or medical discipline information in the Data Bank.

The fact that 40,000 decisions to restrict or refuse to license or credential a physician were made each year doesn't mean that the rejected physicians didn't simply apply elsewhere and get accepted. And you would never know or be able to check records for yourself because you cannot query the Data Bank.

WHAT IS IN THE NATIONAL PRACTITIONER DATA BANK?

What does the federal government know that the AMA thinks you cannot be trusted to know or understand about your doctor? The Data Bank has received legally required reports of all malpractice payments for all types of licensed health care practitioners since September 1, 1990. The Data Bank has similarly received reports of all but the least serious state licensure and hospital or managed care organization and professional society peer-reviewed disciplinary actions for physicians and dentists since that date. Licensure actions for other types of practitioners and certain other types of actions were added later. The Data Bank also has reports on Office of Inspector General exclusions of practitioners from participation in Medicare, Medicaid, and other federal health programs and on Drug Enforcement Administration (DEA) actions limiting the authorization of practitioners to prescribe controlled substances.

As of December 31, 2013, the Data Bank contained 1,051,116 reports. 430,437 of the reports concerned physicians. [10,11] Of these reports:

- 307,961 were reports of malpractice payments (71.5 percent of physician reports).
- 88,070 were reports of state licensure disciplinary actions or modifications of such actions, including reinstatements (20.5 percent).
- 19,129 were reports of hospital or other peer-reviewed, disciplinary actions affecting clinical privileges for more than thirty days or modifications of such actions, including reinstatements (4.4 percent).
- 12,732 were reports of Office of Inspector General (OIG) exclusion from participation in federal health care programs and payment by such programs (e.g., Medicare and Medicaid) or reinstatement reports related to previous exclusions (2.9 percent).
- 1,635 were DEA actions concerning authorization to prescribe controlled drugs (0.2 percent).
- 910 were reports of peer-reviewed professional society disciplinary actions or modifications of such actions, including reinstatements (0.2 percent).

A total of 209,352 physicians, including interns and residents, were responsible for these reports. Many had only one report, but some had dozens or even hundreds. [12]

It should be noted that the Data Bank also receives reports on other types of practitioners in addition to physicians. In fact, it has 606,708 reports on 372,602 other practitioners, but in this chapter we concentrate on physicians.

To what extent are malpractice and miscreant behavior being kept from the public? Some physicians have literally hundreds of malpractice payments, but you cannot find out who they are. The physician with the most payment reports had 251 as of December 31, 2013. Another physician had 206 reports. Six physicians have between 100 and 199 payments reported to the Data Bank. 45,747 physicians have three or more malpractice payment reports. [13]

It should be emphasized that about 85 percent of all licensed physicians have no malpractice payments at all in their records, and another 10 percent have only one malpractice payment. Just over 3 percent have two payments. This means that fewer than 2 percent of all physicians have three or more payments. [14] Clearly anyone in this 2 percent with three or more payments is an outlier whose record is worthy of investigation before you use their services, but you generally have no way of knowing who has any malpractice payments, let alone three or more. And you certainly have no way of getting the information necessary to judge for yourself whether a given physician's particular malpractice payments were something you should be concerned about. In the author's experience in working with actual Data Bank malpractice data and reports, most payment reports represent significant malpractice, but a few do not. [15]

The AMA claims that malpractice payments are a poor indicator of physician quality. [16] Certainly they are not a perfect indicator, but they are important to consider. Malpractice payments are not a random event equally likely to happen to any physician regardless of knowledge or skills. Furthermore, most payments represent serious harm to the affected patient. Only about 3 percent of malpractice payments result from emotional or very minor physical injuries. [17]

Other injuries resulting in malpractice payments are far more serious and can be either temporary or permanent. Almost a third of all payments are made because of the death of the patient. Another 5 percent are cases involving extremely serious malpractice injury resulting in such things as quadriplegia, significant brain damage, or other injury requiring lifelong care. Another 28 percent involve other permanent injuries to the patients. [18]

Before retirement, the author often had occasion to read Data Bank reports for research or while reviewing draft decisions in cases in which practitioners appealed their reports to the secretary of HHS. Many of the cases were appalling.

There were many cases in which surgeons removed healthy kidneys, healthy ovaries, or other organs and left the diseased ones. In some cases the wrong operation was performed on the wrong patient. Procedures were performed without patient consent. Incorrect drugs or improper dosages were administered. There were cases of failure to treat when treatment was obviously required. The list was virtually endless.

Another example publicly reported in various news media is the case of a physician who had a record of drug abuse, malpractice suits, and licensure actions in several states. [19] He moved to Hawaii, where he was licensed and then committed additional malpractice. He began a spine operation without ensuring that the hospital had the titanium rod he needed to implant. Mid-operation he found out that the rod wasn't available. His solution was to cut off a section of the shaft of a screwdriver and insert it in the patient's back! Three days later the patient fell and broke the implanted screwdriver shaft. Another operation was needed to retrieve the broken pieces of the screwdriver and implant the proper rod. Two additional surgeries and various complications followed. The patient died two years later. [20]

Malpractice is not the only issue patients and potential patients need to be concerned with. Licensure or peer reviewed disciplinary reports also were filed against physicians for multiple sexual assaults on patients, fighting, and other misbehavior. In one instance, for example, two physicians got in a fistfight over who was to use the operating room next. In another instance, a physician got so angry in the hospital that he broke a copying machine, dented a door, and threw things on the floor.

There were also cases in which physicians had mental problems rendering them a significant risk to themselves and their patients. One physician, who was not institutionalized, copied the Data Bank on long, handwritten letters threatening to torture and kill members of a state licensing board. Another physician, who was institutionalized, appealed her Data Bank report from the mental institution and then began harassing staff by e-mail. She also filed numerous trivial changes (often involving just punctuation or spacing between words) to the practitioner's statement in the Data Bank report she was appealing. Each change caused a new copy of the report to be sent to the reporting entity and any entities which had queried on her and received the report!

Chances are that if you knew a physician had a significant malpractice history, had sexually assaulted patients, had gotten into fistfights with other medical personnel, had intentionally broken medical or office equipment, or otherwise demonstrated mental instability, you would want to choose another physician for your care. Unfortunately, you are unlikely to be able to find out this information. You certainly cannot get it from the Data Bank.

Even if you could access the Data Bank's information, as good as it is—and it is the best anywhere—you would find it is not comprehensive for either malpractice payments or medical disciplinary actions. There are a few loopholes or exceptions in the reporting requirements.

The most notable loophole concerns malpractice payments. Although payments in any amount must be reported, if a payment is made for the benefit of an institution rather than a named individual physician, the payment is not reportable to the Data Bank. Through what is known as the "corporate shield," institutions may prevent reporting of their employed physicians or other practitioners by making sure that malpractice claims are brought against the institution rather than the employed practitioner who might have been at fault. Depending on the method used by the institutions to make sure their practitioners are not named in the suits and settlements, a report may be legally required. But the Data Bank has no way of knowing about these situations and enforcing the reporting requirement. Use of the corporate shield in some cases might be considered similar to tax avoidance, which is legal, rather than tax evasion, which is illegal. In other cases tax evasion is the better analogy. In any event, use of the corporate shield is contrary to the spirit of the reporting law.

There is no firm data on the extent of use of the corporate shield, but it is probably growing as hospitals increasingly acquire physician practices and create arrangements in which physicians become hospital employees. As part of these arrangements, hospitals become legally responsible for the care provided by their physician employees and provide malpractice coverage for them. This makes it easy to shift claims from the reportable employed physicians to the nonreportable hospitals.

It is important to note that the federal government does *not* use the corporate shield to protect federally employed physicians from being reported. Although under the Federal Tort Claims Act all malpractice actions against federally employed physicians are formally filed against the government and not the individual employee physician, if the standard of care was not met the responsible practitioner(s) are identified and reported to the Data Bank if a payment is made. This ensures that their record will be complete if they later seek to practice in a capacity other than as a federal employee or if they seek new employment within the government.

As significant as the corporate shield is, it is not the ultimate malpractice-reporting loophole. If a payment isn't made, there is nothing to report. As will be discussed in a later section, most malpractice events do not result in a payment, and the gap between the number of malpractice events and malpractice payments is increasing because of tort reform. So fewer and fewer malpracticing physicians are being reported.

Some observers also consider the fact that peer reviewed disciplinary actions affecting a physician or dentist's clinical privileges for thirty days or less are not reported to the Data Bank to be a loophole in reporting. Others claim that minor peer reviewed disciplinary actions do not rise to the level of meriting a permanent report on a physician's record; the law reflects this view, but the thirty-day threshold creates an opportunity for abusive reporting avoidance.

Anecdotally, we know that many peer reviewed clinical privileges actions are imposed for only twenty-nine or thirty days specifically to avoid reporting. This avoidance may be responsible for the fact that after almost a quarter century of required reporting, about 46 percent of hospitals had *never* reported even one clinical privileges action to the Data Bank. Although simple oversight may be responsible for some of this nonreporting, it is likely that the vast majority stems from imposition of nonreportable penalties. It simply is beyond belief that 46 percent of hospitals have never had reason to discipline a physician because of incompetence or misconduct from September 1990 through June 2012.[21]

It is unknown how many practitioners have escaped being reported because of the corporate shield or the thirty-day threshold. What is known is that the Data Bank is the only relatively comprehensive national source for malpractice and medical disciplinary information. There simply are no other "one-stop-shopping" repositories for the kinds of information reported to the Data Bank. Indeed there are no other central repositories at all for most of the kinds of information contained in the Data Bank.

THERE ARE NO PUBLICLY AVAILABLE COMPREHENSIVE SOURCES FOR YOUR DOCTOR'S HISTORY

If you cannot get comprehensive information on your doctor's background from the Data Bank, where can you get it? You probably can't. State licensing boards on their websites provide varying kinds of information and varying levels of detail about what they do provide. Typically they will tell you if the state has taken a licensing action against a doctor and may provide a copy of the board's order. Some states may provide limited malpractice payment or hospital or MCO disciplinary information.[22]

Besides being limited in type and detail, profile information on state board websites almost always suffers from other flaws. Except for information about the state's licensure actions, any other information on state board websites is often self-reported by the physicians, and physicians with problems in their past have an incentive to "forget" these problems when self-reporting. This means that any nonlicensure data on state board websites is often incomplete and unreliable. The state boards are prohibited by law from posting any Data Bank information even if they receive it.

Another problem is that generally the information provided on state board websites will only concern actions or payments in the state. If the physician is licensed in multiple states, which almost a quarter of all physicians are, you would need to check the websites of the boards of all the states in which the physician is licensed—if you can find out where he or she is licensed.[23]

The easiest way to check state board websites is to go to a website operated by Administrators in Medicine, the association of executive directors of state medical boards: http://www.docboard.org/docfinder.html. The site has a "beta" combined search of the websites of twenty-three medical or osteopathic boards from twenty-two states. It also has links to the websites of all the remaining medical or osteopathic boards, but you have to check each remaining board individually.

Various commercial services on the Internet also claim to be able to check a physician's record for consumers. However, since these services cannot access the Data Bank and there are no public sources for comprehensive and reliable information on malpractice payments and clinical privileges disciplinary actions, the author considers them to be of questionable value.

In the long run, the only way for the public to be able to get relatively comprehensive information on their physicians' malpractice and medical discipline background is for Congress to repeal the secrecy provision in the law that created the Data Bank. This will only happen if enough voters demand that their congressional representatives change the law. The AMA opposes any change making the information public on the grounds that consumers will misunderstand the information and that it will hurt good physicians.[24] The secrecy will continue unless there is considerable public pressure for change. HHS cannot make the information public unless Congress amends the law and the president approves the legislation. If you want access to the Data Bank's information, write your congressional representative, senator, and the president.

IF YOU CANNOT GET THE INFORMATION NECESSARY TO PROTECT YOURSELF FROM INCOMPETENT AND MISCREANT PHYSICIANS, YOU HAVE TO RELY ON OTHERS TO PROTECT YOU—BUT DO THEY?

Why should you care that you cannot see the Data Bank's reports? Hospital or MCO peer reviewers and state licensing boards are supposed to protect the public from incompetent or misbehaving practitioners. Unfortunately, experience suggests that you cannot rely on them to protect you from highly questionable doctors. As suggested by the story of the physician who had malpractice cases and licensure actions in several states and was then licensed in Hawaii, where he committed additional malpractice, state licensing boards and peer reviewers may not adequately screen or discipline physicians. (See chapter 3 for more information on peer review.) You need to protect yourself to the extent you can.

Although most doctors are competent and caring, more than a few are not. Virtually every physician I've ever asked has said he knew one or more physicians he'd never go to or refer a family member to. Physicians confirm this. Marty Makary, MD, tells the story that one of his Harvard professors speaking to about three thousand physicians at a conference asked, "How many of you know of another doctor who should not be practicing because he's too dangerous?" "Every single hand went up."[25]

Over a twenty-year period, more than half of all the money paid out for physician malpractice was paid because of the malpractice of only about 1.8 percent of all physicians. That's worth repeating: only 1.8 percent of physicians were responsible for over half of all the money paid for malpractice over a twenty-year period! Malpractice isn't a random event; a few malpractice-prone physicians are responsible for the bulk of it, as reflected in paid malpractice claims. Most of these 1.8 percent of physicians responsible for over half of the malpractice dollars paid out had multiple malpractice payments in their records.

Even more alarming is the fact that malpractice incidents resulting in payments are only the tip of the malpractice iceberg. Only a small proportion (fewer than 13 percent) of adverse incidents resulting from negligence result in a claim,[26] and only a small proportion of claims (about 20 percent) result in payments.[27] This means that less than 3 percent of malpractice events result in a payment. This provides more evidence that the physicians in the

1.8 percent are the worst of the worst, so unsafe, perhaps, that the culture of physicians protecting physicians is less likely to come into play and other physicians are less likely to rally around them to help head off malpractice claims or keep those claims from being successfully pursued.

Did the licensing boards or hospital peer reviewers take action to stop the few outlier physicians responsible for half of the malpractice dollars paid from committing additional malpractice? Not very often. Only about 11 percent of the physicians responsible for half of all the money paid for malpractice have *ever* had even one action taken against their licenses and only 6 percent of them have ever had any action taken against their clinical privileges. Even in the unlikely event that they have had a licensure or clinical privileges action taken against them, they still may be practicing in another state or at another facility. So most of those in this irresponsible, unsafe group of highly questionable physicians are likely to still be practicing, *most likely without any comprehensive notice to the public of their past record.*

If licensing boards and peer reviewers took effective action to restrict practice or revoke the licenses of the 1.8 percent, malpractice costs could be reduced substantially without "tort reform." Tort reform actually only shifts the real costs of malpractice from physicians and their malpractice insurers to the injured patients, their insurers, and the taxpayers rather than reducing these costs. Even more importantly, the number of patients who are injured or killed could be substantially reduced.

THE FAILURE OF HOSPITALS AND OTHER PEER REVIEWERS TO PROTECT THE PUBLIC

Over the first 23-1/4 years the Data Bank collected reports, hospitals and other health care providers with peer-reviewed medical staff took reportable disciplinary action against only 12,449 physicians. In 2013, the most recent year available and also a fairly typical year, only 546 physicians were disciplined for more than thirty days, the threshold for reporting to the Data Bank. This minute percentage (about 0.064 percent) of the estimated total number of licensed physicians means that fewer than 7 of every 10,000 physicians were disciplined. The 546 disciplined physicians include 279 whose clinical privileges were affected for more than thirty days but not revoked completely. Only 287 physicians in 2013 had their clinical privileges revoked or otherwise lost their privileges to practice at a hospital or managed care or similar provider.[28] If we assume 2 percent of physicians are incompetent or miscreant, it would take almost 60 years to revoke their privileges *at even one facility* at the rate of 287 physicians revoked each year. The problem is compounded by the fact that a physician's loss of privileges at one facility may have little or no impact on privileges to practice at other facilities and therefore on the public's safety. Disciplined physicians often simply practice elsewhere.

The situation is simply ludicrous. It is beyond belief that only 287 physicians out of over 850,000 (i.e., fewer than 3 in 10,000) were so incompetent or behaved so inappropriately that they deserved to lose their clinical privileges in 2013.

Further evidence of the failure of peer reviewers to protect the public comes from malpractice payment records. As noted above, only about 6 percent of the physicians responsible for half of all the money paid for malpractice—the very few physicians responsible for the bulk of the nation's identified malpractice problem—have *ever* had an action revoking or even limiting their clinical privileges reported to the Data Bank. Surely if the peer-review system was working properly to protect the public, peer reviewers would have restricted or revoked the clinical privileges of the more than 6 percent of the physicians who cause the bulk of the malpractice problem.

Still another way of looking at the extent of the failure of many hospital peer reviewers to adequately discipline their dangerous peers is provided by the fact that in the Data Bank's years of operation, from September 1, 1990, through June 30, 2012, only slightly more than half of currently operating hospitals have reported even one clinical privileges action to the Data Bank.[29] There has been little change in reporting since mid-2012.

There is no evidence that physicians in any one state are more competent than physicians in any other state, but the extent of the failure of hospitals to take and report disciplinary actions varies widely from state to state. In South Dakota only about 24 percent of hospitals had ever reported even one clinical privileges action by mid-2012. In Louisiana it is only about 32 percent. The failure of hospitals to act is not limited to relatively small states, which often have small hospitals. Only 37 percent of Texas hospitals had ever reported a clinical privileges action to the Data Bank. It simply is not reasonable to believe that over a twenty-two-year period only these very small percentages of hospitals had grounds to revoke a physician's clinical privileges or restrict them for more than thirty days, especially when in other states a much larger percentage of hospitals have taken and reported disciplinary actions.

Why are hospitals and other peer reviewers failing to act? Physicians fill hospital beds and keep hospitals financially viable. Hospitals are especially reluctant to take action against physicians who admit lots of patients, especially patients to high-profit programs such as cardiac surgery. Hospitals often look the other way for such physicians if they possibly can, even to the extent of not taking action when a physician has many questionable admissions and performs unnecessary, but highly profitable, procedures. Hospitals are also reluctant to take action against physicians who are seen as leaders in the community or who are publicly tied to the hospital's image. They do not want to harm their own reputation.

Another factor is fear of litigation. Physicians often threaten to sue or actually file lawsuits if peer-review sanctions are proposed or imposed against them. Even though peer review committee members, hospitals, and other entities with peer review are protected by the HCQIA from having to pay money damages for good faith peer review activity even if a court finds in favor of the plaintiff physician,[30] they may have tens or hundreds of thousands of dollars in legal costs to defend themselves. Furthermore, if the court found they did not act in good faith, they might have to pay damages. So even though hospitals have won most of the cases brought against them for peer-review actions, the legal protection for hospitals and their peer reviewers is not as strong or effective as it might appear at first glance. This only adds to the reluctance of most hospitals to take peer-review actions except in the most extreme circumstances.

Physicians are complicit in the failure to act. Hospital actions are taken by peer review committees composed of physicians. As in most professions, physicians generally tend to be sympathetic to other members of the profession, to give them the benefit of the doubt, to minimize penalties, to suggest retraining is the solution rather than discipline, and so on. Perhaps the unspoken back-of-the-mind thinking of the peer reviewers is that they might be the one in the hot seat the next time and they would not want their career damaged or ended.

The failure of peer review committees to act prevents identification of dangerous physicians to the Data Bank. Often action is taken only in the worst cases when hospitals and peer reviewers think a physician has become more trouble than he is worth.

Examples abound.[31]

- An FBI investigation of unnecessary cardiac procedures at Redding Medical Center (Redding, California) revealed hundreds of unnecessary cardiac catheterizations, cardiac bypass surgeries, and valve surgeries over a ten-year period, which were very profitable for the hospital and the physicians involved. The physicians blocked any peer review of the program. Some patients died.
- In Sacramento, California, a judge found that a physician had been involved in orthopedic surgical procedures which were "unnecessary, bungled, or both" at Mercy Hospital. The judge also found that the surgeon's peers should have "blown the whistle" on numerous occasions, but did not.
- At Edgewater Medical Center in Chicago four physicians and a hospital administrator were criminally prosecuted and found guilty in a scheme to admit patients who didn't need care and to perform unnecessary surgical procedures on at least 1,650 patients. Some patients died. No peer review action had been taken in any of these cases.

- A physician who had been dismissed by the University of California at Irvine for incompetence began practicing at Western Medical Center in Santa Ana, California, where he was sued for malpractice thirty-nine times before he was finally suspended. He then began practicing without restriction at Tustin Hospital Medical Center about a mile away in the town next to Santa Ana.
- An ear, nose, and throat specialist practicing at the University of Kansas Medical Center, Providence Medical Center, and Bethany Medical Center, all in Kansas City, Kansas, was convicted of numerous counts involving unnecessary care, without effective peer review at any of the facilities.
- After an orthopedic surgeon repeatedly tested positive for cocaine and was involved in about twenty malpractice suits over an eleven-year period, a hospital in McAlister, Oklahoma, finally suspended him. He moved to the Dallas, Texas area, where he was also licensed, and began practicing at Garland Community Hospital even though his drug abuse history was known. He became one of the hospital's biggest sources of revenue, and the hospital took no action against him. The Texas medical board eventually revoked his license.

Hospital administrators and peer reviewers may rationalize their failure to act in cases like these by, in effect, passing the responsibility on to the state licensing board. Unfortunately licensing boards only rarely act, too.

LICENSING BOARDS: THE FAILURE OF THE PUBLIC'S FIRST AND LAST LINES OF DEFENSE FROM INCOMPETENT AND MISCREANT PHYSICIANS

State medical licensing boards are charged with licensing physicians to protect the public from incompetent physicians, from physicians whose conduct is unacceptable, and from persons who claim to be physicians but aren't. They are supposed to do this by granting licenses to qualified physicians and taking disciplinary action against those who prove to be incompetent or whose behavior is not acceptable. (See chapter 1 for more details on state medical boards.)

State licensing boards are really both the first and the last lines of defense against questionable physicians. Boards are the first line of defense because they can stop a questionable physician from beginning to practice in their state. Boards are the last line of defense because they can revoke or restrict licenses of physicians already practicing. They can do this even if peer reviewers at hospitals or other providers have failed to act. Their role is crucial because they can restrict the practice of dangerous physicians or keep them from practicing anywhere in the state. Even if peer reviewers have acted, peer reviewers can only protect the patients at their hospital or HMO; they cannot protect the public in general.

The states have various organizational arrangements for the boards, which operate under differing medical practice acts. In all cases, however, the boards are dominated by physicians. While there may be public members—nonphysicians who are supposed to be appointed to represent the public—they may not actually represent the public interest. The Missouri Board of Healing Arts, for example, is composed of eight physicians and one member of the public. The "public" member is an attorney whose biography says he has "defended physicians and physician groups of almost every medical specialty and hospitals in the state courts of Missouri."[32] And this attorney is supposed to represent the public! Even if public members are not tied directly to the medical profession, they often have little impact on the operations of the board. The result is that many of the boards appear to have a culture of protecting physicians from the public rather than protecting the public from incompetent physicians and those with conduct problems.

Even for those medical boards which do conscientiously try to protect the public, lack of adequate funding and adequate staffing is often a problem. In many states licensing fees are part of the state's general revenue and used for other purposes beyond funding the board. If boards do not have adequate resources to investigate complaints and initiate action when necessary, they cannot protect the public even if they want to.

LICENSING—FAILURE TO PROTECT THE PUBLIC WHEN GRANTING LICENSES

The Data Bank's information should be crucial to licensing boards' effectively screening applicants for both new and renewal licenses. Licensing boards cannot protect the public if they do not know an applicant's background. Although they require applicants to report their malpractice and medical discipline history on licensure applications, unless boards query the Data Bank they cannot be sure applicants are telling them the complete story. As noted earlier, entities that query the Data Bank find that applications from practitioners with problems in their past are missing information crucial for decision making about 9 percent of the time.

Nevertheless, with the exception of the Florida board, state medical licensing boards rarely obtain and use the Data Bank's information. Physician licensing boards submitted only 62,916 requests for information to the Data Bank in 2010—a minuscule 1.5 percent of all queries to the Data Bank. Licensing boards submitted only one query for every fourteen physicians and, given that over 190,000 physicians have licenses in more than one state, perhaps only one query for every eighteen medical licenses.[33]

Because the state licensing boards generally aren't getting or using the Data Bank's information, they do not have the information they need either to prevent incompetent physicians or those with behavior problems from being licensed at all in their state or to restrict their licenses if they do grant them a license.

LICENSING—FAILURE TO PROTECT THE PUBLIC BY TAKING DISCIPLINARY ACTION AGAINST LICENSEES

As noted above, licensing boards also are the public's last line of defense from incompetent physicians or those with behavior problems because they can revoke or restrict the licenses and keep these physicians from practicing in the state.

Unfortunately, it appears that licensing boards often fail in this last-line-of-defense function.

The Public Citizen report "State Medical Boards Fail to Discipline Doctors with Hospital Actions against Them" illustrates the extent of this problem.[34] Public Citizen's analysis of data from the Data Bank's Public Use Data File, which excludes any information that would identify individual physicians, found as of December 30, 2009, that there were 5,887 physicians with adverse clinical privileges reports in the Data Bank but no licensure action report from any state. A total of 581 of these physicians had three or more adverse clinical privileges reports. Three had as many as twelve such reports but no action by a state board against their licenses, not even a reprimand![35]

Some clinical privileges actions are taken for extremely serious reasons, such as "Immediate Threat to Health and Safety." Of the Data Bank's clinical privileges reports for physicians with no licensure reports, 243 reports involved 220 physicians judged by their peers to be an "immediate threat to health or safety." They had been judged by peers as an "immediate threat to health or safety," but no licensing board had taken any action against their license.[36] There were another 1,371 clinical privileges reports concerning 1,191 physicians whose peers concluded that they had practiced with incompetence, malpractice, or negligence, or who were judged to be "unable to practice safely," yet no licensing actions had been taken to protect the public.[37]

Licensing boards could easily find out about every clinical privileges action by querying the Data Bank. Even without querying, they find out about clinical privileges actions taken in their state. In accordance with federal law, copies of all clinical privileges action reports filed with the Data Bank are sent to the licensing board of the state in which the clinical action was taken. State laws also generally require hospitals taking clinical privileges action to file state reports to the licensing board. So although the licensing boards know of the peer review actions taken against physicians practicing in their state, in many cases they fail to follow up with licensure action. If a peer review action is taken in another state against one of their licensees who is also licensed and practicing elsewhere, the board won't find out about it unless they query the Data Bank or the physician eventually lists it on a licensure renewal application. Therefore, they often fail to act to protect the public from physicians who get in trouble in one state and move back to another state to practice.

Licensing boards should act even when hospitals and MCOs do not. In addition to receiving complaints directly from the public, licensing boards receive copies of all Data Bank malpractice payment reports for their state either from the payer or from the Data Bank. They also often receive state-mandated malpractice payment reports. But even though they get this malpractice information, boards often do not take any action or take only weak action—even against physicians with blatant or repeated malpractice records. And as noted for clinical privileges reports, since the boards typically fail to query the Data Bank, they typically fail to find out about and take action concerning malpractice payments for their licensees practicing in another state. This leaves the questionable physician free to move back to the state and resume practicing without any review of his record.

California provides some specific examples of weak or nonexistent action by a licensing board. The *Orange County Register* reported that during the three-year period ending June 2011

> doctors negotiated settlements with the Medical Board of California in 62 of 76 cases in which patients had been killed or permanently injured. More than half of those 76 cases—63 percent—were settled for penalties below the board's own minimum recommendations. . . . Among the deals approved: A probation term two years below recommendations for a San Bernardino osteopath who sent a patient home to his death after misreading 'grossly abnormal' EKG readings. No probation at all for a Rancho Palo Verdes anesthesiologist after one of his patients suffered severe brain damage. A public reprimand for a Costa Mesa cosmetic surgeon whose patient died following a liposuction procedure.
>
> State officials defended these settlements as reasonable, and note that the law doesn't require boards and bureaus to follow their own recommendations.[38]

A further indication of the frequent failure of state licensing boards to take any action even when physicians have significant malpractice records is the fact that nationally only 10.9 percent of the 19,364 physicians who from 1990 to 2011 were responsible for over half of all the money paid out for malpractice claims in the United States had ever had *even one* action taken against their license in any state. A few states did better, but even in the most activist state, North Dakota, only 30.2 percent of physicians responsible for half of the money paid out for malpractice claims in the state had action against their license. Other states were often far worse. South Dakota had *never* taken a licensure action against any of the twenty-seven physicians responsible for half of all the money paid for malpractice in that state over the twenty-year period studied.[39] One has to wonder how many of the physicians with the worst records in North Dakota who were disciplined by that state's board simply moved across the border to South Dakota and continued to practice unrestricted and un-retrained.

In any event, the failure of licensing boards to act is critically important. They are both the first and the last lines of defense for a public that cannot protect itself from questionable physicians because they cannot get the information necessary to do so.

FAILURE OF THE MALPRACTICE LIABILITY SYSTEM TO PROTECT THE PUBLIC OR EVEN ADEQUATELY COMPENSATE FOR MALPRACTICE INJURY OR DEATH

The legal system through malpractice suits is another potential protection for the public from incompetent or miscreant physicians. Indeed, at first glance, malpractice suits may be the most significant protection, at least in the sense of compensating victims after the fact. Over 71 percent of all the physician reports in the Data Bank are for malpractice payments. That represents 307,961 payment reports over a twenty-three-year, four-month period, an average of almost 13,200 physician malpractice payments each year.

But it is clear that the effectiveness of malpractice cases as a protector of the public is decreasing. The number of physician malpractice payments reported to the Data Bank consistently decreased from a high of 16,566 in 2001 to an all-time low of 9,370 in 2012. The number of payments increased to 9,682 in 2013,[40] but this is still almost a 42 percent decrease in twelve years. It is extremely doubtful that there has been a 42 percent decrease in actual malpractice injuries nationally during this period. The most significant factor in this decrease is likely that tort reforms enacted in many states over the period have made it increasingly difficult for injured patients or the survivors of patients who died from malpractice to bring and win malpractice suits.

It is also likely that the number of malpractice payments will continue to decrease for several years even if no more states enact tort reforms, since the typical malpractice payment comes between four and five years after the malpractice event and many payments take much longer. Tort reform typically affects only suits brought after the reform is enacted; previously pending cases are handled under the old rules, so it may take eight to ten years or more for the full impact of tort reform to be observed in payment records.

Even the pre-tort reform number of malpractice payments each year was so low as to provide evidence that the legal system was then, and is even more now, inadequate in either protecting the public from malpractice or providing adequate compensation when malpractice occurs. The 1999 Institute of Medicine report *To Err Is Human* estimated that as many as 98,000 Americans—almost 270 people each and every day—died each year as a result of avoidable medical errors.[41] A 2010 study by the HHS Office of Inspector General was the first to obtain a statistically valid national incidence rate for adverse events in hospitalized patients.[42] It found that as many as 1,560,000 Medicare beneficiaries a year were injured in hospitals and that an estimated 180,000 hospitalized Medicare beneficiaries each year "experienced an event that led to their deaths."[43] A 2013 study of all hospital deaths, not just those of Medicare beneficiaries, associated with preventable errors found "the true number of premature deaths associated with preventable harm to patients was estimated at more than 400,000 per year."[44] Thus there are almost 1,100 preventable deaths in hospitals every day—one preventable premature hospital death every 79 seconds!

Although there are as many as 400,000 preventable hospital deaths each year, there are fewer than 10,000 malpractice payments each year—fewer than 30 per day—for all types of injuries, not just deaths, and for all patients, not just hospital patients. Clearly the vast majority of malpractice victims are not being compensated. The cost of their injuries (or deaths) is being shifted from the people responsible for the injury to the victims, their families, their health insurers, and the government through the Medicare and Medicaid programs. Even worse, not only are the people responsible for the errors managing to shift the costs of their errors to others, they are also largely avoiding accountability from licensing and peer review systems. So business continues as usual and patients continue to be harmed or die.

This shifting of malpractice costs to the victims has an unfortunate effect on the safety of the general public. If the physicians responsible for malpractice were forced to pay for it, they might be forced out of practice by their inability to secure malpractice insurance. Furthermore, the increased cost of malpractice insurance might prompt other physicians to press peer reviewers and licensing boards to take action against the few physicians who cause the bulk of the malpractice problem and thus reduce insurance costs the way these costs ought to be reduced—by reducing malpractice itself. Unfortunately the response of the medical profession to date has been to call for more and more tort reform to make it difficult or impossible to bring claims and win cases rather than to take steps to reduce the underlying problem of injuries and deaths resulting from malpractice. It is a sad commentary that when physicians call for malpractice reform they invariably mean reform of the legal system rather than reform of medical practice to increase safety and reduce actual malpractice that harms patients.

The gross failure of the legal system to compensate the vast majority of malpractice victims or their survivors also has a significant impact on the ability of the Data Bank to serve as a comprehensive resource for alerting users about questionable physicians. If no malpractice payments are made, the physicians responsible for the errors are not reported to the Data Bank, so licensing boards, hospitals, MCOs, etc., are not informed of a questionable physician. And, of course, the public cannot be protected by licensing boards, hospitals, and so on—to the extent they act to protect the public—if they are not informed there may be a problem with a physician's care. And certainly the public cannot get the information itself.

WHAT SHOULD BE DONE TO PROTECT THE PUBLIC?

Several actions are needed to protect the public from dangerous physicians.

The Data Bank should be opened to the public. Individuals should be able to go online and search for any practitioner's record at no cost. They should have access to the full details of all reports, with redaction only of identifying information for the physician that could lead to identity theft (Social Security numbers, full birth dates, etc.).

But opening the Data Bank is not enough. Reporting to the Data Bank must be improved so it becomes a fully comprehensive repository.

Licensure action reporting needs to be improved. This can be accomplished by improving the licensure boards. Licensing boards need to be reformed and adequately funded so that they have the resources necessary to protect the public. The culture of many of the medical boards needs to be changed so that their actions are taken to protect the public rather than the profession in all cases, not just the worst cases. A majority, if not all, of the members of medical boards should be nonphysicians; physicians should serve only as expert witnesses in hearings or as staff members. Appointments to boards should be made in a nonpartisan way not solely under the control of the state governor. These reforms would make it more likely that boards would take all (or at least more of) the actions that ought to be taken to protect the public and report these actions to the Data Bank. [45]

Clinical privileges action reporting also needs improvement. As with licensure reporting, this can be done by improving peer review. The peers doing the reviewing should be selected randomly from a qualified pool and should come from institutions other than the one whose practitioner is being reviewed. [46] Peer reviewers also need to be adequately paid for their time. These reforms would allow peer reviewers to operate as independently as possible, without influence by either the institution or the practitioner being reviewed. The law governing reporting of clinical privileges actions to the Data Bank needs to be changed so that if a practitioner has a series of otherwise nonreportable actions, that is, a series of actions affecting clinical privileges for thirty days or less, the series of actions becomes reportable. Perhaps the threshold should be more than two otherwise nonreportable actions in a five-year period. These reforms would make peer review more effective and fair and also go a long way toward ensuring that all peer review actions which should be taken are taken and reported to the Data Bank. Additional ideas for improving peer review in hospitals are given in chapter 3.

For malpractice, loopholes like the corporate shield must be closed. Self-payments and payments made without a written claim must be reported and revealed. Other possible loopholes for malpractice payment reporting should be closed. That includes the biggest loophole of all: not compensating the vast majority of patients injured or killed by malpractice.

The malpractice compensation system needs to be reformed—true reform to appropriately compensate all malpractice, not "tort reform" making it harder to bring or win malpractice cases. Compensating all malpractice victims would ensure that all questionable physicians are reported.

Because the current system fails to adequately compensate (or compensate at all) the vast majority of malpractice victims, it fails to identify to the Data Bank the vast majority of malpractice events and the physicians found to be responsible for them. It also fails to prevent further malpractice. Patients with relatively minor injuries should be given the option to bring cases administratively to an independent state malpractice claims review board composed of nonphysicians with access to medical experts. Barriers to bringing suits should be reduced rather than increased, and plaintiffs' legal fees should be added to malpractice awards so that winning a case results in fully compensating the victim without the necessity of noneconomic "pain and suffering" damage awards to recoup legal fees. Noneconomic damages should not be capped per se but should be limited to what the jury agrees they would individually accept for themselves in similar circumstances. Punitive damages should be prohibited and not included in an award of noneconomic damages. Because of the expense of bringing a case, frivolous claims are few and far between. But if a judge finds a case to be frivolous, the attorney bringing the case should be sanctioned. Such reforms would lead to many more malpractice victims being compensated and many more reports to the Data Bank in the short run, but in the long run, dangerous physicians would be weeded out and malpractice injuries and costs would decrease. Even in the short run, real costs would not increase. Malpractice costs now paid by the victims, their health insurers, and the public would simply be shifted back to the malpracticing physicians responsible for creating the problem and their malpractice insurers.

One legal reform which should not be adopted is to put injured patient compensation programs under the direction of those causing the injuries or responsible for paying the compensation through early offer or mediation programs. As an incentive for admitting malpractice, these programs act to shield the malpracticing physicians from further sanctions or reporting. Thus, although some individual victims may benefit, the general public is not protected and there will be more victims. Putting the fox in charge of guarding the henhouse has never been a successful strategy, except for the fox.

Chapter Three

Failures and Successes of Physician Peer and Performance Review

Gerald Rogan, MD

DEVELOPMENT NEED

Each year thousands of hospital inpatients are seriously harmed due to avoidable errors. Some die prematurely. Medical experts have publicly reported this for years. Recent corrective actions have reduced errors, but some problems persist. Corrective actions include more frequent hand washing to reduce hospital-acquired infections, more comprehensive preoperative planning such as the use of procedure checklists to assure surgical equipment is available, inpatient treatment guidelines so physicians do not need to remember everything, bar coding of patient identification wristbands and drugs to avoid medication errors, double-checking of blood products to avoid transfusion reactions, and the use of patient-activated rapid response teams to promptly assess deteriorating patients before death. The benefit of these actions varies.

During 2000–2008, one required quality improvement process was deficient in several hospitals: effective medical staff peer review. Over the past several years, responsible parties have attempted to institute corrective actions in order to improve the peer review process. Successes have varied. Leaders have developed creative methods, some from other industries, such as aviation, and some hospitals have embraced them.

In this chapter, the author presents follow-up to the stories that took place at Redding Medical Center (RMC) in Redding, California, between 1997 and 2003 and at St. Joseph Hospital, Towson, Maryland, during 2008. This chapter does not identify the best method for successful peer review but focuses on the underlying problem of ineffective peer review.

WHAT IS PEER REVIEW, ITS GOAL AND PROCESS?

Peer review refers to a formal evaluation by physicians of certain selected actions performed by one of their colleagues or expected actions that were not performed. Peer review is performed by the hospital medical staff, not by nonphysician hospital administrators, hospital board members, nurses, or government inspectors. Some physician medical groups also perform peer review for patient care provided in outpatient clinics.

The goal of peer review is not to punish a physician colleague but to educate and improve medical decision making. Its method is to identify individual cases with an adverse outcome (called "trigger" cases), review each for errors of omission or commission, educate the culpable physician regarding the accepted standard of care, and, when needed, implement appropriate corrective actions. Sometimes the privileges of a physician must be limited temporarily or permanently in order to improve patient care. An example of a problem discovered by the peer review process is when a physician orders too much blood thinner and the patient almost bleeds to death.

Typically the hospital medical staff sets forth criteria for case selection. Examples include unexpected return to the operating room, unexpected loss of more than two units of blood, unexpected serious complications, unexpected admission to the intensive care unit (ICU), or postoperative infection. These are called "fallout" criteria or "triggers" because the patient's situation departs from the expected course.

Peer review can also be employed to verify a diagnosis that resulted in a procedure. For example, a sample of cases without complications may be selected to assure the relevant procedure was medically indicated. Under this process, there is no triggering event that prompts a review. Instead, cases free of complications are selected for review to verify the medical necessity of the procedures performed. This type of peer review is important for patient safety and fiscal accountability.

Peer review findings are confidential, locked away from probes by lawyers and even government officials. Confidentiality prevents an error that is discovered during the peer review findings from prompting a medical malpractice lawsuit. If a lawsuit is filed for other reasons, any findings on the same case by a peer review body remain confidential.

The agency that administers Medicare is called the Centers for Medicare and Medicaid Services (CMS). The CMS, the State health officials, the hospital accreditor, or a patient's lawyer may not discover the specific findings of a particular case reviewed. Without assurance of confidentiality, physicians would refuse to provide peer review of their colleagues.

When a peer review committee finds a physician's decision making or behavior departs from the relevant accepted standard of medical care, in addition to other corrective action, the committee may report the finding to the hospital governing body. The governing body, such as a board of trustees, may report the matter to the physician and the relevant state licensing agency and file a report with the National Practitioner Data Bank (see chapter 2 for more on the National Practitioner Data Bank).[1]

When an accrediting company discovers a failure to provide peer review, it reports the deficiency to CMS and to state government authorities. A deficiency report will prompt a second survey by the accreditor which focuses on the deficiencies found. In addition to accrediting companies, the State of California, where the author resides, performs its own surveys of hospitals to assure compliance.

BARRIERS TO EFFECTIVE PEER REVIEW

When peer review is performed within a hospital's medical staff, the names of those performing the peer review are known to the physician being reviewed. This can be a serious barrier to effective peer review when the physicians involved are friends, research colleagues, or longtime professional associates. To mitigate this conflict of interest, private peer-review companies, using experts from other hospitals, offer confidential reviews to client hospitals and their medical staffs. The reviews, usually performed on de-identified medical records and de-identified physicians, assure the absence of bias. The private peer-review company reports the findings to the hospital medical staff peer-review committee for further action. Only the committee knows the names of the physicians and patient cases reviewed.

MEDICARE'S PEER REVIEW REQUIREMENTS

In order to participate in the Medicare program, Medicare requires all hospitals to implement a physician peer-review process. The CMS (government) requirements are called Conditions of Participation. One of these conditions is the performance of inpatient peer review. The requirement for peer review is contained in Federal Regulation 42CFR482.21.[2]

In California, the state agency responsible to license hospitals is the California Department of Public Health, Licensing and Certification Program.[3] Independently of Medicare requirements, California state law also requires medical staff peer review in order for a hospital to qualify for a license to provide health care services.

VERIFICATION OF THE PERFORMANCE OF PEER REVIEW

CMS is organized under and is part of the Department of Health and Human Services of our federal government.

Peer review confidentiality poses a dilemma for oversight. There is no way for CMS, a state, or an accreditor to look at the casework performed by the peer review committee in order to validate that peer review is actually performed or that it is effective. The peer review committee may claim it is performing peer review, but the assertion cannot be directly verified. The peer review committee can falsely assert that peer review is being performed. When peer review is ineffective, only the physicians directly involved with the review know.

Both the CMS and the Office of Inspector General of the Department of Health and Human Services (OIG/HHS) are empowered with the responsibility to enforce Medicare's peer review requirement by virtue of its granting or denying provider status to hospitals that care for Medicare patients.

The performance of peer review is partially verified by the hospital accreditation process. Every hospital in the United States applies for accreditation. CMS does not accredit hospitals directly but relies instead on accreditation by private companies to verify that government requirements for hospital participation in Medicare are met.

VALIDATION OF PERFORMANCE OF PEER REVIEW

Because individual case files are confidential, evidence of ineffective peer review must be developed from reports from informed whistle-blowers or through indirect measures, such as an unexpectedly low rate of disciplinary action, absence of reports to the National Practitioner Data Bank, an unusually small percentage of cases reviewed, or findings from a qui tam (whistle-blower) lawsuit.

A medical malpractice lawsuit can identify a physician's repetitive negligence. Then the substandard medical care subsequently discovered can be correlated with a concomitant accreditation status. However, an individual case is not likely to show a pattern of negligence. Accordingly, a successful medical malpractice lawsuit is not likely to discover a failure of the peer review system.

Basically, to verify the performance of medical staff peer review, the government and the accreditor must accept the word of the committee members. In the case of RMC, the responsible parties lied.

ENFORCEMENT OF PEER REVIEW REQUIREMENTS

CMS or the OIG may revoke a hospital's provider status when peer review is not performed or is ineffective. If this happens, no Medicare payment can be made to that hospital, effectively causing it to close. This situation essentially occurred at RMC around 2003[4] and at Martin Luther King Memorial (MLK) Hospital in Los Angeles around 2007.[5] RMC was sold, and the hospital stayed open under new ownership. MLK hospital closed.

Rarely is failure to perform peer review a sufficiently severe violation to prompt CMS to revoke a hospital's provider status. Instead, the hospital is required to file a plan of correction with CMS but is not required to follow it. If the problem is not corrected, the state's inspection process is repeated until peer review is performed or the government gives up. In the case of RMC, in 2000, when the peer review deficiency was discovered, our governments, both state and federal, gave up. Enforcement was delayed until 2003 after a dismayed patient filed a qui tam lawsuit and the FBI became involved.

HOSPITAL ACCREDITATION

Probably all hospitals in the United States agree to submit to an accreditation process, which is voluntary. The three companies in the United States that accredit hospitals are The Joint Commission (TJC), the Health Care Facilities Accreditation Program, and Det Norske Veritas Healthcare, Inc.[6] TJC formerly enjoyed a monopoly for all hospitals except osteopathic hospitals.

Hospitals pay their accreditors for each accreditation. Prior to 2008, whenever TJC accredited a hospital, CMS was required to accept the accreditation and not challenge the hospital's provider status. This authority is called "deemed status." TJC was deemed to stand in the place of our government to assure the hospital's compliance with Medicare provider requirements.

The accreditation process is between the hospital and the accreditor and is protected from discovery. The details of the interaction are not shared with our government. This means that should the accreditor ignore a failure of the hospital to comply with a government requirement, or meet the accreditor's own standards, our government and the public may not discover the hospital's failure directly.

The accreditation process includes a review of the peer review process. The accreditation findings are confidential between the hospital and the accreditor. The accreditor may or may not report whether a particular deficiency is present. With respect to peer review, the government is not informed about the details of any physician negligence discovered. CMS may know only whether the peer review process requirements are met or not met.

THE REDDING MEDICAL CENTER (RMC) STORY

In Northern California in 2003 a qui tam lawsuit was filed against RMC. The complaint came from a patient who knew the care he received was negligent. The case was presented to the government, who accepted it because of a reasonable likelihood RMC was abusing the Medicare program: providing unnecessary services for which it received unjustified Medicare reimbursement. The FBI stepped in, filed a search warrant, and sent over forty agents to RMC and physician offices to retrieve hundreds of patient files. Shortly thereafter, medical experts hired by the Department of Justice identified negligent care provided to more than 700 patients. The negligent physicians were Dr. Chae Hyun Moon, an internist who called himself a cardiologist, and Fidel Realyvasquez Jr., a board-certified cardiovascular surgeon. Patients identified were treated between 1997 and 2003. During this period, TJC accredited RMC.

The RMC case was closed around November 2005. Settlement details are available on the Internet.[7]

During three government surveys in 1999, three years before the negligence was stopped, state surveyors discovered peer review was not being performed but did not know why or that the care delivered at RMC was negligent. TJC also reported to the state that RMC failed to provide peer review. The California Medical Association's Institute of Medical Quality, which tagged along with TJC accreditors, confirmed the peer review deficiency.

Yet months later, after no correction to the peer review process was made, RMC was fully accredited. CMS and the State of California gave RMC permission to operate for three more years as a fully accredited hospital and without another survey to verify performance of peer review, which the state knew had not been corrected.

The documentation in the state and CMS files suggests that neither CMS nor State of California officials believed the absence of peer review was significant enough to impose its requirement. One CMS official stated to the author, by telephone, that the peer review requirement is only an element of a condition of participation and, therefore, not important enough to restrict the hospital's provider status. On the other hand, there is evidence RMC lied to regulators by falsely claiming peer review was being performed by a contracted external entity created for this purpose, an entity that never existed. RMC kept most of its medical staff uninformed about the peer review process in the cardiac services sections, including the medical staff chief of patient safety, Dr. Ian Grady. Details are in the disaster analysis.[8,9]

But CMS has enforcement powers. For example, CMS could have denied Medicare payment for the cardiac services at RMC for elective cases until the peer review deficiency was corrected. Instead, CMS chose to do nothing effective to impose its provider requirements on the hospital or its medical staff. The State of California could have closed the department. The RMC hospital administrators and physicians who controlled the medical staff refused to permit the required peer review. TJC, the state, and CMS simply dropped the ball.

The refusal to comply was driven by Dr. Moon and his colleagues, who were making millions of dollars from provision of unnecessary services, with the cooperation of hospital administrators, who were reporting record profits to the hospital's parent, Tenet Healthcare. Drs. Moon and Realyvazquez, respectively, were in charge of the peer review for their sections.

As a result, patient safety at RMC was not assured. CMS knew it was not assured. In a letter in 2000 from CMS to the RMC administrator, CMS explicitly cited RMC's inability to assure patient safety as a reason RMC must correct its medical staff's peer review deficiency. Yet a few months later, CMS gave RMC unrestricted provider status without validated evidence that peer review was being performed.

To be fair to CMS, until the findings of the qui tam lawsuit became public, CMS did not know that care at RMC in its cardiology services sections was negligent, or that the absence of peer review allowed the negligence to continue for at least six years and damage over 700 patients. CMS could not have known the details about cases of negligence, because the peer review findings are confidential.

ROOT CAUSE ANALYSIS OF THE RMC MEDICAL DISASTER

When 700 patients are damaged at one institution, it is like a 747 jetliner crashing into a sea wall in front of a runway. Yet by 2007 there was no disaster analysis of RMC, unlike the jetliner crash at San Francisco International Airport on July 6, 2013.[10] The author asked several agencies of government, including the OIG, as well as a Medicare quality assurance contractor, to provide one. All refused. So the author, with the help of two RMC physician insiders and armed with the Freedom of Information Act (FOIA), performed the disaster analysis as a public and professional service. What happened at RMC was shameful to the medical profession. Its root cause could not be ignored.

But even after the RMC case was settled, around 2005, the absence of peer review was not identified as the critical cause of the system failure at RMC. Instead, no one really knew what caused the RMC safeguards failure. It appeared to the author that our government believed that its punishment was enough. Institutional culpability that might show a failure of institutional design, impotent patient safety regulations, or government inaction was not worth discovering.

In November 2007, after the FBI investigation was finished and RMC sold, the author filed a request for records under the FOIA with both CMS and the state. The documents found in the state's files confirmed that both our state and federal governments knew there was no peer review during the year 2000 and did nothing to enforce the requirement. CMS told the author the requirement of peer review was only an element of the Medicare Conditions of Participation, not important enough to force the hospital to comply. A state official explained that their lack of enforcement was due to limited survey and enforcement personnel and the need to prioritize scarce resources. The agency had no desk-level procedure to weigh one reported deficiency against another. The state staff simply made a bad judgment call that allowed ongoing negligent care for hundreds more patients over the subsequent three years. The staff, including at least one physician expert, did not believe the absence of peer review was important enough to enforce on a priority basis. It was not until three years later that the FBI's physician experts provided the missing peer review, after hundreds more patients were irreparably damaged.

The disaster analysis found that the details about TJC's remedial requirements from its 2000 accreditation survey, which retrospectively were not imposed on RMC, were not shared with CMS and were not available to the public, despite a request under the FOIA. CMS had no details on file because they never received them from TJC, as was the custom and practice at the time. It was not that the FOIA request could not legally compel the release of protected records. There were no records and never were.

By accident, a letter from TJC to RMC was found in the state's file. The state official claimed it was left there through error. The question of why it would ever be in the file was not answered. The document seemed to embarrass the state official, because for a time she demanded its return, even though the state has no obligation to protect the confidentiality of TJC documents from an FOIA request. After a few days, the state formally released the record.

The document showed TJC knew RMC did not provide peer review, yet gave RMC provisional accreditation. TJC stated it expected the hospital to eventually comply, which we know in retrospect it never did. No documentation is available to know why TJC fully accredited RMC despite the failure of its medical staff to perform peer review. From review of the available documents, it appears that TJC failed to enforce its accreditation requirements, during which time it fully accredited RMC for three years, without justification.

One can assert that the failure of CMS to impose ongoing correction action on RMC was negligent. CMS officials at Regional Office 9, San Francisco, who were in charge, could have had faith in and required enforcement of its own conditions of participation (COP) requirements, by virtue of giving more weight to the need to provide peer review as a critical element to assure patient safety. Instead CMS treated the element of peer review as a minor requirement, not as a critical unmet need to protect patients. It was like flunking algebra yet graduating with a degree in electrical engineering. Now, in hindsight, we all know better.

The absence of peer review was to RMC as the failed O-rings were to the Challenger space shuttle explosion. The difference is that officials investigated the Challenger disaster for its root cause, but not the RMC disaster.

DEEMED STATUS

In 2008, Congress revoked the deemed status of all accrediting organizations, including TJC, which subjects their accreditation activities to CMS oversight.[11] The new statute was signed into law on July 15, 2008. The new law removed automatic deemed status for TJC, effective July 15, 2010.[12] This change means that CMS now has the authority to determine whether TJC's accreditations are sufficient to assure Medicare's COP are met.

This change may result in greater accountability of accrediting organizations to the government, and thereby to the people, depending upon how well CMS reviews the accreditors' performance. Prior to this change, compliance with the Medicare law was assured by an organization whose income came from those institutions that allegedly complied with Medicare rules—a clear conflict of interest, over which our federal government had no control until the statutorily authorized "deemed status" was revoked and made subject to government oversight. Empowered by the new law, effective in 2010, should an accreditor falsely accredit a hospital and have the falsehood discovered, CMS may revoke the accreditor's deemed status. Then the accreditor's hospital clients would have to find another accrediting company which would have the necessary delegated authority to verify to our government that Medicare's provider requirements are met.

One reported reason for this change in law was the alleged negligence of TJC found by our root cause analysis of the RMC disaster. It was our disaster analysis, developed during 2007–2008, that found the improper accreditation of the RMC by TJC during 2000. During 2008, when the legislation was considered by the Senate Committee on Finance, Subcommittee on Health Care, one of its staff members contacted the author to request our preliminary findings about the root cause of the RMC disaster. We reported our documentary evidence that TJC had accredited RMC despite the hospital's ongoing violations of Medicare COP, based on the TJC letter left in the state files, reportedly by error.

HOW TO IMPROVE PEER REVIEW

Experts discuss how to improve patient safety and have identified barriers to effective peer review. Some have implemented insightful corrective methods.

Peer review is so important, one would think it would be measured and reported to the public. Effectiveness of peer review might be measured with the following data:

- Number and percent of medical records reviewed to validate medical necessity
- Number and percent of records reviewed per number of discharges
- Number and percent of problem cases reviewed
- Number of records reviewed per number of discharges
- Number and percent of errors of physician judgment, for example, unnecessary stent placement
- Failure of system support: number and percent, for example, lack of audit of image interpretation
- Types of corrective action taken by the peer review process: number and percent

  - No action
  - Education and monitoring
  - Restriction of privileges
  - Hospital system correction
  - Number of physicians reported to the National Practitioner Data Bank
  - Number of physicians reported to the state medical board per number of cases reviewed, such as is promoted by Public Citizen [13]

PEER REVIEW AS A TOOL FOR MEDICARE PROGRAM INTEGRITY

Services provided that are not medically indicated may not be reimbursed by Medicare. Unfortunately, Medicare contractors may miss medically unnecessary services and, therefore, pay for them by error. Only 1 percent of claims are audited. Typically, auditors accept the interpretations of medical image findings without challenge: without auditing the images themselves. Peer review can identify cases of improper image interpretation and take corrective action early, before CMS requires an audit and demands repayment. Image audit standards are required for mammograms [14] and Pap smears, [15] but not for cardiac imaging. Therefore, peer review of cases that are without complications has precedence. It can be performed to verify medical necessity, to verify patient safety, and to assure that Medicare pays only for medically necessary services, as intended by statute.

Initially, peer review for medical necessity can be focused on procedures that pose a conflict of interest in a fee-for-service payment system: procedures in which the need for the procedure is determined by the physician who performs and interprets the test used to verify that the procedure is needed. One example is the placement of a stent into a coronary artery. The need to place a stent is determined by a coronary angiogram. The angiogram image will show a narrowing in part of the artery that must be opened in order to allow adequate blood flow to the downstream heart muscle. Once the artery is opened, a stent is placed across the treated area to prevent closure. The critical physician interpretation is based on the amount of narrowing seen on a 2-D image of a 3-D vessel: is the amount sufficient to impair blood flow so that a heart attack is threatened? In such cases, the artery must be opened. In cases of mild narrowing, the patient may be treated with medicine alone.

Typically, the angiogram image is interpreted by the cardiologist in real time during the angiogram. When the narrowing is severe, the artery is immediately opened with a high-pressure balloon (an angioplasty) followed by placing a stent across the narrowed area. Should the cardiologist interpret a severe narrowing when it is minimal, the error causes an unnecessary opening and stent placement. Some evidence suggests that an unnecessary angioplasty and stent placement can make a patient worse over time, compared with medical treatment alone.

A cardiologist who is reimbursed by a fee-for-service method is paid extra for each artery segment that is opened and each stent placed. This payment method sets up a conflict of interest. To mitigate this conflict, the angiogram interpretations can be reviewed by peers to verify the medical necessity of each opening and each stent, in real time, or upon audit. This process will assure a severe narrowing was not overlooked and that an insignificant narrowing is not aggressively treated. In this manner, peer review can detect errors of commission: too many procedures done; and errors of omission: a needed procedure that was not performed. The mistakes found can enlighten the physician and halt the perpetuation of the same error on subsequent patients.

Note that in such cases, the patient may have no complications. In fact, performance of medically unnecessary services can result in claims data which perversely implies the hospital is top quality. By treating normal patients with unnecessary procedures, the complication rate may be lower because healthy patients do better than sick patients. The data then would imply the hospital is a center of excellence, when, in fact, it is a center of abuse. The key variable is identified by routine audits for medical necessity. During the period RMC was abusing patients, its staff claimed it was a center of excellence. Three days before the FBI stormed RMC with over forty agents, a highly placed RMC official bragged to the author about the high quality of cardiac services RMC provided.

PERVERSE INCENTIVES IN FEE-FOR-SERVICE

Self-referral in a fee-for-service payment system inherently poses a financial conflict of interest. The physician can be financially motivated to order an unnecessary angiogram, misinterpret the image, assert the disease is worse than it actually is, and place an unnecessary stent, without anyone ever discovering the abuse. RMC is the "poster child" for this kind of abuse. The safeguard for patients is effective peer review. But the peer review must not be limited to cases in which complications arise. The peer review must be performed on random cases as well in order to be sure the services provided are appropriate, not too many and not too few, even when the patient does well. Reliance on review of cases triggered only by complications is insufficient to assure services are medically indicated.

PEER REVIEW WILL HELP PHYSICIANS AND HOSPITALS

Peer review can be very helpful. In 2007, the Medical Board of California revoked Dr. Moon's license to practice medicine.[16] Dr. Realyvazquez completed probation and maintains his medical license.[17] Reportedly, because the hospital administrators colluded with members of the medical staff to thwart the peer review process, the hospital was kicked out of Medicare. The owner, Tenet Healthcare, sold its RMC hospital, one of its most profitable. The hospital became a Medicare provider under new ownership. Had peer review been performed, these complications may have been avoided. RMC's medical staff could have provided effective peer review and constrained the negligent physicians in a timely manner. Instead, the FBI called in experts who performed the missing peer review for the first time, after the damage was done.

CLAIMS DATA IS NOT EFFECTIVE

Between 1997 and 2000, health care researchers found that an extraordinarily high number of cardiac procedures were being performed in Redding, considering its population. However, this detailed health care statistical information had no impact on the poor quality of care in Redding. There was no government investigation based on the statistical findings. The academic data was unable to help protect patients. RMC claimed the high volume of services discovered by researchers was due to the high quality of its physicians. Dr. Moon reportedly asserted he was finding disease that other, less intelligent physicians simply overlooked. When the coronary angiogram was normal, Moon relied on imaging of the wall thickness of the coronary artery using ultrasound to detect otherwise hidden disease. Unfortunately, Dr. Moon was interpreting ultrasound artifact as disease—spontaneously dissecting coronary arteries. Dr. Realyvasquez would bypass arteries when the arteriogram showed no disease.

ONGOING FAILURE OF GOVERNMENT OVERSIGHT

The California legislature investigated the alleged statewide peer-review problem in 2008. It held an all-day hearing. A quality improvement company and Medicare contractor, Lumetra LLC, conducted research ordered by the Medical Board of California. Lumetra found deficiencies in peer review at many hospitals. At the legislative hearing, the California Medical Association testified that Lumetra's report was flawed and its findings should be ignored. The "flaw" was that many hospitals refused to report whether or not their medical staffs provided peer review. Lumetra reported the anecdotal case of RMC and several other California hospital cases. Despite this, the State of California legislature did nothing effective to improve enforcement of the performance of peer review in order to better protect patients. Refusal of a hospital to report whether or not peer review is performed is a good reason to require the performance of peer review as a quality measure.

In the Redding case, several doctors practicing in other cities discovered individual patients who had been treated at RMC with unnecessary coronary artery bypass graft operations. For example, one cardiologist in a nearby community reported her patient had received bypasses of three coronary arteries, all of which were normal at the time of the operation. She saw the angiogram that the RMC cardiologist, Moon, had performed. It was normal in her opinion, which opinion was confirmed by other experts. Yet the patient had the surgery anyway. According to an OIG investigator, six patients at RMC who had received unnecessary treatment were reported to the Medical Board of California (MBC) by physicians from outside the Redding community. The MBC reviewed none of them, reportedly because the patients refused to release their medical records to state reviewers. Allegedly, these patients believed their treatment was top quality (see chapter 1 for more on medical boards).

CMS does not report the presence of peer review on its hospital quality website.[18] Patients cannot know whether a hospital medical staff provides peer review or whether it is effective. There is no measure of effectiveness of peer review because the experts in charge of measures have not yet created one.[19] CMS does not require the medical staff peer review process to provide routine audits of cases for medical necessity. Instead CMS relies upon post-pay recovery based on data analysis or patient complaints. When Medicare contractors perform audits of cardiac cases, rarely are the images themselves reviewed to confirm the subsequent procedures are medically indicated. In the RMC case, the Medicare contractor reviewed a sample of Moon's cases and missed his negligence, because the images themselves were not reviewed. Even though the Medicare contractor, NHIC, was suspicious of Moon's behavior because of the volume of his services, it found no evidence of negligence or unnecessary services.

Our anecdotal report about RMC, as well as many other failures of peer review throughout the United States, is available to the public.

MARK MIDEI, ST. JOSEPH HOSPITAL STORY

In 2008, a similar case to the RMC story was discovered at St. Joseph Hospital in Towson, Maryland. Dr. Mark Midei inserted unnecessary cardiac stents into the arteries of hundreds of patients whose diseases did not require them. He interpreted the cardiac images he performed, without peer review oversight. His interpretations were used to justify the angioplasties and stents he placed. In some cases, he overstated the severity of the coronary narrowing. Many patients needed medical treatment only, without an angioplasty. As at RMC, Midei's negligence at St. Joseph was discovered by medical experts who had been hired by the FBI pursuant to a qui tam lawsuit. Midei was in charge of his own peer review. His conflict of interest was not mitigated. Midei made more money for every stent placed, plus the stent manufacturer provided kickbacks. The reason Midei was in charge of his own peer review is unknown. But at RMC, Moon was in charge of his own peer review because he was a high admitter and made a lot of money for the hospital. Likewise, Midei was a high-volume doctor for St. Joseph. Midei lost his license.[20,21]

SENATE COMMITTEE INVESTIGATION

The US Senate Subcommittee on Health Care investigated the matter of Midei's peer review failures and reported its findings to the public.[22] Its "disaster analysis" discovered the root cause of the damage. Its report may have been the first disaster analysis ever performed by a government agency for a health care disaster. Unlike airplane disasters, health care disasters are not routinely examined to discover their root cause, such as the failure to perform effective peer review. As a result, the public has no way to know why so many patients have been damaged at one hospital over several years before the negligence is discovered. Simply, our government does not consider a medical disaster to be a sufficient justification for routine root cause analysis.

One important reason that peer review may be ineffective is that it has traditionally been an "in-hospital" activity controlled by those being reviewed. Methods are under review to mitigate this problem. Recently, peer review problems in some Veterans Administration hospitals have been flagged for improvements by the General Accounting Office. The primary concern found was that the peer review process was not assessing the roles of individual physicians in creation of the adverse event that instigated peer review.[23]

The culture of medicine must embrace effective peer review in order to help reduce errors of omission and commission regarding diagnoses and patient management. Physicians must support peer review as educational rather than to promote "blame and shame." Some experts report that peer review has been embraced in the Korean Airlines, the Israeli military, the National Aeronautics and Space Administration, some hospital systems, and many other institutions, but not routinely in hospitals. Government must assure robust enforcement of peer review requirements in order to protect patients. Effective peer review as an audit tool can contain payment for unnecessary services. Websites describing hospital quality measures do not tell patients where peer review is effective and not effective. The public has no way to know whether their hospital medical staff enjoys the benefit of effective peer review.

The current peer review system depends on the occurrence of an adverse event before it is set in motion. From a patient's point of view, this process is inadequate. It allows patients to be damaged before the substandard care is identified. It would be better to discover the potential problem before damage occurs. Most hospitals attempt to assure a physician is qualified through the credentialing process. Each physician must prove qualification for each procedure performed in a hospital. Some hospitals have higher standards than others, but all have a credentialing process.

Unfortunately, the credentialing process is not sufficient to assure patient safety. This conclusion is supported in other articles.[24] Some doctors overstate their experience. Some understate their problems. Some develop problems over time which may remain hidden. Therefore, ongoing effective peer review is required in addition to credentialing.

THE CULTURE OF PHYSICIANS

Effective peer review requires a change in the culture of medicine. Physicians must learn that peer review can be helpful. In the case of RMC and St. Joseph Hospital in Towson, Maryland, effective peer review would have saved the hospitals and the culpable physicians Moon, Realyvasquez, and Midei from public rebuke, as well as protected hundreds of patients from harm. External peer review of de-identified treating physicians and patients, performed by qualified nonconflicted expert physician peers, can help remove the parochial impediments to effective peer review. Reliance on hospital accreditation to assure patient safety is not enough to assure patient safety.

REMEDIES

1. Medicare requirements to perform peer review must be clarified and effectively enforced.
2. Accrediting organizations that fail to identify missing peer review should be effectively disciplined by CMS and state agencies so that inadequate accreditation is not profitable.
3. CMS should require the committee that develops quality measures to create a quantitative measure of peer review effectiveness.
4. The measure must be reported by each hospital and the information made available to the public.
5. Hospitals should establish a patient safety officer to assure peer review is effective.
6. Medicare should require routine audits for medical necessity for selected procedures that carry an unmitigated conflict of interest, such as cardiac procedures, wherein the need for the intervention is determined by the interventionist without oversight, particularly under a fee-for-service reimbursement payment method.
7. Medicare should support methods to improve the effectiveness of peer review.

In summary, effective peer review remains an unmet need in many hospitals. Peer review is needed to learn from errors and to validate medical necessity. Without effective peer review, patients will continue to be at avoidable risk of medical negligence that is potentially harmful. Medicare will continue to pay for unnecessary care. Without robust automatic analysis of medical disasters, the root causes, such as failure to perform effective peer review, will remain hidden. We will not benefit from the knowledge that could be taught by our mistakes. Medical disasters warrant routine root cause analysis just as we do for airplane crashes.

Author's Comment

I hope the information in this chapter will help in the following ways:

1. Hospital board members will ask more questions.

2. OIG officials will discover the need to regularly provide medical disaster investigations.
3. CMS officials will find the need to require routine audits for medical necessity by the peer review committee rather than relying completely on Medicare contractors to discover unnecessary services.
4. Leaders of accrediting organizations will understand patients are watching and must rely on accreditation excellence.
5. Rank-and-file physicians will figure out ways to make peer review work.
6. Performance measure creators at the Institute of Medicine will consider peer review for a quality performance measure.
7. Industrial psychologists will continue to find ways to make effective peer review acceptable to physicians.

Comment by Editor, John James

Experts are working on methods to make peer review effective. Here is one example:

A proactive way to mitigate ineffective peer review, which comes *after* the harm, is for hospitals to implement periodic 360-degree reviews. These are multisource feedback (MSF) exercises in which a physician's performance is *anonymously* reported on a periodic basis by subordinates, peers, and department heads. Behind these feedback evaluations is the reality that many physicians perform their healing art while effectively burned out or otherwise impaired. Physicians are no different from other human beings working in a high-stress environment.[25] The second fact of life with physicians is that they are known to have a poor ability to discover their individual weaknesses that need improvement.[26] Under these conditions, it seems obvious that anonymous performance and behavioral reviews by those working closely with a physician are the best way to determine where a physician needs improvement.

Particularly in Canada, 360-degree review instruments have been evaluated and applied to hospitals since the late 1990s. The province of Alberta has had a mandatory review process called Alberta Physician Achievement Review since 1999. The process involves self-evaluation of physicians along with evaluations by patients, peers, referring physicians, consulting physicians, and nonphysician coworkers.[27] There was not good correlation between physician self-assessments and the collective assessments of others. Interestingly, physicians' self-evaluations were less favorable than the evaluations by their peers. The primary goal of these reviews is to provide data on which the individual physician can act to improve the quality of his care and interactions with coworkers; however, under some circumstances additional actions may be needed to expedite improvements. The information is not intended to be available to patients.

A decade later it seems that the 360-degree reviews of physicians in Canada has had little impact on other jurisdictions or countries. The barriers to adopting this approach seem to be (1) the need for a high-trust environment in the hospital, (2) the need for anonymity of physicians' and coworkers' comments, and (3) those being reviewed must be assured of confidentiality of the collective results.[28]

More recently three MSF tools have been evaluated in twenty-six nonacademic hospitals in the Netherlands. The MSF reporters included secretarial assistants and patients. The investigators found that self-ratings did not correlate with coworker or patient ratings; however, ratings by peers, coworkers, and patients correlated with each other. The team of investigators deduced that to acquire minimally reliable data, evaluations were necessary from five peers, five nonphysician coworkers, and eleven patients.[29] In a review article involving analysis of forty-three published studies, investigators found slightly different numbers for validity; eight physician colleagues, eight coworkers, and twenty-five patients were necessary for valid data.[30] In my opinion the MSF approach holds great promise to help physicians improve the quality of their services.

Chapter Four

Dangerous Medical Devices

John T. James, PhD, and Stephen S. Tower, MD

INTRODUCTION

We have all come in contact with medical devices. These can include inert objects as simple as bandages and tongue depressors or machines as complicated as a mechanical heart. For many Americans, medical devices have been life prolonging; however, others' lives have been shortened or the quality of their lives has been substantially diminished because a device has been inserted in their bodies. The US Food and Drug Administration (FDA) is responsible for "approving" or "clearing" devices for use in patients. The process by which devices are "approved" is called premarket assessment (PMA), and the process by which devices become "cleared" is called the 501(k) process, so named because of the applicable section of the law creating the process. The former process is much more rigorous, involving carefully controlled new studies, than the latter process, which clears new devices that are "substantially similar" to ones already in use. Because of harm associated with some devices cleared for use, the Institute of Medicine (IOM), which is the medical branch of the National Academy of Sciences, was asked a few years ago to review the 501(k) process and make recommendations. Much was at stake here because device manufacturers want freedom to innovate without costly studies, but patients want assurance that devices placed in their bodies are safe and effective.

The FDA's development and approval process for new devices includes several tracks. The goal of government regulation is to provide the public with reasonable assurance of safe and effective devices while avoiding overregulation of the industry. FDA's authority over devices was given by Congress in 1976 after many women were rendered infertile or died from use of the Dalkon Shield and other intrauterine birth control devices. Two routes for approval were created: (1) the PMA process, under which the manufacturer had to demonstrate scientific evidence that the device was safe and effective for the intended use and (2) the 501(k) process, under which the manufacturer had only to assert that the device was "substantially similar" to another device that was already on the market as of 1976 or later. This latter process was intended for devices that were not to be inserted inside a person—for example, a hearing aid would fall into this category. As time went on, more devices with more substantial risk fell under the 501(k) process. A law in 2002 directed the FDA to "take the least burdensome approach in all areas of medical device regulation." Due to resource limitations, the FDA shifted approval so that now less than 1 percent of medical devices come through the PMA process.[1]

The FDA designates devices into three categories as follows:

- Class I devices involve little risk to the patient, for example, bandages.
- Class II devices have intermediate risk, such as an electrocardiograph machine.
- Class III devices pose the highest risk to patients and are implantable and lifesaving. These include implantable pacemakers, stents, and heart valves.

Class III devices were supposed to go through the more rigorous PMA process, but a report from the US General Accountability Office found that most of the Class III devices cleared through the 501(k) process were implantable and life sustaining.[2] Although the FDA had committed in the mid-1990s to stop accepting Class III devices through the 501(k) process, the agency was still doing this as of 2009.

An IOM report, published in 2011,[3] did not fully settle the matter of how the goals of patient safety and rapid device innovation can be reconciled. The IOM committee determined that "the 501(k) clearance process is not intended to evaluate the safety and effectiveness of medical devices with some exceptions. The 501(k) process cannot be transformed into a premarket evaluation of safety and effectiveness as long as the standard for clearance is substantial equivalence to any previously cleared device." What the public does not understand is that when the FDA finds that a device is "substantially equivalent" to a device on the market, there is no assurance to the public that the device is safe and effective. The IOM further concluded there is no evidence on which to determine whether the 501(k) process facilitates or inhibits innovation. The IOM made it clear that innovation involves improving upon what is already out there, something the 501(k) process does not do. Ultimately, the IOM concluded that the 501(k) process must be replaced by a system that combines premarket and postmarket performance data to regulate devices based on sound evidence. Until this happens, it is the opinion of the present authors that the public must be cautious when the time comes to consider implantation of a device for which there is no reasonable assurance of safety or effectiveness; in essence, it has been cleared (not approved) through the 501(k) process.

In the opinion of the present authors, unsafe devices can be cleared for marketing to the public in three major ways. One is that a new device is "substantially equivalent" to a previous device that is *not* safe or effective. Thus a new device enters the market that is no better than another cleared device, which itself may have come on the market through the 501(k) process because it is "substantially equivalent" to yet another device. One can envision a cascade of marginal devices, each like the other, being placed in patients. The second way a device can be mistakenly cleared is that it is *not* "substantially equivalent" to a device that has a track record of apparent safety and effectiveness. The third way is that a device was put through an inadequate PMA process. If the clinical trials are too short to reveal the shortcomings of the device or if the trials are performed by physicians invested in the technology, then there is a perverse incentive to overlook problems. These three major gaps in the process should reinforce the patient's wariness in choosing to have a device implanted in their body.

This chapter is divided into two parts: cardiovascular devices and hip replacement devices. Stories will be told of how cleared devices led to rather extensive harm to many patients. We will examine the routes to that harm, which not only include flaws in the devices themselves but also medical misapplication of the devices in ways that were not intended. We provide a checklist that patients can use to protect themselves from harm due to insertion of a medical device and then suggest ways that advocates for improved patient safety can exert influence on legislators and the FDA that should be making and implementing laws, respectively, to protect the public from harm.

CARDIOVASCULAR DEVICES

Cardiovascular devices include a remarkable collection of mechanical and electronic contraptions. Mechanical devices are designed to prolong the life of a patient by supporting the flow of blood in veins and arteries by removing or opening blockages and by filtering blood to prevent clots from reaching vital organs such as the lungs. Mechanical devices also include replacement parts for the heart, particularly mechanical heart valves, heart support devices, and probes that facilitate visualization of blood flow within the heart or ablation of troublesome areas near the heart that contribute to atrial fibrillation. Electronic devices include those that monitor the beating of the heart, regulate the beating of the heart (pacemakers), or shock the heart when its

beating becomes erratic (automated external defibrillators, AEDs). Obviously, such devices have saved many lives, but failure of these devices or failure
to properly manage their use may quickly lead to patient harm and death.

The history of the development of devices that provide "electrical management" of the heart provides insight into how cardiac devices were developed over several decades and ultimately imparted renewed health to many
patients, but with missteps along the way. By electrical devices we mean
those that control the heart through electrical impulses that are small and
localized (pacemakers) and those that provide a substantial shock to restore
normal electrical rhythm to the heart (implantable cardioverter defibrillators,
ICDs). Experimental pacemakers were produced as early as 1932 in the
United States and used therapeutically in Sweden in 1958 for temporary
heart pacing. By the late 1960s permanent pacing was available, but the
devices suffered from poor reliability and bulky size.[4] These early pacemakers ignored the natural heart rhythm, so pacemakers were developed to sense
natural heart rhythm so the pacemaker would not impose its "will" over
useful, natural heart impulses.

The 1980s saw worldwide standardization in pacemaker design and con-
nectivity to the heart, and ablation (tissue destruction) techniques were developed to eliminate electrical pathways that interfered with normal heart
rhythms. The 1990s saw development of evidence-based guidelines as the
cardiology community found more uses for pacemakers and ICDs. However,
it has been noted that local practices tend to dictate which patients receive
pacemakers rather than the evidence-based guidelines. Overuse of pacemakers became the standard in many places. By the turn of the millennium large
clinical trials were performed to foster genuine evidence for guideline writing. Sometimes the investigations turned up evidence that the pacing was
harmful to patients, as for example when dual-chamber ventricular pacing
was found to actually increase the risk of patient death.[5] What we observe in
this history is decades of clinicians gradually developing devices that help
their patients, but this morphs into a period of somewhat reckless overuse,
followed by a period of reconciliation based on demands from regulators for
high-quality clinical trials. What we also know is that sometimes clinicians
take their patients into harm's way with their untested contraptions.

In his book *Collateral Damage* Dan Walter tells the story of harm that
came to his wife, Pam, when she was being treated for atrial fibrillation.[6] She
was supposed to have an ablation procedure to "burn" tissues in the walls of
the atrium that were causing the arrhythmia. The inexperienced cardiologist
performing the procedure had a new type of Lasso mapping catheter that can
uncoil to position itself in the atrium, but the cardiologist turned the probe the
wrong way and the thing got stuck in Pam's heart. A senior cardiologist
scrubbed in and gave the stuck probe a hard yank, and it did come loose with
part of Pam's mitral valve hanging on the end. Pam was going into heart

failure, and her blood pressure was dropping. She underwent emergency open-heart surgery to repair her damaged heart. The device used in Pam's heart was FDA approved through the 501(k) process because it was alleged to be "substantially equivalent" to an earlier form without the coil that had already been approved through the 501(k) process. Even a casual observer could see that the two devices were quite dissimilar. A few years after Pam's ordeal, doctors at Harvard would publish a study showing how to deal with mitral valve entrapment of this type of catheter.[7] It is not to give the catheter a hard yank. This story is an example of a poorly regulated, potentially dangerous cardiac device placed in the hands of an inexperienced cardiologist. This is a recipe for patient harm.

When evidence of problems with devices appears, the FDA, sometimes after prolonged deliberation, issues warnings about the device or recalls its approval. These warnings and recalls fall into three categories as follows:

- **Class I recall:** This is the most serious type of recall. A device has a high risk of causing harm or death.
- **Class II recall:** The device has some chance of having a serious problem. But most problems may be short-term and can be fixed.
- **Class III recall:** The device has a low risk of causing a health problem.

Dr. Zuckerman and her colleagues, searching FDA databases, found that there were 113 Class I recalls in the years 2005 to 2009.[8] The recalls were based on information provided by doctors, researchers, patients, and device makers. Of these 113 Class I recalls only 21 had gone through the PMA process, 80 had gone through the 501(k) process, and 8 had been exempted from FDA regulation. Thirty-five of the Class I recalls (the most in any category) were for cardiovascular devices. The majority of Class I recalls of cardiovascular devices cleared through the 501(k) process were for AEDs. It is estimated that hundreds of people have died from malfunctioning AEDs. The point is that the FDA's process of regulating cardiovascular devices has failed many persons, and it seems that pressure is mounting to further relax the FDA's scrutiny of medical devices. Dr. Zuckerman and her colleagues (2011) recommended four changes to the FDA processes of device regulation, which can be summarized as follows: (1) Class III devices must go through the PMA process; (2) high-risk designation depends on the severity of the outcome if the device fails; (3) the FDA should have additional authority to inspect production of 501(k)-cleared devices; and (4) there should be additional postmarket surveillance and postmarket performance standards. However, to quote Dr. Zuckerman (personal communication, January 2014), "Early in the Obama Administration, the FDA's efforts to strengthen laws and regulations regarding devices were blasted by members of Congress. The device lobbyists were out in full force in the House and Senate, claiming that any safeguards would "cost Americans jobs"—although there was no evidence to support that claim. By 2014, an effort was under way—this time by the FDA—"to weaken the regulation of devices even more."

Part of the blame for this situation, which leaves the public at risk, is the relative cost of the PMA process versus the cost of the 501(k) process and the reluctance of Congress to appropriate enough money for the FDA to use the PMA process more often. The government has estimated that review of a 501(k) submission costs about $19,000, whereas review of a PMA submission costs about $870,000.[9] User fees provided by law from the companies submitting applications pay no more than one-fourth of these costs. Congress hears the voices of the lobbyists, but they seldom hear the voices of harmed patients. If you or someone you know has been harmed or has died because of a device failure, then report this to the FDA and make certain your senators and representative hear from you. Your silence says you do not care about harmed patients.

Patients not only must worry about the risk of cardiovascular devices when used as intended, but they must also be aware that improper use of such devices can place them at additional risk. Blood normally flows from veins into the heart, where it is pumped to the lungs to be oxygenated and give up carbon dioxide. Clots that form in veins (venous thromboembolisms) can easily work their way through the large chambers of the heart and lodge in the tiny vessels of the lung, causing respiratory distress and death. It is reasonable in a patient at high risk of a venous thromboembolism to place a filtering device into the inferior vena cava (IVC) to keep any clot from advancing to the lungs if more conventional anticoagulant therapy is not appropriate. Many of the IVC filters are retrievable, and the FDA recommends that these should be removed as soon as possible.

Although no randomized control trials (the gold standard for making medical guidelines) have demonstrated long-term safety of IVC filters, they continue to be inserted in increasing numbers. As of 2012 approximately a quarter of a million filters were in patients, and most of these were retrievable filters. Unretrieved, removable filters left in place pose a risk to the patient, yet only a third of the filters are retrieved. The FDA has recommended that retrievable filters be removed once the risk of a pulmonary embolism subsides.[10] The approval of such filters occurred through the 501(k) process, and in the opinion of three physicians it is unclear how such filters ever were approved in the first place, except through this much less rigorous process. They point out that complications include hematoma, air embolism, device migration, embolization of broken parts, and perforation of the IVC.[11] They emphasize that clinicians have a responsibility to inform patients that IVC filters have a known harm profile and no demonstrated benefit.

HIP REPLACEMENTS

Hip replacements are big business in the medical industry. Most of us know friends, coworkers, and family members who have had hips replaced without any untoward complications. However, certain kinds of hip replacement devices have caused substantial harm to many patients because of their design. Hip replacement devices were first marketed in the 1970s with a design that involved metal-on-plastic. Over the years it was apparent that the plastic wore out well before the metal did, so designers came up with a metal-on-metal (MOM) hip replacement device that was cleared through the 501(k) process. Estimates suggest that about one million MOMs have been implanted worldwide since 1996; however, registries maintained in the United Kingdom and Australia suggest that the failure rate of MOM implants is two to three times that of non-MOM replacements.[12] Current recommendations in the United Kingdom are that metal-on-polyethylene hip bearings are suitable for most patients, and recent improvements have mitigated the wear properties of the plastic.[13]

By 2010 the British Medicine and Health Registry issued a safety alert about MOM implants, calling for anyone with such a hip that is found to have a cobalt or chromium level above 7 parts per billion in their blood to have imaging studies of the hip to determine the cup orientation and whether the adjacent bone is decaying or there is loosening of the joint. In addition, if the patient is experiencing pain, then imaging studies are recommended.[14] Such studies may also reveal "abnormal tissue reactions" in tissue adjacent to the implant and various types of masses, including solid masses and cystic masses. At least it seems that cancer may not be associated with the use of MOM hips when compared to other types of hip replacements, including metal-on-polyethylene. Based on a study of more than 10,000 patients with MOM implants and 18,000 non-MOM-implanted patients in the Finnish Arthroplasty Register from 2001 to 2010, and from the Finnish Cancer Registry of 2010, the investigators found no difference in the incidence of cancer in the two groups.[15] This study has important limitations, including a control group older than the MOM group and the short period of review. Older patients have higher rates of cancer than younger patients, and it can take many years of exposure (latency period) to a carcinogen before a cancer is diagnosed.

The picture in the United States is somewhat more muddled because it seems that the FDA has not been able to keep track of the performance of MOM hips compared to other replacements. For example, the FDA rightly assumes that Americans would like to know an answer to the question "What are my chances of developing a reaction to my metal-on-metal hip implant and having medical problems?" The agency's answer is "The FDA does not know at this time how often adverse local tissue reactions occur in patients with metal-on-metal hip implants." The agency does identify those types of persons that are more likely to have an adverse reaction to metal ions, to include the following: bilateral implant patients, females, persons with drug or natural immune system limitations, persons with sensitivity to metals (cobalt, chromium, or nickel), overweight patients, and athletes engaging in intense physical activity.[16]

In an interesting twist to logic, the FDA seems to favor MOM hip implants. Patients are urged to ask their orthopedic surgeon abut MOM hip implants.[17] The first question to ask is "What are the benefits and risks of each type of hip implant system (metal-on-metal, metal-on-polyethylene, ceramic-on-polyethylene, ceramic-on-ceramic, and ceramic-on-metal total hip systems . . .)?" The next question is "Why is the metal-on-metal hip implant the best for my situation?"

Evidence is mounting that MOM implants with cobalt heads can lead to cobaltism—a systemic poisoning of the patient due to excess cobalt in their blood. One of the authors of this chapter, an avid Alaska outdoorsman and physician, has had direct experience with this illness as a result of a MOM hip replacement. His story and insights follow:

> In 2006 I required a hip replacement. As an orthopedic surgeon with thirty years of experience in training, research, and practice relating to hip replacements, I was ideally positioned to make informed choices about the timing, technique, surgeon, and implant selection for this operation. I chose Johnson & Johnson's (J&J) MOM "ASR" hip because I fit the profile of a patient that might most benefit from a MOM hip with a ball the same size as the original.

My need for a hip had gradually become apparent to me over the previous decade. My symptoms had progressed to the point of disturbed sleep and an inability to continue cycling for recreation and fitness. I had already set aside running, skiing, and contact sports but had continued to cycle on and off road at a competitive level. Generally conservative in choosing implants for my patients, I decided to roll the dice with my own device. If my experience was favorable, I might adopt the technology for my younger, more active patients that were historically at risk to either wear out the implant or dislocate a traditional metal-on-plastic hip using a smaller ball.

I had been following the evolution of the MOM and MOP hips expectantly over fifteen years of their development, testing, and marketing. I had concerns about the elevated levels of cobalt and chromium in the blood of most patients implanted with that technology, but I felt that if the devices had been blessed by the FDA they were likely safe.[18] I was wrong. As a reasonably connected research arthroprosthetic surgeon, I had opportunity to quiz one of the designers of the model I chose. My concerns about heavy metal exposure were preoperatively satisfied by that doctor several years before my operation: "Steve, how can something measured in parts per billion in the blood possibly hurt a patient?"

I discovered as a patient what my colleague had missed in his foundational research into MOM hip bearing surfaces. Chrome-cobalt metallosis (metal bits from wear or corrosion) can destroy tissue and initiate pseudotumors around the hip implant and also poison the patient as dissolved metals reach the blood. Within forty-two months of my ASR implantation, my blood cobalt level had peaked at over one hundred times the level tolerated for cobalt-exposed industrial workers. My ears were ringing, I was partially deaf and losing some vision, and I was experiencing subtle heart failure. Worse yet, a tremor, mood instability, and mild cognitive dysfunction were threatening my career.

Replacement (revision) of my ASR hip replacements became necessary. Hip pain was again keeping me up at night and was precluding anything more than a short bike commute. Over three years I had made constant inquiries to J&J and its consultant surgeons about my high blood cobalt levels, neurological problems, and deteriorating hip function. I was repeatedly reassured that no one else was noting such problems.

My revision surgeon found a mass of metallic sludge and destroyed ligaments around the failed ASR. The chrome-cobalt ball was exchanged for a somewhat smaller ceramic one, and the chrome-cobalt socket exchanged for a plastic one. My hip pain resolved, and, more surprisingly, so did my neurologic, cardiac, and psychological issues. Although this might be explained by freak improbable coincidence, the only patient in whom I had implanted an ASR had a similar recovery when I revised his failed ASR. I had only implanted six MOM hips, and one of the six patients, like myself, became sick because of high blood cobalt levels. It seemed likely that although rarely recognized and reported then, high cobalt levels (hypercobaltemia), cobalt poisoning (cobaltism), and hip tissue damage from metal wear particles were common in patients with MOM hips after several years of wear and tear.

Concerned that a million American patients implanted with similar technology may be condemned to the same experience, I attempted to get the attention of my colleagues, the industry, and the FDA. I first approached the Centers for Disease Control (CDC) in Atlanta. They were interested in spreading the word nationwide in their weekly newsletter, but that was nixed by the FDA: ". . . Medical devices are our turf, and we are studying the problem." I directly approached the FDA but was rebuffed: "Dr. Tower, we do not consider you as an expert because you are not employed by industry or forwarded to us by your professional organization." I wrote up my own and my patients' experience and persisted against a peer review process dominated by industry consultants. "Arthroprosthetic Cobaltism: Neurological and Cardiac Manifestations in Two Patients with Metal-on-Metal Arthroplasty: A Case Report" was published in late 2010 with an unusual commentary by the presidential line of the American Academy of Orthopedic Surgeons (AAOS) that downplayed arthroprosthetic cobaltism as likely a freakishly improbable occurrence.[19,20]

Then, three of four of the immediate past AAOS presidents were or had been well-compensated consultants to the companies that were marketing the MOM hips. The FDA's policy of listening only to industry or industry's surgeon consultants remained a nearly insurmountable catch-22 for me over four years of continued efforts to increase awareness of the potential complications of MOM hip replacements. I submitted seven proposals for presentations at the annual meeting of the AAOS on MOM hip complications. All were rejected by a program committee composed primarily of surgeons that consulted for companies marketing MOM hips.[21] Although frustrated in my attempts to relay concerns through "appropriate channels," I achieved some success in raising awareness of MOM hip replacement harm through publications in the lay press and the peer-reviewed general medical journals in which I reported additional Alaskan patients that had been poisoned by their MOM hips.[22,23,24,25]

In early 2014, almost four years after my initial series of publications, guidelines endorsed by the AAOS and other American orthopedic professional organizations for monitoring patients implanted with MOM hips were published. The guidelines almost matched those I had proposed four years earlier.[26] The AAOS guidelines stop short of recommending systematic annual surveillance of patients with MOM implants with an annual blood cobalt level and a review by the patient's primary provider for potential symptoms of cobaltism, a practice recommended by me and by the National Prescribing Service (NPS). The NPS is a nongovernmental organization that advises Australia's doctors on best medical practices.[27]

WHAT IS BEHIND TOWER'S EXPERIENCE?

Australia, like Alaska, appears to be years ahead of the rest of the world in describing the complications related to MOM hips.[28,29] Why did Australia and Alaska lead the charge to remove the MOM hips from the marketplace? Both are relatively isolated markets where previously unknown problems are more prone to stick out like a sore thumb. When a doctor like Tower that cares for a comparatively small number of patients stumbles over a "rare" problem again and again, it suggests that the problem is not rare. Australia has an additional advantage of having a national total-joint registry. The ASR was pulled from the Australian market years before J&J recalled it worldwide. After several years of common use, the Australian Registry noted that ASRs were being revised at a rate significantly greater than hips employing 1970s-era hip technology.[30,31]

Most patients likely have little knowledge of the brand and type of hip that they have been "fitted" with. Of the roughly one million metal-on-metal hips implanted in the United States only about 90,000 ASRs have been formally recalled. Tower believes that this equates to industry abandoning those patients with unrecalled metal-on-metal hips. When the ASR was voluntarily recalled in August 2010, J&J did not know the identities of the patients implanted with each ASR hip but did have record of the surgeon, hospital, and date for each surgery. Because of this deficiency in record keeping, the onus of identifying and notifying the at-risk patients was placed upon the surgeon without a confirmation process notifying J&J which patients had been contacted and appropriately evaluated. There are no guarantees that a patient with a recalled ASR will be notified that they are at risk for elevated blood cobalt levels, hip tissue damage, and damage to the brain, nerves, and heart. Most patients implanted with MOM hips have levels of blood cobalt greater than that allowed in industry, but most patients and primary medical providers are unaware that this can result in an insidious progressive illness associated with the prosthetic hip that is outwardly functioning well.

This potential for insidious illness and suffering was recently illustrated in a case report in the *New England Journal of Medicine* of a woman who required a heart transplant because of high blood cobalt levels related to bilateral ASR hips. The cause of her heart failure was only noted a year after the transplant, when her graft began to fail. Once her ASR hips were redone, her blood cobalt plummeted and her second heart recovered.[32] The same week a case report of hip-implant-related cobalt poisoning with heart and thyroid failure, deafness, and blindness appeared in the respected medical journal *The Lancet*.[33] The diagnosing clinician credited an episode of *House* with his awareness of "arthroprosthetic cobaltism." Dr. John Sotos had coined the term "cobaltism" for Tower's first publications; he was also medical advisor to *House*. Previously Sotos had weighed in on the "nosology" of cobalt poisoning. Tower had preferred the acronym CRAP (cobalt-related arthroplasty poisoning). That attempt at gallows humor was not lost on Sotos, but he felt that the typically stodgy medical journal editor might not be amused.

Tower believes that the MOM hip debacle illustrates the weaknesses of both the PMA and 501(k) processes of American premarket medical device regulation. The system is fundamentally imbalanced, with all allowed inputs coming from self-interested parties with a stake in the marketing success of the implant. This amounts to self-regulation, a concept repeatedly proven to fail in the medical industry.

The postmarket surveillance system is nearly nonexistent in the United States. And if a critical flaw is successfully recognized and acknowledged, a reliable process for identifying, notifying, and monitoring the patients at risk does not exist in the United States. That task appears to be delegated to law firms and late-night TV, a quality-and-assurance process grievously lacking in efficiency and fairness. Tower's professional organization, the AAOS, remains firmly opposed to any reform of the medical device regulation other than further deregulation. In the meantime, Consumers Union is pressing the hip and knee replacement industry to offer warranties on their devices. There is some hope for the patient in these efforts, but the patient remains a guinea pig until patients with MOM hips are periodically evaluated and postmarketing surveillance of the performance of joint replacement devices is taken seriously by the FDA. For example, ad hoc monitoring of blood cobalt levels has already proved fruitful in American patients.

Although traces of cobalt are essential for life, it does not take much to cause poisoning. The general threshold for normal cobalt levels in the blood is 1 ppb, but using a definition of greater than 14 ppb as a level indicative of MOM-implant-induced cobaltism, a group of eighteen patients has been identified. Collectively, their symptoms include the following: mental decline, disordered mood and sleep, rashes, neurological difficulties, and heart problems. Extreme cases can lead to numbness, weakness, deafness, blindness, heart failure, and hypothyroidism.[34] Pseudotumors also appear at the site of the implant. Although the FDA is aware of cobaltism as a result of MOM implants, the agency has not developed a systematic surveillance program to detect early cobaltism before the patient has been harmed. In contrast, the UK Medicines and Healthcare Products Regulatory Agency recommends annual blood cobalt determinations for most patients with MOM implants with the idea that revision of the implant may be necessary.

As a result of a recent federal court action, J&J agreed to pay $4 billion in a settlement with 8,000 patients, if they approve the settlement, to compensate for their suffering caused by failed MOM implants and for medical care associated with revision of the failed hips. The failed hip device, introduced in 2005 without clinical testing, originated with the DePuy Orthopedics division of J&J. In 2011 that division estimated that the implant would fail in five years in 40 percent of the recipients.[35] The device was cleared for market by the FDA through the 501(k) process. The predicate hip was another MOM hip that fell out of favor around 1975. That design never underwent any form of controlled clinical trials, and its eventual extinction was a clue that MOM hips are fundamentally flawed. In the opinion of the present authors far too many patients suffered from this flawed device because the FDA did not have a rigorous mechanism to capture patient complaints. All ASR hips were recalled by J&J in August 2010. At this writing the plaintiffs have yet to approve the $4 billion settlement with J&J, and it is not known how many of the 90,000 patients implanted with ASR hips are aware that they are at risk to be poisoned by their replaced hip.

The patients implanted with the ill-starred ASR are relatively fortunate compared to the 900,000 implanted with unrecalled MOM hips, because the ASR recall has been high profile and it is likely that most patients with that device are aware of its potential complications and are being monitored. In Tower's experience most patients do not know the type of hip they have been "fitted" with. Patients and primary medical providers are unlikely to recognize that progressive neurologic, psychological, and cardiovascular problems might be caused by an asymptomatic hip replacement.

WHAT SHOULD THE CAUTIOUS AND
EMPOWERED PATIENT DO?

The empowered patient should ask many questions when a device is to be placed into their body:

- How long has the *exact* device proposed for me been on the market?
- What are the known risks and benefits of the specific device? Ask for quantitative information—and not on like devices, just the one they want to stick in you.
- What are the alternatives to placement of the device and what is their risk-benefit profile?
- Has anyone verified that the device has not been recalled or a warning issued by the FDA?
- Has the device been recalled or is its use restricted in other countries?
- Does the medical provider have a vested interest in the device being considered?

Write down the answers for your records and be certain your surgeon knows you are recording his answers. You are not a guinea pig.

Finally, when you become aware of potential failure or harm caused by a medical device, report this to the FDA and make certain that your federal legislators are aware of your report. Do not be satisfied with silly form letters from the sources you report to. Demand to hear what they are doing to improve the protection of patients from poorly regulated devices. You are not a guinea pig.

Chapter Five

A Contemporary Review of Health Care-Associated Infections

Daniel M. Saman, DrPH, MPH, CPH

It is not difficult to make microbes resistant to penicillin in the laboratory by exposing them to concentrations not sufficient to kill them, and the same thing has occasionally happened in the body. —Alexander Fleming (Nobel Lecture, December 11, 1945)

SAFETY FROM INFECTION

In 1847 the twenty-eight-year old obstetrician Dr. Ignác Semmelweis, who has been called a "failed genius" by best-selling author Atul Gawande,[1] was instrumental in initiating a movement of medicine toward a germ theory and away from the contemporary miasma (bad hospital air) theory. Semmelweis is responsible for attributing the many deaths of newborns and mothers, called bedside fever at the time, to no hand hygiene by physicians. They would work in the morgue on cadavers and go straight to the delivery room without washing their hands. He nearly eliminated bedside fever and its associated mortality with his epidemiological study suggesting that if doctors and nurses on his ward scrubbed with a chlorine lime solution between patients the mortality would be reduced from 18 percent to only 3 percent.[2] However, this unpublished proof did not change the way the majority of physicians practiced obstetrics, and the nonresponse infuriated Semmelweis, who spent some years in a mental institute. The "failed genius" label is mostly because of the harsh attacks on his contemporaries for their refusal to believe his theory: "You Herr Professor have been partner in this massacre," ". . . I declare before God and the world that you are a murderer and the 'History of Childbed Fever' would not be unjust to you if it memorialized you as a medical Nero."[3] These raw attacks led him and his theory to be dismissed by other physicians. His story offers advice to current patient safety advocates and infectious disease researchers on how *not* to achieve wide adoption of lifesaving advancements such as hand hygiene, and mirrors much of the current struggle patient safety advocates have with hospitals and infectious disease specialists in getting hospital staff to adopt proven hand hygiene practices. While the great improvements in patient safety, hand hygiene, germ theory, and microbiology cannot be overstated, at present, hospitals still struggle to achieve anything close to 100 percent hand hygiene compliance and have had only limited success at reducing preventable infections and associated harm.

The field of patient safety is maturing fast, with striking new research consistently changing perceptions of safety. No longer does the field cling to the old paradigm of infections as an inevitable consequence of medical care; rather, according to the newer understanding—substantiated with great evidence—the majority of infections and ensuing harm are preventable. The Centers for Disease Control and Prevention (CDC) estimated that about 1.7 million health care–associated infections (HAIs) occur in US hospitals with nearly 100,000 deaths, of which 35,000 deaths were from pneumonia, 31,000 from bloodstream-associated infections, 13,000 from urinary tract infections, 8,000 from surgical site infections, and 11,000 from infections of other sites. Though the magnitude of HAIs is astonishing, there is still a lack of transparency for HAI reporting and reluctance among health care facilities to implement proven mechanisms that reduce HAIs despite HAIs having been estimated as one of the top ten causes of death in the United States.[4] Recently, however, HAI reporting has been mandated by Centers for Medicaid and Medicare Services (CMS) via the National Healthcare Safety Network (NHSN).[5,6]

Behind the legal mandates are stories like that of Kathy Day, RN, that have compelled the medical industry, especially hospitals, to take more seriously the harm caused by infections that they give to patients. Kathy's story is as follows: "My father, John P. McCleary, fell getting out of bed on September 26, 2008. His rural community hospital ER doctor diagnosed a minor tibia fracture and recommended rehabilitation. The local long-term-care facility did not offer rehabilitation, so he stayed in the hospital for twelve days and was discharged home in good condition on October 8. He walked into his house with a walker that afternoon. The morning of October 10, he was stricken so severely that he couldn't sit up in bed. He was rushed back to the hospital and later was diagnosed with hospital-acquired methicillin-resistant *Staphylococcus aureus* (MRSA) pneumonia. He became a totally dependent, bed-bound patient overnight, and he never walked again. He suffered through sepsis, an MRSA urinary tract infection, hearing loss, thrush, a fifty-pound weight loss, and skin ulcers. But his greatest loss was his independence and the ability to live at home with his beloved wife of sixty-two years. It broke his heart and his will to live. My mother and my family mourned the loss of my father after he died in a local nursing home isolation room on January 9, 2009. Later we discovered that dad's hospital had an MRSA outbreak that also took the lives of two other beloved community seniors just before my father's first hospital admission. Because we were not informed about the risk of MRSA there, my father was not given the opportunity to make safer choices for his care."

Achieving dramatic reductions in HAIs is possible, and we know this because hospitals have implemented patient safety mechanisms that have dramatically reduced HAIs. The Michigan Keystone ICU project headed by Dr. Peter Pronovost led to a 66 percent reduction in catheter-related bloodstream infections. The most important part of the intervention was implementing a five-procedure checklist, in which each procedure had independently been shown to reduce catheter-related bloodstream infections: hand washing, using full-barrier precautions during insertions of central venous catheters, cleaning the skin with an antiseptic, avoiding the femoral site if possible, and removing unnecessary catheters.[7] Though the intervention has been described as relatively simple and easy to implement, it must be noted that achieving good results is greatly more complicated than just a simple checklist to guide the insertion of venous catheters. In their 2009 paper rebuking the media spin of a *simple* checklist in *The Lancet* entitled "Reality Check for Checklists," Bosk et al. state that "when we begin to believe and act on the notion that safety is simple and inexpensive, that all it requires is a checklist, we abandon any serious attempt to achieve safer, higher quality care. . . . The answer to the question of what a simple checklist can achieve is: on its own, not much."[8]

In addition to the checklist, the Michigan Keystone intervention included education, training, and coaching. A designated physician and nurse team leader were educated on patient safety, thoroughly training the team leaders via conference calls and coaching, plus providing education to the team on the efficacy of the five-point checklist. Partnering with team leaders and infection control practitioners was also necessary while advising the CEOs to stock antiseptics before the implementation of the intervention. The intervention is remote from what continues to be spun as a simple checklist. More accurately, the intervention was intended to shift the culture of patient safety and depended on buy-in from key stakeholders in participating hospitals. Changing the culture in a health care facility requires resources and personnel investments, not *just* a checklist.

A necessary prerequisite to improving patient safety is the acknowledgment that reductions in HAIs are achievable, regardless of the patient population and facility type. As another, yet more recent, example of the preventability of HAIs, Saman et al. (2013) performed a study that found 23.4

percent of hospital intensive care units (ICUs) in the United States reported zero central line associated bloodstream infections (CLABSIs). [9] Other studies have also found that a variety of interventions can indeed reduce almost all types of associated infections in many different types of health care facilities. The nature of the interventions include the following: interdisciplinary team rounds, thorough surveillance of infections, collaboration between medical staff, well-vetted protocols, and additional training. [10,11,12,13] In the aggregate, the evidence supports preventability of most HAIs.

Proven strategies and interventions support the contention that reductions can be achieved and negate dogma on HAIs as natural consequences of care. Despite the advancements in patient safety, there are stories that elucidate some of the inherent challenges to the current medical system and what the public may initially think of as "simple" problems to solve. At Brigham and Women's Hospital in Boston, Atul Gawande along with infectious disease specialists and microbiologists played pivotal roles in reducing the spread of MRSA, wound infections, and bloodstream infections. [14] Given the high-tech medical scene at Brigham and Women's, one of the most difficult problems faced by infectious disease staff may have seemed out of place: hand hygiene compliance. Though hand hygiene lacks the intellectual appeal of state-of-the-art medicine and lifesaving surgeries, according to the World Health Organization (WHO), it is essential to preventing infections and has been shown to be clinically efficacious in reducing MRSA and all HAIs. [15,16] In spite of this and the huge body of literature devoted to the science of increasing hand hygiene compliance among hosptial staff, [17] hospitals around the country still struggle with improving hand hygiene. [18] In fact, some patient safety research has focused on empowering patients to ask physicians to wash their hands, [19] though there is general discomfort among patients doing the asking. [20] Empowered patients understand the risk of HAIs and should have no hesitation to respectfully ask all who come in contact with them to confirm that they have washed their hands.

A multitude of in-house strategies have been attempted at Brigham and Women's Hospital, including the posting of warning signs, repositioning sinks, and installing more sinks that are often automatic. They bought special five-thousand-dollar "precaution carts" that store everything for washing-up, gloving, and gowning in one ergonomic, portable, and aesthetically pleasing package. They gave away free movie tickets to the hospital units with the best compliance. Even with all these smart interventions, Brigham and Women's still has major issues with their hand hygiene. The hospital was successful in improving compliance from 40 percent to 70 percent. However, this increase did not reduce infection rates, because, as Gawande notes, "If 30 percent of the time people didn't wash their hands, that still left plenty of opportunity to keep transmitting infections"[21] Moreover, hand hygiene alone is likely .insufficient for widespread and dramatic improvements for patient safety. For example, the ties that physicians wear in hospitals have been implicated in spreading infections, and in some facilities they have been banned.[22] Overreliance on improving hand hygiene compliance rates for reducing HAIs without a more comprehensive culture of safety may not bring the desired change that hospitals and patients are seeking. A comprehensive culture change incorporating hand hygiene, a desire to improve patient safety at every level of the organization, implementation of proven bundles and checklists, and transparency about HAIs may be what makes the biggest difference in hospital infections and patient safety.[23]

UNDERREPORTING OF HAIS

The national burden of HAIs has been challenging to quantify given that hospitals were not required to report their infections until recently. Even after government reporting mandates, studies have found examples of states in which underreporting of CLABSI cases reached 33 percent[24] and wide variation in validity of infectious disease data has also been demonstrated.[25] The current numbers on the incidence of HAIs are all estimates because true population incidence is unknown given that all HAIs are not uniformly reported. Without a census of how to track infections, estimates are developed as a gauge of true population incidence. Arguably, counting HAIs is difficult for reasons of definition, feasibility, economic constraints of hospitals, and time commitment. In contradistinction to medicine—where HAIs are not uniformly tracked and surveillance is slow and immature—the agricultural industry requires farmers to count cows per farm; thus, humorously (or tragically), more is known about cow density per US county than the number of HAIs by county or health care facility. Since my initial *cow* article in early 2012,[26] more data have been made publicly available and transparent through the Hospital Compare website, which currently tracks HAIs including CLABSIs, surgical site infections (colon and abdominal hysterectomy), and catheter-associated urinary tract infections. However, other health care harms associated with hospital care, such as falls and injuries, objects accidentally left in the body after surgery, air bubbles in the bloodstream, mismatched blood types, and severe pressure sores by facility (only a partial listing), were listed at one time, but currently the data have been taken off Hospital Compare.

Even the wealthy and powerful are not immune to HAIs. One example is the tragic death of US Representative John Murtha of Pennsylvania in 2010 at the age of seventy-seven. He was a respected member of Congress. Mr. Murtha had surgery for gallbladder problems at the National Naval Medical Hospital in Bethesda, Maryland. He was sent home, apparently in good condition; however, two days later he began to suffer complications and was taken to the Virginia Medical Center in Arlington, Virginia, where he died surrounded by his family. It seems that Mr. Murtha's intestine was nicked during the laparoscopic surgery; this resulted in an HAI.[27]

Research has been performed utilizing the Hospital Compare database, showing variation among hospitals with respect to infection rates and showing the importance of patient-reported levels of hospital staff responsiveness and CLABSIs.[28] New efforts to determine accurate numbers of each type of HAI are desirable. Knowing the precise magnitude of the epidemic of HAIs is not just some useless academic exercise. The medical care community must ask itself if prevention efforts have been successful (reduced infections over time), and which ones are the most cost effective. Reducing suffering of patients and reducing the costs of medical care are major targets for the US health care industry, or at least they should be. Treating the consequences of an HAI can easily reach into the hundreds of thousands of dollars. Though Hospital Compare data is still not perfect (not validated at every state), this type of transparency and public reporting can assist patients, hospitals, and physicians.

UNJUST TREATMENT OF PATIENTS

Given our understanding that HAIs are mostly preventable, our attention is drawn to the injustice of acquiring such infections. Suffering people seek medical care to be healed, not to be given an infection that debilitates or kills them. Other causes of death on the top ten list include cardiovascular disease, cancer, injuries, and cerebrovascular disease. From a patient's view, knowledge of such unintended consequences of care leading to harm, regardless of preventability, can make the hospital experience one to be feared. One of the current movements to reduce infections is to empower patients to ask questions about the delivery of care and to tell physicians and health care providers to wash their hands.[29] However, few patients feel comfortable asking physicians and nurses whether or not they washed their hands,[30] and if the patient is seriously ill, this approach is obviously not feasible. Expecting patients to "look out" for themselves when it comes to infection prevention in a hospital is simply unrealistic and unjust.

The greatest opportunity for injustice occurs when a hospital or medical facility refuses to acknowledge responsibility for giving an infection to a patient. Such a case is well documented for scores of patients that were infected with the hepatitis C virus while seeking care for cancer in an outpatient oncology facility in Nebraska (see chapter 6).

ACQUIRED EMERGING THREATS

In this chapter infections acquired in hospitals are referred to as health care–associated infections, or HAIs. Several terms have been used to mean new infections acquired in health care facilities: nosocomial infections, hospital-associated infections, and health care–*acquired* infections. *Acquired* may best describe reality with HAIs, while *associated* is less blaming toward the facility. When the infection clearly originated in the facility, it is not as reasonable to say the infection was *associated* with the facility as the infection was *acquired* from the facility. Though patients may well have bacterial strains on their skin (*S. aureus*) or be MRSA colonized *before* presenting at the facility, facilities can still prevent those bacteria from entering the bloodstream through preventive surveillance and decolonization,[31] not using a razor for hair removal,[32,33] and thoroughly cleaning the surgical site with an antiseptic before incision, to name a few preventive steps.[34] Infectious agents that harmlessly reside on the skin of a patient, but through actions inside a hospital reach the bloodstream or invade the surgical site, should be called *acquired* rather than *associated*, even though the patient brought the pathogen into the hospital.

Many of us are currently colonized with *Staphylococcus* (*S.*) bacteria.[35] A nationally representative survey in 2003–2004 of *S. aureus* nasal colonization found 28.6 percent of the people sampled were colonized with *S. aureus* and 1.5 percent with MRSA, an increase from 0.8 percent in 2001–2002.[36] Yet the development of staphylococcus infection requires breaking the most important barrier to infection, the skin, and preventive measures such as the Michigan Keystone intervention to reduce venous catheter infections have been proven to reduce bloodstream infections originating from the skin. Though it remains that susceptibility to infections varies from patient to patient due to immune function differences, systematic facility-wide patient safety interventions can reduce the risk of acquired infections.

New emerging threats originate from bacteria that we do not normally carry on our skin, such as *Clostridium difficile* (*C. diff*) and carbapenem-resistant *Enterobacteriaceae* (CRE). Both *C. diff* and CRE represent increasingly common, highly antibiotic-resistant bacteria. According to the CDC, *C. diff* infection is at historically high levels, causing severe diarrhea and dehydration, and has been linked to about 14,000 annual deaths. To reduce *C. diff* infections, the CDC recommends that clinicians avoid unnecessary antibiotic prescriptions, identify and isolate *C. diff* patients, and wear gown and gloves.[37] According to a 2008 study, CRE infections are very difficult to treat and have up to a 50 percent mortality rate.[38] The CDC reports that in the first half of 2012, 4 percent of US hospitals had at least one CRE-infected patient, while about 18 percent of long-term acute care hospitals had at least one CRE-infected patient.[39] Untethered use of antibiotics in the United States facilitated the emergence of these deadly threats. The empowered and cautious patient will not take an antibiotic unless it is clearly needed to resolve a bacterial infection. Empowered patients should ask for a microbial culture-and-sensitivity test to determine the optimal antibiotic to attack their specific pathogen.

Ann Chellis tells the story of her father's battle with HAIs, including *C. diff*: "On April 26, 2010, my dad had back surgery in the Bay Area, and then he was transferred to a rehabilitation facility in Northern California with the expectation of returning home in approximately one week. He did well for approximately two days and then began to deteriorate. During the next two months he contracted MRSA and *C. diff* at the rehabilitation facility and the local hospital to which he was transferred when he became septic. My mother and I were constantly at his side, wiping down beds, sinks, and toilets with Clorox, but not once did I see a housekeeper at either facility. I didn't realize my father had *C. diff* until I read his autopsy report and all his medical records. My father lost twenty pounds in two months, developed bedsores, and was treated as though he were ignorant. We observed that patients with MRSA were placed in rooms with healthy patients. Nurses would come in and not wear gloves or wash their hands between treating their patients. My father was transferred back to the hospital for a colonoscopy, and as the RN was preparing him by orally administering a liquid, he was actually aspirating the liquid into his lungs and drowning on it. When I questioned the RN, she told me the gurgling sound was the air mattress! Shortly thereafter, he coded and was removed from life support. The following day he died. Each day I see my father's face as he slowly died in his hospital bed."

ANTIBIOTIC STEWARDSHIP

Only eight bacterial pathogens account for 83 percent of all HAIs: *Staphylococcus aureus* (16 percent), *Enterococcus* species (14 percent), *Escherichia coli* (12 percent), coagulase-negative staphylococci (11 percent), *Candida* species (9 percent), *Klebsiella pneumonia* and *Klebsiella oxytoca* (8 percent), *Pseudomonas aeruginosa* (8 percent), and *Enterobacter* species (5 percent).[40] About 20 percent of all HAIs are multidrug-resistant organisms (MDROs), which means over time they have developed the ability to withstand the destructive power of many antibiotics as a result of overuse of those antibiotics. The broad-spectrum antibiotics for last-resort treatment—carbapenems, colistin, vancomycin—have issues with nephrotoxicity, though current thinking on the degree of nephrotoxicity has changed (e.g., vancomycin may only increase risk of nephrotoxicity in patients who are already at increased risk of nephrotoxicity).[41,42] With about 20 percent of all HAIs caused by an MDRO, and with broad-spectrum drugs inducing nephrotoxicity, a new class of antibiotics is necessary to curtail MDROs.

In response to the growing MDRO problem, the Infectious Diseases Society of America (IDSA) advocated for the creation of "10 new, safe, and efficacious systematically administered antibiotics by 2020." As of early 2013, only two antibiotics have been developed and approved since the IDSA's 2009 advocacy for new antibiotics.[43] With few drugs being developed against MDROs, another tactic is practicing antimicrobial stewardship. According to IDSA, "Antimicrobial stewardship programs optimize antimicrobial use to achieve the best clinical outcomes while minimizing adverse events and limiting selective pressures that drive the emergence of resistance and may also reduce excessive costs attributable to suboptimal antimicrobial use."[44] The microbial culture and sensitivity tests mentioned above can help in this stewardship.

In lieu of new antibiotics, reducing unnecessary antibiotic prescriptions may be one of the best ways of limiting the spread of antibiotic resistance. A 1998 study by Nyquist et al. found that children between 0 and 4 years old received 53 percent of all antibiotic prescriptions, with antibiotics needlessly prescribed to 44 percent of patients with common colds, 46 percent with upper respiratory infections, and 75 percent with bronchitis, for which antibiotics have not been shown to improve outcomes.[45] Prescribing rates have dropped since the CDC's antimicrobial stewardship campaign began in 1995, though antibiotic prescribing patterns for persons fourteen years and younger for acute respiratory infections, pharyngitis, bronchitis, and the common cold are still high. Acute respiratory infections, which do not generally require antibiotics, accounted for 58 percent of all office-based antibiotic prescriptions for persons fourteen years old and younger.[46] Such unnecessary prescriptions can reduce the effectiveness of antibiotics for entire populations. The reason stewardship is of public health concern is because the organisms that can grow resistant in one patient because of an unnecessary antibiotic can spread to other people.

Interestingly, prescribing patterns also vary greatly by region; the South in the United States has the highest antibiotic prescribing rates in the nation, with 936 prescriptions per 1,000 persons compared to 639 prescriptions per 1,000 persons in the West.[47] Without attention to stewardship, antibiotic resistance has no natural barrier to slow its spread. New antibiotics will unquestionably be developed by 2020, though even these newer ones will likely be ineffective long-term, as pathogens will continue to grow resistant unless physicians reduce the unnecessary prescribing of antibiotics and patients stop demanding antibiotics for viral infections.

Another opportunity for improving antibiotic stewardship outside the health care industry is to curtail the massive overuse of antibiotics in food animals. About 80 percent of the antibiotics sold in the United States are used in the meat and poultry industries.[48] The additional risk of harm reaches humans because antibiotic-resistant bacteria (called superbugs) can reach humans in the meat they eat or through environmental contact. *Consumer Reports* demonstrated the presence of superbugs in commercial poultry, and distinct outbreaks in humans who have eaten contaminated meat have been reported. Workers in the meat and poultry industries are especially likely to acquire superbugs as part of their biome and can pass these on to those with whom they associate. Several respected organizations called for stopping the use of antibiotics at subtherapeutic doses in food animals for growth promotion.[49] The meat industries continue to argue that any of the above concerns are not posing significant risk to human health. The wise consumer will ensure that any meat they eat is thoroughly cooked to destroy antibiotic-resistant pathogens.

EPIDEMIOLOGY OF HAIS

In 2010 the Society for Hospital Epidemiologists of America (SHEA) set forth guidelines on a national research agenda on HAIs. In their agenda, the top five issues of priority were "(1) preventing the spread of multidrug-resistant aerobic gram-negative bacilli (e.g., *Acinetobacter* species and *Pseudomonas* species) in health care facilities; (2) implementing effective strategies to ensure antimicrobial stewardship in health care settings; (3) preventing the spread of MRSA infection in health care settings; (4) developing effective strategies to ensure adherence to hand hygiene standards; and (5) developing strategies to prevent *C. diff* in health care settings." Improved research and funding in epidemiology can thoroughly address SHEA's priority areas. In fact, SHEA also addressed some areas in medicine *believed* to be evidence based, but are not. For example, the use of bundles (i.e., a set of evidence-based practices that when performed together improve patient safety and outcomes) for controlling urinary tract infections is not evidence based.[50] Universal screening and isolation of patients colonized with MRSA is still controversial and not completely substantiated by the epidemiological literature.[51]

There are currently some estimates, though not recent, demonstrating the public health impact of HAIs in the United States. A report from the CDC estimated an annual HAI incidence of 1.7 to 2 million people, though data that informed this estimate is from 2002. The report also estimated "33,000 HAIs among newborns in high-risk nurseries, 19,000 among newborns in well-baby nurseries, 418,000 among adults and children in ICUs, and 1,266,000 among adults and children outside of ICUs."[52] A more recent study using Hospital Compare,[53] found 11,000 CLABSIs among all reporting US hospital ICUs with at least 1,000 central line days.[54] However, this is only among ICUs and does not include all US hospitals. As such, data from Hospital Compare is still limited but does present opportunities addressing the research gaps in the epidemiology of HAIs.

Only four types of infection are responsible for most HAIs: CLABSI (14 percent), ventilator-associated pneumonia (15 percent), catheter-associated urinary tract infection (32 percent), and surgical site infection (20 percent). A great number of deaths are associated with these types of infections, with CLABSIs accounting for 30 percent of all HAI deaths.[55]

CONCLUSION

There is great complexity in the field of patient safety and a need for better epidemiological studies that can fill in the gaps of knowledge and lead to improved care and better health outcomes for all patients. Health care providers and patients must drive this change, demanding that safety be a top priority. Providers can recognize the burden of HAIs, work as a team with all providers, immediately convene when an infection has occurred, and apologize to patients when HAIs occur. Patients can also drive the change by bravely asking questions about hand hygiene and hospital infection rates. Hospitals should welcome patient input at the policy-making level in the health care process (see chapter 9 for the role patients played in forming legislation to improve control of HAIs). Though patient safety advocates have nudged many hospitals toward a culture of safety, it is the responsibility of each hospital to ensure the safety of patients that have entrusted their lives to it. As the section on antimicrobial stewardship outlined, the health of populations can be drastically reduced when there is little effort to mitigate unnecessary antibiotic use and few new drugs developed to combat new drug-resistant strains. The difficulty of changing the culture of medicine—or any culture, really—should not be downplayed. It is a significant challenge and has to be understood as that. In spite of the challenges, we can all be moved by the fact that at least 100,000 lives are lost each year due to infections that were *acquired* in health care settings, and we *should* be moved to improve patient safety and demand better outcomes. Given the burgeoning patient safety movement, a drive toward accountable care, and new prevention paradigms toward HAIs, the challenge is recognized and being pursued. Though the number of lethal HAIs has significantly decreased in the past few years, when in the hospital, constant vigilance will be necessary to keep infection risk to a minimum. Strategies for patients can be found at http://www.cdc.gov/HAI/patientSafety/patient-safety.html.

Chapter Six

Oversight of Physician Offices: Dr. Welby or Dr. Applebee?

Evelyn V. McKnight, AuD

How are doctor's offices and restaurants alike? Certainly both are important components of the service sector of our economy. They are places where basic human needs are met, often quickly. And when we walk into the office or restaurant, we trust that we will be safe in the service we seek. But if we believe that both are carefully regulated for safety, we would be wrong. Applebee's Restaurants, indeed all restaurants, are inspected regularly for safety, whereas doctor's offices are not. This was true when the popular *Marcus Welby, MD* television show ran in the 1970s and still holds true today.

Most people are surprised to learn that their doctor's office is not subject to regular review to see if it meets minimum safety standards. It is a situation that has confounded physicians, patients, and policy makers for years. When the New York legislature considered legislation for safety standards in physician offices almost a decade ago, chairman of the assembly's health committee Richard Gottfried (D-Manhattan) stated, "I think the average citizen assumes that there must be Health Department regulations governing physicians' offices and believes that they are periodically inspected like restaurants."[1] Although bills to regulate office-based procedures failed to pass, PHL230-d, "The Office-Based Surgery Law," went into effect in 2013. Under this law in New York State, private physician practices that perform some types of office-based surgeries are required to maintain accreditation from an accrediting agency and report selected adverse events resulting from office-based surgery. Multiple aspects of the private practices are evaluated and surveyed as part of the accreditation process.[2] As of 2011, only twenty-three states have some sort of regulation for office-based surgery. The vast majority of offices lack accreditation by one of the major accrediting agencies.[3]

In contrast to private physician offices, restaurants have been inspected for many years. The passage of the Pure Food and Drug Act of 1906 was in large part due to the graphic descriptions of the unsanitary process by which animals became meat products in Upton Sinclair's *The Jungle*.[4] Since the initial passage, food handling laws have continued to be expanded to ensure food safety for the public.

Local public health departments regularly inspect businesses serving food to ensure restaurants and other food retail outlets are following safe food handling procedures. Local laws regulate how frequently these inspections take place and what specific items are inspected. In general, environmental health inspectors check that safeguards are in place to protect food from contamination by food handlers, cross-contamination from combining food, and contamination from other sources in the restaurant.[5]

Medicine can learn about providing quality service efficiently from the restaurant industry. Atul Gawande, an American surgeon and journalist with an interest in optimizing modern health care systems, compares a large restaurant chain to our medical system. Both strive to deliver a range of services to millions of people at a reasonable cost and with a consistent level of quality. The restaurant chain is able to do so, but the medical system is not. He states, "Our costs are soaring, the service is typically mediocre, and the quality is unreliable. Every clinician has his or her own way of doing things, and the rates of failure and complication (not to mention the costs) for a given service routinely vary by a factor of two or three, even with the same hospital." But he found that the restaurant chain (The Cheesecake Factory) was able to produce thousands of quality, attractive meals with little waste to customers across the entire country every day. Gawande spent some time in the kitchen of one of the restaurants. He found a bevy of cooks, utilizing a standardized set of instructions and procedures. But perhaps more importantly, he found that the meals had to pass inspection by the kitchen manager, who commented on the praiseworthy aspects of the meal as well as the parts that needed improvement. The kitchen manager used a strict grading system and declared some meals unacceptable; they would have to be redone. Gawande goes on to say, ". . . the oversight is tight, and this seemed crucial to the success of the enterprise."[6]

I learned the hard way that my personal "Dr. Welby" was no "Dr. Applebee"! In the fall of 2000 I was living a charmed life. I had a loving husband, three healthy sons, a rewarding career, and a comfortable home in the Midwest. But after a cancer diagnosis, the medical care I received in my doctor's office changed my life in a profound and permanent way.

My husband Tom and I were shocked when I was diagnosed with breast cancer. I was a healthy forty-five-year-old with no risk factors. Immediately we turned to the only oncologist. Tom was well acquainted with him, since Tom had referred to him many of his own patients through his work as a family physician in our small town; we were confident I would receive quality care. The doctor assured us that this breast cancer diagnosis was only a "little bump in the road of life" and I would resume my charmed life after six months of chemotherapy in his private clinic.

The six months of chemotherapy, which involved a potent infusion every three weeks, were challenging but not defeating. During the months of recuperation I continued to experience fatigue, but we were assured that I would soon be able to rejoin all the activities of family life. Within seven months I felt a lump grow over the mastectomy incision site, and we were terror stricken. The biopsy came back positive, and the doctor had tears in his eyes when he informed us that I was now facing stage III breast cancer.

The doctor urged us to consult with the Mayo Clinic and the University of Nebraska Medical Center. When we decided I would have high dose chemotherapy and stem cell rescue, I underwent extensive testing in preparation. Once again we were shocked when results came back positive—this time for hepatitis C virus (HCV). Once again I had no risk factors and no explanation for how I had contracted this disease, which is typically associated with risky behavior such as illicit drug use. The doctor seemed equally mystified by this enigma. We were terrified of this disease because it is the leading cause of chronic liver disease, cirrhosis, and liver transplantation in the United States[7] and were so stigmatized by the diagnosis that we told no one else about it. We had one life-threatening disease to face—cancer—and we decided that we would put HCV in the back of our minds and devote all our energy to surviving the stem cell rescue and beating the cancer.

But being an astute clinician, Tom could not let the puzzle go unsolved. After the successful stem cell rescue, he let his thoughts turn toward solving the conundrum. Finally, he shared his puzzlement with Jean, his office nurse of twenty-one years.

The nurse was dealing with her own set of challenges. Her oldest son had been diagnosed with testicular cancer and had gone through chemotherapy at the same time and place that I had—Dr. Javed's oncology clinic. Immediately she shared Tom's concern and offered this observation: "You know, Doctor, when I sat with my son during chemotherapy, I saw some nursing procedures that I did not think were safe. When I mentioned it to the doctor, he assured me everything was done properly. But I'm not sure it was."

What happened next was a set of unbelievable events, a true story that is stranger than fiction.

Here is a quick synopsis of the debacle:[8]

- Tom and his nurse diagnosed four more patients with hepatitis C (including Jean's son), all cancer patients at the oncology clinic we used.

- Tom went to the clinic director (Dr. Javed) with this news. He suggested they do a chart audit, using his oncology clinic charts as controls so that "we can see what's going on in *your* clinic, Tom," insinuating that Tom's office was the source of the infections. The doctor absconded to his native Pakistan within days with the explanation that he was leaving to care for his sick mother but promised to return in two weeks.
- The doctor did not return, but instead organized a political campaign and was elected to the Punjab provincial legislature in Pakistan. He was then appointed Minister of Health for Punjab province.
- The Nebraska Department of Health and Human Services and the US Centers for Disease Control and Prevention (CDC) investigated and determined that at least ninety-nine Nebraskans contracted hepatitis C at this clinic during chemotherapy.

The HCV was transmitted when a nurse reused syringes to access a large saline bag numerous times for port flushes. A patient with known HCV came to the clinic for treatment. After a blood draw the nurse used the same syringe to access the saline bag, contaminating the bag with HCV. Subsequently, patients who were given flushes with saline from the bag were exposed to HCV.

The outbreak had huge repercussions for the patients, their families, the medical system, and the community at large. We suffered physically, emotionally, socially, and financially. At least six people died from HCV, not the cancer that brought them to the doctor in the first place.[9] The resulting eighty-nine lawsuits dragged on for years, and the community was divided between supporters of the victims and supporters of the medical community. I would venture to say that many are still struggling to recover from the disaster. I know that I am.

Perhaps the most unbelievable part of this story is that many people knew about the reuse of syringes in the clinic. Through testimony given during litigation we learned that the doctor knew about it (in fact, he kept the names of patients diagnosed with HCV on a sticky note inside a cupboard door and cautioned the nurses to "be extra careful around these patients"). Doctors, nurses, lab personnel, housekeepers, and administrators of the adjoining hospital knew about it for several years. An audit done by a local community clinical oncology program documented five pages of violations of standard infection control measures, and these findings were given to the oncologist and the administration of the associated hospital in 2001, more than a year before the outbreak was investigated.

And yet nothing was done to stop the dangerous practices. The hospital took the position that the clinic was a private physician office and merely rented space from the hospital; therefore it was not responsible for the outbreak. The hospital further claimed that they were not responsible for overseeing the independently owned clinic's infection-control practices and had met their responsibilities by forwarding concerns to the clinic oncologist. The infection-control breaches were never reported to state health authorities. Since there was no oversight mechanism or inspection by a public health entity, unsafe practices continued unchecked for at least fifteen months, exposing more than 600 patients to deadly diseases.[10]

CURRENT STATUS OF THE PROBLEM AND HOW IT IS AFFECTING PUBLIC HEALTH

Was the Nebraska outbreak an incredibly tragic one-time fluke? Unfortunately not.

Researchers at the CDC studied forty-eight recognized outbreaks due to unsafe injection practices in the United States since 2001. Like the Nebraska outbreak, patients were infected with blood-borne or viral diseases in doctor's offices due to a potential exposure to inappropriate use and handling of supplies (e.g., syringes, needles, intravenous tubing, medication vials, and parenteral solutions) for administering injections and infusions. As a result of these outbreaks, 150,000 Americans have been advised to be tested for deadly diseases. Ninety percent of these outbreaks were associated with outpatient settings, including physician offices, specialty clinics, and alternative medicine clinics, and the remaining 10 percent were ambulatory surgery centers or hospital-based settings. The authors state, " . . . unlike acute care hospitals, most outpatient facilities do not fall within the purview of state or federal licensing/certification agencies and are not routinely inspected for adherence to recommended practices."[11]

Without regulation of physician offices, patients may be put at risk in many different ways, especially when doctors provide services in which they have no formal training. Dr. Carol Roberts was a prominent advocate of alternative medicine in Tampa, Florida, giving speeches and writing a book on the subject. She had graduated from Harvard University and the University of Texas Medical School, specializing in otolaryngology and emergency medicine. She practiced ear, nose, and throat medicine for ten years and then practiced emergency medicine[12] before establishing a holistic health clinic. She was self-taught in the practice of holistic health, had written a book about it, and had a weekly radio show,[13] but she had no formal training in holistic medicine.

The Florida Department of Health investigated the holistic health clinic and the state epidemiologist, Roger Sanderson, presented its findings to the Association for Professionals in Infection Control and Epidemiology (APIC) Annual Meeting in 2010. The investigation found multiple violations of infection control and injection safety that could have resulted in HCV transmission. His report confirmed that the clinic used single-dose vials of medi-cations as multidose vials for multiple patients and that blood from intrave-nous (IV) lines was spread to the tabletop and patients' clothing. The patients and staff who were interviewed reported that the clinic workers used a sy-ringe for drawing up medications from multiple vials for intravenous infu-sions, and then used the *same* syringe to draw up medications for other patients' IVs. In addition, the nurse used a syringe to flush a port and then used the same syringe to access a heparin vial. In all nine patients were diagnosed with HCV through unsafe practices[14] in the private physician's clinic.

Melisa was one of the patients harmed in the holistic health clinic. Melisa went to the doctor seeking better health but came away with life-threatening HCV. She endured long months of treatment throughout 2010 and describes them as the worst days of her life. She felt terrible most days and felt even worse if she did not drink a gallon of water daily to rid her body of the toxins introduced by the taxing treatment regimen of a combination of ribavirin and interferon. She came to know where every rest area was between her home and her doctor's office two hours away. Even her dog understood that she was miserable and offered her comfort by licking her face and not leaving her bedside. Her suffering grew worse when she wrenched her back while picking up the small dog. Her husband then had to carry her everywhere, even to the bathroom. Every month her credit card was charged $5,500 for drugs and medical visits; the total bill was over $55,000. She grew to under-stand why many choose not to undergo treatment for HCV; it is too difficult physically, emotionally, and financially for many people.[15]

The harm caused by infecting patients in outpatient clinics elicited inap-propriately small punishment for the magnitude of pain and suffering caused by irresponsible behavior. For infecting nine patients with HCV in her pri-vate clinic, Dr. Roberts was merely reprimanded by the Florida Board of Medicine and fined $15,000. At the licensure hearing, Florida Board of Med-icine member Dr. Onelia Lage expressed concern that Roberts was providing treatments that aren't "fully evidence-based" (such as chelation therapy) and added, "It's important that you not put patients at risk."[16] Dr. Lage's state-ment had no regulatory power, and the disciplined doctor is free to practice integrative medicine for which she has no formal training or board certifica-tion. She is currently practicing in Naples, Florida.[17] See chapter 1 for further review of state medical boards consistently failing to discipline physicians in proportion to the harm they have caused to patients.

Medical injections are just one of many medical procedures that are pro-vided in physician offices. In fact, the number of procedures and complexity of procedures performed in nonhospital settings continues to grow due to decreased cost and increased convenience for patients. By some estimates, at least fifteen million procedures are performed annually at more than 50,000 office-based locations in the United States, but as of 2010 only twenty-three states had any kind of regulation of such offices.[18]

Private offices are often not staffed with qualified anesthesia personnel who are trained to respond to complications and emergencies. In addition, they often do not have an infection preventionist (a professional with specific training in infection prevention) on staff. When unqualified or missing safety personnel are in facilities that are substandard and/or inadequately equipped, the result may be disaster. One study analyzed data from incident reports to the Florida Board of Medicine to compare outcomes of procedures in physician offices versus ambulatory surgery centers. It found ten times more adverse incidents and death in the office compared to ambulatory surgery centers. The data showed the death rate per 100,000 procedures was 9.2 in offices compared to 0.78 in ambulatory surgery centers. More deaths were related to cosmetic procedures than any other procedure.[19]

Although comprehensive oversight of all physician offices does not exist, there is a patchwork of some oversight mechanisms, intended to assure safety in discrete sectors of health care provision.

The Occupational Safety and Health Administration (OSHA) is charged with assuring safe and healthful working conditions for employers and employees. When a complaint about working conditions is filed, OSHA may conduct an unannounced inspection. If a violation is found, a citation with possible fines will be levied and a follow-up visit may take place.[20] Although OSHA regulations are intended to ensure the health and safety of workers, a safe environment for workers may have some spillover for patient safety.

Some private physician offices have a Clinical Laboratory Improvement Amendment (CLIA)–regulated laboratory. The purpose of CLIA certification is to ensure quality laboratory testing, and labs must be certified to receive Medicare and Medicaid payments.[21]

The Health Insurance Portability and Accountability Act (HIPAA) was passed in 1996 to protect confidentiality of patient records in physician offices and other medical settings. The Office for Civil Rights enforces HIPAA by investigating complaints, conducting compliance reviews, and educating medical professionals to foster compliance. The HIPAA Privacy Rule protects the privacy of individually identifiable health information; the Security Rule sets national standards for the security of electronic protected health information; the Breach Notification Rule requires covered entities and business associates to provide notification following a breach of unsecured protected information; and the Patient Safety Rule protects identifiable information being used to analyze patient safety events and improve patient safety.[22]

The Office of Inspector General Medicaid Fraud Control Unit investigates and prosecutes Medicaid fraud as well as patient abuse and neglect in health care facilities,[23] while the Centers for Medicare and Medicaid Services' Recovery Audit Program identifies improper payments made on claims of health care services provided to Medicare beneficiaries.[24] These deal only with monetary fraud, not cases where patients' lives are endangered.

Many insurance companies require physician offices to participate in the Healthcare Effectiveness Data and Information Set (HEDIS) on a variable basis. The comprehensive tool measures performance on important dimensions of care and service on eight domains of care through eighty measures.[25] The findings are generally shared with the providers to allow for performance feedback and quality improvement opportunities.

The restaurant industry also must comply with federal standards, but inspections differ from the health care delivery sector in that the food industry has regular and comprehensive inspections by the local health department, often unannounced. Local laws regulate how often these inspections take place and what is inspected. Inspections are very thorough and look at such things as safe food sources, handling, and storage; employee hygiene; facility and utensil sanitation; fly and vermin control; lighting; ventilation; water supply; and waste disposal.[26]

HOW PATIENTS CAN MINIMIZE RISK TO THEIR HEALTH FROM DOCTORS' OFFICES

Johnny owns a small, family-run business, is a loving husband and father, and is an active community volunteer. He was shocked when the Red Cross rejected his blood donation in February 2008 because he had hepatitis C. He had donated blood just three months earlier without incident, as he had done every three months for a decade. Some detective work by the North Carolina Health and Human Services epidemiologist showed that he was infected at his cardiologist's office through reuse of syringes[27] during the three months in between blood donations. Johnny would have to endure eighteen months of grueling treatment to clear the disease and suffered debilitating headaches, crippling fatigue, crushing joint pain, and frightening blood clots.[28]

After the North Carolina outbreak, the One and Only Campaign, a public health campaign about safe injection practices, was established. If Johnny had had access to the resources available through the One and Only Campaign, he could have talked with his providers about safe injections during his medical visits. The Safe Injection Practices Coalition and the CDC launched the campaign to eradicate outbreaks resulting from unsafe injection practices. The One and Only Campaign suggests patients ask their providers these questions before receiving an injection:

• Will there be a new needle, new syringe, and a new vial for this procedure or injection?

- Can you tell me how you prevent the spread of infections in your facility?
- What steps are you taking to keep me safe?[29]

Although this chapter has highlighted unsafe injections in physician offices, many other types of harm may happen. A watchful and engaged patient is a necessary component of safe health care. "Questions Are the Answer"[30] is a campaign fostering communication between patient and provider, sponsored by the Agency for Healthcare Research and Quality. The campaign lists questions to ask for improving health care through a partnership between provider and patient. The questions are a starting point for a discussion that empowers patients to be knowledgeable partners in their health care decisions. Perhaps the most important question to ask is "What's your backup plan?" Patients have died within physician offices after being administered anesthesia by a nonanesthesiologist and even from a reaction to an allergy shot, all because there was no emergency plan in place.[31]

Some private physician offices participate in voluntary accreditation to assure patients, insurers, and governmental agencies that they are providing quality care. The major accrediting agencies are Accreditation Association for Ambulatory Health Care, the American Association for Accreditation of Ambulatory Surgery Facilities, and The Joint Commission. To be accredited, a medical practice compares itself to nationally recognized standards and also undergoes a site inspection from the accrediting organization. Areas of review include infection prevention, facilities and environment, clinical records management, and quality of care. The accreditation process is thorough and time intensive, and voluntary accreditation shows that a particular clinic has done a careful review in its effort to provide quality care.

Patients may consult the findings of external agencies that rate physicians, such as Press Ganey, the National Committee for Quality Assurance, and The Joint Commission. These ratings tend to report general trends and do not give information about individual practitioners. State health departments, however, post current licensure disciplinary actions against individual practitioners. These are of limited value in many states (see chapter 1).

County clerk's offices, state health departments, and state insurance departments have records on claims against individual doctors that can be accessed by the public. When reviewing suits against health care providers, it must be recognized that while numerous malpractice lawsuits against an individual physician may be an indicator of competency, some malpractice suits lack merit and are dismissed without settlement.

To discover information about an individual physician, the first step is to access the website of the state's medical licensing board and search for the doctor by name (be aware that there may be more than one physician with the same name). This search will indicate if disciplinary action has taken place in that state (but not other states) and the date of action. If the physician has practiced in more than one state, this process must be repeated for each state. The second step is to enter the physician's name (in quotation marks to keep the phrase intact) in a search engine with additional identifiers such as "malpractice," "lawsuit," "blog," or "news."[32]

Many robust review websites for restaurants have changed the industry for the better. This is not the case for physician-owned clinics. Review sites (such as HealthGrades, RateMDs, and Angie's List) exist, but the listings are often sparse and lack substance. Patients are reluctant to post reviews because they fear reprisal from their physician, through litigation or dismissal from the practice. In addition, review sites are often incomplete—they may rate attractiveness of the front office and timeliness of appointment but not rate the physician's skill and competency.[33]

Until review sites exist that are well populated and contain data that are fair and useful, patients must do their own investigation. *Consumer Reports* lays out a thoughtful approach to selecting a physician that combines understanding your own needs, referrals from trusted sources, and checking of credentials.[34]

FORCES THAT WORK AGAINST "FIXING" THE PROBLEM

The solution to the problems caused by lack of regulation seems simple: pass a law requiring all physician offices in the United States to be inspected and audited for safe practices.

It's not that easy, however. Under our current US health care system, there is no mechanism for enforcement of such a law.

Even the Food and Drug Administration (FDA) does not have this jurisdiction. The FDA is responsible for assuring the safety, effectiveness, and security of drugs, vaccines, and other biological products and medical devices,[35] but it does not have any jurisdiction in health care provision.

Although private medical practices are loosely regulated in the United States, hospitals come under much greater scrutiny. To receive Medicare and Medicaid reimbursement, hospitals must pass a comprehensive audit and inspection (usually through The Joint Commission). Medicare and Medicaid reimbursement through the Centers for Medicare and Medicaid Services (CMS) is a very sizable portion of hospital revenue and is very important for a hospital's financial health. In addition, most if not all other health plans adopt CMS guidelines in determining reimbursement rates. So why not require physician offices to pass a comprehensive and coordinated audit and inspection for Medicare and Medicaid reimbursement, similar to hospitals?

A huge increase in staff and resources would be needed for CMS to carry out oversight of private physicians. According to the American Hospital Association, there were 5,724 hospitals in the United States in 2011.[36] In contrast, there were 850,085 physicians with active licenses in the United States in 2010, according to a census done by the Federation of State Medical Boards.[37] Although this number reflects the number of physicians, there is no data on the number of physician offices. This lack of data adds to the complexity of the problem. How can we regulate physician offices if we don't even know how many there are? It is safe to assume that there are many more physician offices than hospitals. It would seem that at this time of fiscal challenge it would be very difficult to make the necessary increase in funding to CMS for oversight of private physician offices. In addition, creation of a federal regulatory body that enforces quality health care provision would be a national culture shift toward more centralized health care. Given the current controversy and resistance surrounding a national health system in the United States, the creation of such a body seems unlikely to take place soon.

If all of the above challenges were addressed, there remains the small but significant number of physicians who do not accept Medicare reimbursement and would therefore not be under CMS regulation. According to a *Wall Street Journal* article, the number of doctors who opted out of Medicare in 2012 nearly tripled from three years earlier. According to CMS, 9,539 physicians opted out, compared to 685,000 physicians who do participate in Medicare. Even more physicians do not accept new Medicaid patients.[38]

A different tactic would be for individual states to take on oversight responsibilities. There is some precedent for this in that most states require or recognize accreditation of certain types of ambulatory surgical facilities.[39] Generally, accreditation is necessary for the facility to receive Medicare and Medicaid reimbursement. However, simply having a regulation in place may not completely ensure safety if the regulation is weak or incomplete. Despite an inspection mandate in Nevada, where inspections of ambulatory surgical centers (ASCs) by the Nevada licensure bureau under contract with CMS are required every six years under federal guidelines, an ASC was the site of the largest outbreak of HCV in US history in 2008. Nevada inspections focus on interviews with staff on how they perform procedures but do not involve observing the delivery of medical care.[40]

Medical lobbying groups have a huge presence in Washington, DC. The American Medical Association, along with hundreds of other medical groups, spends millions of dollars to gain passage of bills that benefit their members and to sideline legislation that might harm them.[41] In contrast, grassroots patient safety organizations face challenges in educating the public about dangerous health care situations and in finding resources and funding to advocate for improved oversight.

RECOMMENDATIONS ON HOW THE PROBLEM CAN BE FIXED

There are two general ways of approaching improvement of patient safety in private physician offices—safety by incentive and safety by culture.

Incentives can be negative (fines or reduced reimbursement if unsafe practices are found) or positive (increased reimbursement or attaining a level of accreditation if the practice attains a recognized standard). If these incentives fail and a patient is seriously harmed by negligent practices, then charges of criminal negligence may be in order. In 2010 a former hospital technician and admitted heroin addict was sentenced to thirty years in prison for infecting at least eighteen patients with HCV when she took drug-filled syringes intended for patients and replaced them with syringes contaminated with her strain of HCV.[42] In 2013 a Las Vegas physician was sentenced to life in prison after one of the more than 100 patients who were infected with HCV through reuse of syringes in his clinic died.[43]

The highest level of regulatory incentive would be the creation of a federal program that would regulate and enforce a comprehensive patient safety program in nonhospital settings, including private physician offices. This would become a comprehensive and standardized approach, rather than a patchwork of requirements enacted by different insurance companies, government programs, and state regulations. A patient in Alaska would in theory be just as safe as a patient in Florida. Such regulations must include much more than effective infection control. Outpatients must be afforded rights parallel to those proposed for inpatients that make the patient an informed participant in her medical care.

As discussed before, the states could enact legislation requiring accreditation of private physician offices. An audit of the practice could be part of the accreditation process. This was suggested as far back as 1991, when the Office of Inspector General recommended that the Public Health Service provide funding for a demonstration project that would include state medical boards using random practice audits as preventive, quality assurance measures.[44]

The health care insurance industry could incentivize safety in physician offices by basing reimbursement on performance ratings during practice inspection/audits. Malpractice insurance providers could allow a discount on yearly premiums in the same way.

Although board certification is a voluntary process in the United States, historically 80 percent of doctors in the United States obtain certification.[45] The qualifying examinations for professional board certification could include questions not only on best practices for direct clinical care, but for all aspects of running an office, such as best practices for facilities, record management, patient care, infection control, staff oversight, and education. This could even take the form of a separate board certification for physicians who manage practices. Frequent, rigorous "maintenance of certification" programs must be established to ensure that certified physicians maintain at least minimal competency to run a safe outpatient facility.

Educational programs foster a culture of safety in physician offices. The Government Accountability Office acknowledged this in its recent report on injection practices: "The One and Only Campaign is especially important because CMS's oversight of health and safety standards—one primary way for the Department of Health and Human Services to influence clinicians and health care facilities to use safe practices—is only statutorily authorized for certain settings, such as ASCs. Therefore, the One and Only Campaign represents a unique opportunity to reach clinicians and facilities, such as physician offices, that are not subject to CMS's standards . . . additional targeting of the campaign's efforts to settings that are not overseen by CMS, such as physician offices, could help to focus available resources on the best opportunities to improve patient safety."[46]

Much can be done to create and foster a culture of safety in physician offices. Physician offices could designate a safety specialist to be responsible for surveying and implementing safety improvements in the practice. The safety specialist would be conversant in principles of root cause analysis, quality improvement, and process redesign so that s/he could spot problem areas and enact change.[47]

Physicians may enroll with a patient safety organization (PSO). The Patient Safety and Quality Improvement Act of 2005 authorized creation of PSOs to encourage clinicians to voluntarily report patient safety events without fear of legal discovery. PSOs collect, analyze, and aggregate clinical data to develop insights into the underlying causes of patient safety events. A PSO can provide expertise to physicians so that they may understand and prevent the causes of patient safety events.[48]

To fully embrace patient safety, physicians and practice leaders must adopt and promote a culture of patient engagement, accepting and encouraging patients to be equal partners in their health care experience. Don Berwick, the former director of Medicare and Medicaid, summarized this attitude in a speech to the British National Health Services in 2008, when he was the president and CEO for the Institute for Healthcare Improvement:

> First, put the patient at the center—at the absolute center of your system of care . . . for everything that you do. . . . It is not focus groups or surveys or token representation. It is the active presence of patients, families, and communities in the design, management, assessment, and improvement of care itself. . . . It means equipping every patient for self-care as much as each wants. It means total transparency—broad daylight. It means that patients have their own medical records and that restricted visiting hours are eliminated. It means, 'Nothing about me without me.' It means that we who offer health care

stop acting like hosts to patients and families, and start acting like guests in their lives.[49]

I would welcome a "Doctor Applebee," a physician whose practice is regulated for safety, as a guest in my life any day. Maybe I'll even take him out to eat!

Chapter Seven

Prescription Drugs—To Heal and to Harm

John T. James, PhD, DABT

It was ten in the morning, and one of my coworkers had not come to work, nor had she called to say that she would be late. Abby was uncommonly dedicated to her work, so my co-workers and I began to fear that something could be seriously wrong. Abby was a worrier and had often described to me how difficult it was to get medical care for her youngest son, now in his early thirties. Charles had been living with her since his accident. He had been seriously injured in a car wreck that had left him suffering from chronic back pain. This pain was disabling to the point that he could not hold a job for long. He was not insured for medical care, so he and his mother had to settle for minimal treatment, which his mother could hardly afford. There was no chance that Charles's back injuries would be healed by the type of medical care to which he had access; instead his doctor had been prescribing potent painkillers to mask his disabling pain so he could periodically function at a minimal level. On this morning several calls to Abby's friends soon disclosed the sad news that in the dark hours before dawn Charles had died of an accidental overdose of his pain medication. Charles was one of the increasing number of Americans, now accounting for at least 16,000 deaths each year, that have had their lives snuffed out by overdose of prescription opioid pain medications.[1]

A patient's ingestion of any prescription drug is the final step in a long process that brings drugs from the mind of the pharmacologist envisioning the structure of a useful drug into the patient's body, where the drug exerts a positive effect—usually. This process is a winding trail with many poorly marked turns, slippery rocks, and steep slopes. Drug companies have been fined billions of dollars for deviating from the proper trail and placing patients in harm's way. The latest and largest-ever fine ($3 billion) levied by the federal government was against GlaxoSmithKline for hiding safety data and marketing drugs off-label so that doctors would prescribe the drugs to more patients—whether there was a benefit to patients or not—to bring more revenue to the drug company.[2] Overpromotion and misrepresentation of the addiction risks of the long-acting, opioid pain reliever OxyContin got its maker, Purdue Pharma, fined $634 million in 2007.[3] The proper process of introducing a new drug requires years of scientific investigations, lengthy reports to the Food and Drug Administration (FDA), a means to make prescribers aware of the drug's positive effects, and inspection points that assure safe manufacture of the approved drug. There are important weaknesses in this process that can leave the patient seriously harmed or dead, such as the irresponsible oversight of compounding companies that led to fungal contamination of an injectable drug made by the New England Compounding Center (NECC). This chapter identifies weaknesses in the current process with the hope that action can be taken to shore up those weaknesses to reduce harm to patients.

OFF-LABEL PRESCRIBING

Therapeutic drugs have become a part of life for most Americans, and most patients benefit from the use of medications. Unfortunately, all drugs have side effects. These may be so slight as to go unrecognized, only slightly annoying, seriously disabling, or life ending, even when prescribed appropriately and taken as recommended. Ideally drugs are not prescribed off-label; that is, for illnesses and patient populations for which the FDA has not approved the drug. However, since the regulatory approval process for drugs is onerous, clinicians must be able to meet the medication needs of their patients by prescribing drugs off-label. This can leave patients in harm's way as guinea pigs. For example, drugs approved for use in middle-aged people may be too dangerous for use in children or the elderly. An example of this is Zyprexa, an antipsychotic drug approved for use in adults but marketed for off-label use in children and the elderly by Eli Lilly. The company was fined $1.4 billion for this behavior and for failure to disclose the drug's side effects.[4]

Similarly, a drug may be approved for treatment of a specific disease, but doctors prescribe it to patients to treat other medical conditions, placing the patient at inordinate risk of harm; as of 2008, 97 percent of recombinant factor VIIa, approved *only* for use in hemophiliacs, was being used in US hospitals off-label for bleeding prevention in nonhemophiliacs, and appeared to offer no advantage over standard drugs while creating the harm of excess blood clotting.[5] For many common categories of drugs, off-label prescribing is nearly as common as on-label prescribing.[6] Perhaps one of the most concerning off-label uses of drugs occurs in neonatal intensive care units, where more than 90 percent of the drugs used are not FDA approved for the prescribed indication.[7] The experts making this observation noted that such babies are being placed in an uncontrolled and unapproved medical trial that will not lead to useful data.

The solution to exposure of patients to off-label drug use lies in the hands of four parties: patients, clinicians, drug manufacturers, and legislators. Patients must ask their clinician if the drug they have been prescribed has been approved for use by the FDA for their specific medical condition and age group. If the prescription is off-label, then the patient must inquire about expected benefits and potential side effects, both short-term and long-term. Clinicians must be required *by law* to warn patients that they are receiving an off-label prescription and present in writing to the patient and in the medical record why the drug could be of benefit to the patient. For example, a clinician's personal experience with a drug may be the basis for an off-label prescription, but that must be made clear in the medical record. The final two parties to improved management of off-label prescribing are legislators and the drug manufacturers that they regulate. Government's huge fines on companies for off-label marketing of drugs has not stopped this practice; however, individual representatives and executives engaged in or encouraging off-label marketing that ultimately results in harm to patients must be held legally and *personally* responsible for that harm. Prescription drugs are an invasion of a patient's body, and that invasion should never take place without the patient's *informed* management of risk.

POSTMARKETING DANGERS

The FDA approves drugs for marketing to clinicians and patients based on data presented to it by the drug manufacturer. That data seldom provides assurance that the drug is safe and effective in the long run. Failure of the FDA and drug makers to follow up once a drug is marketed on-label may place patients at serious risk. Twenty drugs, approved by the FDA since 1993, appear on a list of drugs whose approval was withdrawn an average of three years after approval because of potential to harm patients.[8] Many years can pass from the approval of a drug until the FDA acts on serious side effects. For example, in May of 2012 the FDA issued an alert that azithromycin (Z-Pak) caused approximately a 2-1/2-fold increase in heart-related deaths when compared to another commonly used antibiotic (amoxicillin). Azithromycin was originally approved in 1992. The alert was based on a study of data from 1992 to 2006 and published in 2012.[9] Similarly, ten years after FDA approval and $1 billion in sales, a commonly used drug for sepsis

(Xigris) was withdrawn from the market because it does not do what it is supposed to do—reduce mortality in patients with severe sepsis. [10]

In 2007 Congress passed a law giving the FDA power to require drug companies to perform postmarketing studies to protect the public from serious adverse effects that were not evident at the time of approval. Three investigators asked how compliant drug companies have been in performing the studies required by the FDA. [11] They found that as of the end of 2011 the FDA had required 368 such studies of which 271 had not yet been started. One does not have to be brilliant to appreciate that drug manufacturers may not want to conduct studies that reveal serious side effects of drugs they are marketing. The authors assert that the FDA must start enforcing the law against companies that do not comply to improve prescription drug safety. The Institute of Medicine (IOM), the medical arm of the US National Academy of Sciences, has issued a report calling for the FDA to be more vigilant in its postmarketing drug safety efforts to ensure that a drug's adverse effects do not outweigh its benefits. [12]

The problem of postmarketing drug safety can only be fixed by legislation with assertive penalties for noncompliance with laws and by the FDA taking its legally mandated, postmarketing role more seriously. In the meantime, patients and prescribers should be wary of any drug that has not been on the market at least three years; furthermore, both parties have an ethical obligation to report side effects of drugs they prescribe or use. [13]

POLYPHARMACY AND MEDICATION RECONCILIATION

Polypharmacy refers to the use of multiple drugs more-or-less simultaneously with limited knowledge of how the drugs might interact to place the patient at risk of harm. Reconciliation means that someone with expertise evaluates the collection of drugs an individual is taking and recommends changes and deletions to reduce the risk of harm. Sometimes there is a preemptive strike against dangerous polypharmacy. A woman I know with kidney and heart problems was receiving prescriptions from a nephrologist and a cardiologist to manage her high blood pressure, cardiac arrhythmias, and risk of gout. This woman had marginal kidney function, so the choice of drugs to benefit her was limited. Not long ago her cardiologist recommended a new drug to reduce her blood pressure. Being a cautious patient, she waited to fill her new prescription until she discussed the new drug with her nephrologist. That physician told her point-blank, "Don't you dare take that medication." She took the nephrologist's advice against adding one more drug and was doing well the last I heard.

One risk of polypharmacy is an increased risk of falls. Although the risk of falls in elderly persons taking multiple drugs is well documented, a recent study from New Zealand found that persons aged twenty-five to sixty who were taking two or more prescription drugs were two-and-a-half times as likely to experience a serious fall that led to hospital admission or death as those taking no more than one drug.[14] In one study the investigators asked if the underlying disease rather than polypharmacy was behind the excess falls, and they found that the underlying diseases could not explain the excess falls. Statistically, half of persons over sixty-five take five or more medications and almost 20 percent take ten or more. Looking at the other age extreme, hospitalized babies in the United States experienced a median of four distinct drugs during their first day of hospitalization, and by the seventh day, at the ninetieth percentile, twenty-nine to thirty-five drugs had been given.[15] The authors of this large study, which included 20 percent of all pediatric admissions in 2006, suggested that widespread polypharmacy in the young raises patient safety concerns.

Reconciliation of polypharmacy can have a remarkably positive effect on reducing the number of drugs in use and on the well-being of patients. When multiple doctors and multiple medications are in play, patients and doctors struggle to keep track of medications that should be discontinued, have interactions with other drugs, or are not working. Elderly, community-dwelling adults who were taking eight medications on average were subjected to a medication-reduction algorithm, by which the average number of medications was decreased to four per patient. The average follow-up time after reconciliation was 1-1/2 years, during which no adverse events or deaths were attributable to medication discontinuation and 88 percent of the patients reported global improvement in health.[16] The message to patients taking four or more drugs is to ask your doctor(s) to work with a pharmacist specializing in drug reconciliation to reduce the number of medications you are taking. The message to legislators and those "in control" of medical systems is to require that patients subjected to polypharmacy undergo annual drug reconciliation. The only losers in this will be the drug companies who sell less of their stuff. Patients can learn about the prescribing habits of their doctor from a link provided by ProPublica.[17]

ERRORS OF OMISSION: FAILURE TO USE DRUGS

Patients can be seriously harmed or can die prematurely because of failure to prescribe useful drugs. A classic example of this is the failure to prescribe β-blockers for patients with heart failure. The number of premature deaths in the United States attributed to this omission was estimated at 100,000 per year even eighteen years after demonstration in 1982 that such drugs were lifesaving in heart failure patients.[18] More recently the epidemic of hypertension in the United States seems to escape consistent treatment with suitable medications, although there are some isolated success stories in well-integrated health care systems. The elements that made a treatment campaign successful within a group of 2.4 million health-system members in Northern California included (1) electronic medical records available to all caregivers, (2) tracking blood pressure control rates in the entire population, (3) having consistent guidelines that still enable physician decision-making autonomy, (4) medical assistant follow-ups, and (5) simple, generic, single-pill therapy.[19] In this effort the goal was to control blood pressure to below 140/90 mmHg, which was achieved at the 80 percent level by 2009, up from 44 percent in 2001.

The news was not so good across our nation. Using a database called the National Ambulatory Medical Care Survey (NAMCS), which is designed to be representative of all patients seen in nonfederal facilities by office-based physicians, a team of five investigators asked how often patients received new blood pressure medications if their blood pressure was not controlled to 140/90.[20] The time period covered was 2005 through 2009. In patients receiving no blood-pressure-lowering medications with a blood pressure more than 160/100 (well above the recommended treatment level) only 60 percent received a medication if the reason for their visit was high blood pressure. If the reason for their visit was something else, only 30 percent received medication to lower blood pressure. High blood pressure is a well-known cause of treatable cardiovascular death. This is clearly a ripe target for improved patient care because of underuse of drugs.

Potassium is critical for normal functioning of the heart muscles and can be lost through a variety of mechanisms. One example is the story of a young runner who had become potassium depleted while running for months in a hot climate.[21] He collapsed while running, self-recovered, but was taken to a hospital for evaluation. At admission his potassium was well below guideline requirements that potassium be replaced when the patient has heart arrhythmias, but no potassium was given to him despite several heart arrhythmias.[22] His magnesium, also critical for heart function, was also borderline low. Instead of potassium replacement, a series of progressively invasive and inconclusive tests was administered. After five days he was released with no diagnosis or treatment, and three weeks later he died while running. His heart was found to have lesions consistent with potassium depletion. Annabelle Volgman, MD, medical director at Rush Heart Center for Women in Chicago, noted after reading this story: "On a daily basis I struggle with many patients who have arrhythmias, since I am an electrophysiologist. One of the most important, although seemingly mundane to most physicians, is the potassium and magnesium levels of patients. When I hear that a patient has arrhythmias, that is the first question I have, since it is the most common cause of increased irritability of the heart. This is not emphasized enough in medical training. I have thought about recommending that the normal range for potassium be increased to make arrhythmias less common in hospital patients. Your book encouraged me even more. However as you point out, it takes a lot to change the practice of medicine. I may have a tall task ahead of me" (e-mail communication to author, September 21, 2013).

One recent example of the difficulty of changing physician practices comes from a report in which the use of optimal medical therapy (OMT) was examined in patients with stable coronary artery disease who received percutaneous coronary intervention (PCI), an expensive and invasive procedure that mechanically opens up one or more coronary arteries using a stent.[23] Some combination of aspirin, a β-blocker, and a statin comprise OMT. Guidelines call for use of OMT before any PCI is attempted. A definitive study published in 2007 demonstrated that stable patients do no better when given PCI and OMT when compared to those receiving only OMT. Before the study was published, OMT was used 44 percent of the time, and afterward it was used 45 percent of the time before any PCI was attempted. The results of a major trial showing the value of OMT alone were largely ignored by the cardiology community.

If underuse of the simplest and least expensive drugs is commonplace, then many patients may be suffering from widespread failure to receive optimal care. Clinicians in a well-integrated health care system with quality benchmarks and accountability for care, such as the one in Northern California mentioned above, are most likely not to overlook a patient's need for simple drugs. Outpatients should seek integrated care systems that emphasize accountable care, and they must ask about potentially useful drugs if they have an illness. Patients, whether in or out of a hospital, must not assume that their doctor is always going to be following optimal use of drugs. Underuse of drugs may be as serious a problem as overuse. All clinicians must be held accountable for optimal use of drugs for their patients and receive feedback when they fail to do this.

CRITICAL TIMES IN A HOSPITAL

There are critical times in the care of a hospitalized patient when the risk rises due to a change in medications or deletion of medications. Administrative records of nearly 400,000 patients aged sixty-six years or older receiving drug treatment for chronic conditions in Ontario, Canada, from 1997 to 2009 were studied to determine if there was an increased likelihood that drugs, which had been taken by the patient for at least one year, would be discontinued at admission to a hospital or at transition from ordinary care to the intensive care unit (ICU).[24] The records of patients not hospitalized served as controls. The team of nine investigators looked at five classes of drugs and found that the odds of discontinuation of anticoagulant/antiplatelet drugs was almost twice as high in patients admitted to a hospital as in those never admitted. The likelihood of discontinuation of this class of drugs in patients admitted to the ICU compared to controls was slightly above two. A one-year follow-up of the patients whose anticoagulant/antiplatelet drugs were discontinued showed that an increase in a composite measure of death, ER visits, or new hospitalization was about 10 percent.

Editorialists commenting on the study above noted that the patients were possible victims of polypharmacy.[25] The median number of prescriptions in the year prior to hospitalization was twelve. This invites risk of harmful interactions of the drugs and also creates challenges when it comes to continuing the medications during hospitalization. Indeed, the editorialists observe that hospital care can be as much about managing medications as combating the acute illness that brought the person to the hospital.

The message here for patients and their advocates is clear: inspect your medical records and ask if a drug you have been taking was discontinued for a good reason or simply overlooked. The message for providers, especially hospitalists, is to take responsibility for elimination of unintended medication deletions at times of transition. The message for legislators is that the law must state that hospitals are required to offer patients or their advocate a chance to inspect their medical record for changes in their medications that seem unwarranted—especially at times of care transitions. Some hospitals are already voluntarily offering improved patient access to medical records, including physician notes.[26]

One source of medication review after a hospital discharge is at the level of the pharmacy dispensing the drugs. A study from the Netherlands asked whether interventions by community-based pharmacies reduced the frequency of drug-related problems over a one-year period after discharge from a hospital compared to patients without interventions.[27] Patients were over sixty years of age. All patients in the study were taking at least five drugs, and the intervention included medication review, treatment analysis, patient interview, and counseling. The proportion of patients with increased drug-related problems was 8 percent in the intervention group and 20 percent in the control group. The benefit of medication intervention was most effective for patients with heart failure or high blood pressure. If you are taking a host of drugs after hospitalization, ask your pharmacist to review the drugs you are taking and alert you to the most prevalent side effects and potential interactions. This could save you readmission to a hospital and the consequences that go with that risk.

CANCER TREATMENT DRUGS

Cancer is the second leading cause of death after heart disease. Many patients with a diagnosis of cancer are subjected to powerful and expensive drugs to destroy the aberrant cells or to at least cause the cancer cells to regress. These drugs can debilitate a patient and make their final days on earth miserable. Several of the practices surrounding the prescribing of chemotherapy tend to turn patients into victims rather than persons whose care is patient-centered.

Potentially invasive breast cancer is an awful disease. I have seen the fear in the eyes of women who have just been told that the results of a biopsy show a potentially invasive form of breast cancer. I have listened to their struggles as they try to understand the best form of treatment, and then I have seen their debilitation as the chemotherapy attacks more than just the cancer cells. I have heard the stories of women as they struggle with metastatic breast cancer that has invaded vital organs and cannot be cured. I have shared in the reserved joy of those who have experienced a "cure" from this disease—reserved only because it could attack again. Medications to reduce the risk of breast cancer are among the most sought-after, and there have been some measures of success.

Two drugs for reducing the risk of breast cancer have proven effective for women that are at high risk of breast cancer—tamoxifen and raloxifene. A metabolite of tamoxifen blocks estrogen receptors and thereby reduces the risk of hormone-receptor-positive breast cancer. Raloxifene was originally developed to reduce osteoporosis in postmenopausal women but was found to be effective in reducing breast cancer through its action on estrogen receptors. A recent systematic review of these drugs' effectiveness and side effects has been published.[28] When compared to a placebo, the drugs reduced the risk of invasive breast cancer by eight cases per one thousand women over five years, with more recent data suggesting that tamoxifen is more effective. However, tamoxifen caused more thromboembolic events (blood clots) than raloxifene, and it also caused more endometrial cancer and cataracts. The choices for a woman at high risk of breast cancer are daunting: do I need a preventive mastectomy, do I take my chances with drugs, or should I just do nothing? According to the Mayo Clinic, there are lifestyles that reduce breast cancer risk: limit alcohol to one drink a day, do not smoke, avoid obesity, exercise, prolong breast feeding, use hormone therapy guardedly, and avoid radiation from medical testing.[29]

Some experts called for more patient-centered development of oncology drugs and reforms in the way cancer drugs are developed and used in the overall treatment of cancer. An MD points out that of the fifteen hematology-oncology drugs approved by the FDA in 2011 only one had side-effect information on the label.[30] Obviously drug companies have an interest in not parading side effects before the public in deference to positive survival-time data. The author calls for "a fundamental shift in culture orientation among drug developers and regulatory reviewers." The goal of this culture change is implementation of processes, such as placing patient-reported outcomes on labels that make drug development more patient-centered. In my opinion, legal mandates are required from legislators—specifically that information must be given to the cancer patient so that she can make an informed decision about whether to use a drug. The patient has a right to know how a given drug will make her feel as well as the positive effects. Waiting for a culture change has seldom if ever worked in medicine. Of course, waiting for legislative action to protect patients is also a slow process.

The warning here for cancer patients is that they must use all resources to explore and understand the side effects and potential gains from chemotherapy drugs. I know of several people with terminal cancer that have eschewed chemotherapy. The vast majority (70 to 80 percent) of almost 1,200 patients with terminal lung or colon cancer that were participating in a national study did not understand that the chemotherapy they were taking had no chance of curing their cancer.[31] This suggests that oncologists are not communicating the information needed by patients to make informed treatment decisions.

The current paradigm for treatment of cancer patients contains perverse incentives that tend to work against patient-centered care. Three MDs have suggested three principles for reforming this paradigm.[32] First, the fee-for-service model must be abandoned in favor of one that avoids any link between an oncologist's income and treatment choices. Second, care must be in accordance with evidence-based guidelines. Third, a feedback mechanism must be in place to create a database from which providers and patients can quickly learn how effective a drug has been and how cost effective it is compared to other choices (e.g., radiation or surgery). All this was envisioned to happen under "cancer care groups," which are panels of experts involved in care of cancer patients, and who receive compensation for their involvement as part of bundled payments for treatment of each patient with a certain stage of cancer. This framework should also control costs.

According to a "Viewpoint" article in the *Journal of the American Medical Association*, the median *monthly* cost of chemotherapy drugs (in constant 2010 dollars) has grown from $400 in the 1980s to $4,000 for drugs approved from 2000 to 2005.[33] This increase motivated Medicare in 2005 to limit physicians' markup to 6 percent, but recently this percentage has eroded. For example, the author of the "Viewpoint" article points out that adjuvant treatment for breast cancer patients according to guidelines can involve costs that range from $3,000 to $22,500 for the full course of treatment. Obviously, 6 percent of the latter amount ($1,350) is much more than 6 percent of the former ($180). In fact, Medicare data have demonstrated that oncologists chose chemotherapy in order to increase income to their practices.[34] Noting that the current method for physician-administered oncology drugs is not sustainable, experts propose new expected behaviors and payment systems that would uncouple oncologists' incomes from the high cost of cancer-treatment drugs. These changes are long overdue; in the meantime cancer patients have an important role in probing effectiveness, side effects, and cost-effectiveness of the drugs they are offered. While the "system" pays most of the cost of an individual's chemotherapy, it is individuals through taxes and insurance-company premiums that feed the "system." Patients must become informed and cost-conscious.

OVERUSE OF DRUGS IN NURSING HOME RESIDENTS

One of the great tragedies of our society may be the way we are forced to live out our final years. When I was a kid, I remember visiting a relative who was taking care of my great-grandmother. I remember her as a small, bedridden, white-haired, old woman who only talked about her desire to die as soon as possible. She was under the care of relatives, not strangers in a nursing home. Times have changed, and the majority of elderly folks today live out their days in an assisted-living arrangement. In such a place they are highly vulnerable to abuses, and the weapon of abuse can be overused drugs.

In 2011 a federal government audit of nursing homes revealed that half of antipsychotic drugs prescribed to Medicare beneficiaries were medically unnecessary. The inspector general of the Department of Health and Human Services testified late that year before a Senate special committee that half of the 300,000 drug claims received for antipsychotics were *not* prescribed for medically accepted indications.[35] In addition, the standards for prescribing these drugs were often ignored. Doses were sometimes too high or given for too long to individual patients. It seems that the provider community that had been overprescribing these drugs heard the message, because a recent press release from the Centers for Medicare and Medicaid Services found that the rate of prescribing of these drugs has declined about 10 percent.[36] This came about because in 2012 the Center for Medicare and Medicaid Services launched the National Partnership to Improve Dementia Care. The goal of that partnership was to reduce overprescribing by 15 percent by the end of 2013. Four of the five key recommendations for "Choosing Wisely" in the care of nursing home patients specify reductions in the use of drugs, including antipsychotics.[37]

The lesson of the situation with antipsychotic overuse and nursing home residents is that prescribers often do not follow guidelines, and they are not held accountable for this. Antibiotics to combat infections are also overprescribed to nursing home patients, as described in a commentary from the "Less Is More" section of *JAMA Internal Medicine*.[38] In general, antibiotic treatments should not last more than seven days; yet one study showed that almost half of the nursing home prescriptions were for longer than seven days. Overuse of antibiotics, in particular fluoroquinolones, can promote the dangerous and often lethal growth of the bacterium *Clostridium difficile*, which leads to severe gastrointestinal distress (see chapter 5). The writers also note that antibiotics are often prescribed without an examination by the physician. Until *all* prescribers are held accountable for following reasonable standards for prescribing medications, those who look after family members living in a nursing home need to be aware of the risk of too many drugs in this vulnerable population and should inspect medical records for this possibility.

GROSS REGULATORY FAILURES

The stories and evidence described above show that there are many cracks in the regulatory pathways through which drugs are developed, approved, monitored, and prescribed. Because of those cracks, patients should feel no assurance that the drugs prescribed to them are consistently safe and effective. Once in a while one of those cracks dramatically splits wide open, revealing that many patients have been harmed and killed. The most recent example of this occurred in September 2012 as reports of fungal meningitis began to appear in a few states, and the source was soon traced to supposedly sterile preparations of methylprednisolone acetate manufactured by the NECC.[39] This preparation is typically used to relieve back and joint pain. The NECC story is told by Kevin Outterson, a lawyer, and he shows in effect how the small regulatory crack in which compounding pharmacies had been operating for decades gradually widened and finally split wide open to reveal egregious harm and irresponsible oversight. The root cause of that can be traced to the highest court in this country, which decided that compounding pharmacies were not to be prohibited from advertising, because this would violate their First Amendment rights.

The magnitude of the disaster seemed incredible, given that the victims simply wanted relief from their joint pain. As of March 2014, according to the CDC, there have been 64 reported deaths and 751 total cases associated with this outbreak.[40] Regulatory bodies have focused intense scrutiny on this event, belatedly looking for a root cause.

Compounding companies were created to prepare special drug formulations in response to the needs of a specific patient; however, companies were allowed to prepare drug formulations in anticipation of orders. The regulation of these companies, presumed to remain small operations, was relegated to the state where each was located. Compounders gradually grew and wanted to advertise their products, but the law as of 1997 did not permit this.[41] In 2002 the Supreme Court ruled that this law was not constitutional because it violated the compounder's right to free speech. In response the FDA released a compliance guide without the advertising ban, and inspections of NECC by the FDA in 2002 revealed contamination of methylprednisolone acetate. As a result, the FDA and Massachusetts ordered compliance with the rules, but NECC remained generally noncompliant. The Senate held hearings in 2003, and various safety violations by NECC were found in the years from 2004 to 2006 by the state of Massachusetts or the FDA. According to Kevin Outterson, a law drafted by the Senate in 2007 to better regulate compounding companies was successfully stopped by the companies.[42] Five years later the current tragedy began to unfold. Outterson makes three points regarding the striking down of the law in 2002 by the Supreme Court. First, it would have constrained NECC to make only small quantities of the drug; second, it may have totally precluded any compounding because the drug was no more than a copy of a widely available drug minus preservatives; and third, the drug could not have been shipped in large quantities across state lines as was done to generate the catastrophe. The root causes of the harm to patients appear to be as follows: (1) a Supreme Court more focused on free speech in a form never intended by the writers of the Constitution than on protecting patients from unregulated drugs, (2) a compounding company more focused on making money than making safe drugs, and (3) an ambiguous and weak regulatory environment shared by the FDA and the State of Massachusetts.

In November 2013 President Obama signed the Drug Quality and Security Act into law to improve the regulation of drug compounding companies; however, the law fails to protect patients from dangerous preparations.[43] The law creates a new type of license for sterile drug compounders (now called outsourcing facilities) for whom the FDA will assume regulation, but obtaining such a license is *voluntary* on the part of compounding companies! The regulation is not as stringent as for mainstream drug manufacturers. One can anticipate that most compounding companies will not seek such a license, and those that do not will have a competitive advantage over those that are willing to subject themselves to stricter regulation and the costs that go with it. As a patient about to receive a drug from a compounding company, you must ask if that drug originates from an FDA-regulated manufacturer.

WHERE ARE THE UNSEEN DANGERS NOW?

Is there another tragedy like the compounding company tragedy waiting to harm hundreds and kill scores of unwitting patients because the road that leads to patients receiving drugs has unpatched cracks? One way to answer this question is to ask what changes the IOM has recommended because they see some "cracks" that could lead to patient harm. The IOM acts under congressional charter through the National Academy of Sciences to advise the federal government on policy matters pertaining to public health. In 2007 it published a book called *Preventing Medication Errors* as part of its series on how to cross the chasm from where we are to where we need to be in health care delivery. In 2012 it published a book called *Ethical and Scientific Issues in Studying the Safety of Approved Drugs*. The IOM does not deal with nonproblems—there are a lot of cracks to be patched in the pathways that lead to the introduction of prescription drugs into one's body.

The IOM in 2007 estimated that hospitalized patients experience on average one drug administration error per day.[44] Based on limited data, twelve to fifteen errors per one hundred doses of medication occur in nursing homes. In the ambulatory setting the error rate in prescription writing is about the same as in nursing homes. For the care of children the error rates vary widely depending on the service, but seem to range from 4 to 30 percent. Overall, the IOM committee estimated that 1.5 million *preventable* adverse drug events occur in the United States each year, and this does not include errors of omission—failures to prescribe medications that would help patients—which are especially common for patients with heart disease. The IOM writers point out that "millions of Americans take prescription drugs each year without being fully informed by their providers about associated risks, contraindications, and side effects."

The IOM book published in 2007 emphasized as its first recommendation that by law patients must have the right to sufficient information about the drugs that have been prescribed to them to make informed decisions on whether to use them. The IOM's second recommendation charged government agencies with ensuring that trustworthy information is made available to the public. Slowly that has been happening through improved web-based information tailored to patients' understanding level.[45] However, in 2012 the IOM found that "FDA's current approach to drug oversight in the post-marketing setting is not sufficiently systematic and does not ensure consistent assessment of benefits and risks associated with a drug over its lifecycle."[46] Despite this and other shortcomings, *Consumer Reports* offers one source of evidence-based, cost-conscious information on drugs.[47] Rxisk.org provides a place to report drug side effects and find out about side effects that have already been reported. It offers the advantage of international reporting rather than single-country reporting as with the FDA.

Aside from web-based information, the crux of a patient's understanding of the benefits and risks of drugs is going to come from professionals that write prescriptions and from those who fill those prescriptions. I believe this is a serious crack in the system that must be patched. Where do such professionals get their information, is it reliable, and can they apply it safely to patient care? With all due respect to the IOM, their approach to a potential crisis tends to be mollified by proper discourse and widespread recommendations to government agencies. The systemic "cracks" have been pointed out much more forcefully by at least five MDs who have written books with the following titles: *Death by Prescription—The Shocking Truth behind an Overmedicated Nation* (2003),[48] *The Truth about the Drug Companies—How They Deceive Us and What to Do about It* (2004),[49] *Bad Pharma—How Drug Companies Mislead Doctors and Harm Patients* (2012),[50] *Pharmageddon* (2012),[51] and *Deadly Medicines and Organised Crime—How Big Pharma Has Corrupted Healthcare* (2013).[52] These quite unpleasant titles, which speak for themselves, clearly suggest that there are widening cracks in the processes that deliver drugs into the bodies of human beings.

Four MDs have recently addressed the physician's responsibility to "get it right" in an article entitled "Accountable Prescribing."[53] Their primary target is the clinician's tendency to treat numbers rather than bring the patient to improved health—often taking the easy road. For example, the first approach for emerging high blood pressure or diabetes should be improved diet and exercise, not a convenient drug. Additionally, the writers propose quality measures that are met when the clinician prescribes simpler, safer, and proven medications rather than the last one approved by the FDA. For example, given that diet and exercise have been tried, initial use of metformin for diabetes would be rewarded, whereas drugs that do not have proven benefit or have a black box warning should be penalized. The MDs point out that despite this information, more than a half million prescriptions were written in 2011 for a drug (rosiglitazone) banned in Europe and restricted in the United States because of safety issues.

More evidence of the cracked processes involves the overuse of proton pump inhibitors to reduce the production of gastric acid and relieve "acid reflux." This class of medications is among the top ten most prescribed medications, yet data emerging in the past decade show that it has serious side effects, including an increased risk of infection by *Clostridium difficile*.[54] The rationale for ongoing use of this class of drugs is often undocumented in the patient's medical record and can lead to a cascade of additional drugs—inviting the risks of polypharmacy. Criteria are available to protect patients against preventable adverse drug events. In a sample of 600 consecutive elderly patients admitted to a teaching hospital a team of investigators, using a new tool they called "STOPP," discovered 329 adverse drug events of which two-thirds were considered contributory to the reason for admission to the hospital.[55] Almost 70 percent of these were preventable or potentially preventable events. Sticking with Medicare beneficiaries, the Office of Inspector General of the Department of Health and Human Services asked how many "questionable prescribers" there were in the Medicare Part D program.[56] A prescriber must be far out of the norm to be identified as questionable. For example, of the 87,000 general care physicians who prescribed an average of thirteen drugs per beneficiary, a physician must have prescribed an average of seventy-one or more per beneficiary to be considered a "questionable prescriber." There were four other ways to become a questionable prescriber; the most common way was to have prescribed more than seven times the average prescribing percentage of Schedule II drugs, which have high potential for abuse leading to psychological and physical dependence. By applying all five categories of questionability, approximately 0.85 percent of general care physicians were identified as questionable prescribers.

The prescribing paradigm is further confounded by the need for specialized training for doctors who prescribe potentially dangerous drugs, but that training appears to be lacking. To emphasize prescribing concerns, the FDA requires companies that produce drugs with a significant risk of serious or lethal harm to place a "black box" warning on the label. You might suppose that such high-risk drugs would require additional training of physicians before they prescribe these to patients, and you would be wrong.

The safety platform ensuring optimal safety and efficacy of the prescription drugs that get into your body is as cracked as the mud-crisp left behind in a dried-up lake bed. Let's add some water:

- Drug company executives must be held criminally accountable for serious harm to patients (1) if the results of all premarketing trials were not disclosed to the FDA, (2) if the FDA-mandated postmarketing studies were not performed within three years, or (3) if the company engaged in aggressive or misleading off-label marketing.
- The FDA must receive adequate funding from Congress to regulate the safe manufacture of prescription drugs to include (1) foreign-made drugs, (2) drugs made in compounding formularies, (3) generic drugs, (4) drugs placed on fast-track approval, and (5) drugs commonly prescribed in combinations.
- The FDA must be funded to take intentional action to educate and involve the public concerning the advantages and risks of prescription drugs to include (1) educational modules for high school and college students, (2) optimal websites addressing patients' need for definitive information on drug safety (including drug interactions), (3) the risks and benefits of chemotherapy, (4) the advantages of lifestyle changes over drugs, and (5) improving the capturing of patients' reports of side effects.
- The FDA must be given the responsibility and resources to ensure that physician knowledge is sufficient to safely prescribe drugs by (1) providing mandatory training for those physicians planning to prescribe black-box drugs, (2) providing training on use of IT resources to avoid dangerous polypharmacy, (3) working with state medical boards to require mandatory, annual prescribing updates to mitigate the underuse, overuse, and misuse of medications, and (4) creating national databases in which neo-

natologists and gerontologists can share information about appropriate medications for their extreme-aged populations.

- The physician-patient relationship must be strengthened to provide more transparency for the patient to make informed decisions by (1) discussing the risk-benefit of any prescribed medication, (2) warning the patient when a drug is prescribed off-label or is black box, (3) engaging pharmacists in an attempt to reconcile (reduce the number) of medications if the patient is taking more than five medications, and (4) always offering non-medication solutions where these are possible. Physicians' prescribing patterns must be systematically reviewed and progressively stern measures taken to ensure that guidelines are being followed unless there are mitigating circumstances for individual patients.

- The patient should become an integral member of the team trying to ensure the safety of medications for their personal use and for use by *all* other patients by (1) reporting all serious adverse effects into the FDA database and Rxisk.org, (2) knowing why they are taking each medication and what side effects to look out for, (3) asking for medication reconciliation, (4) living a lifestyle that minimizes the need for medications, and (5) demanding the legal right to full transparency from all parties involved in testing, manufacturing, marketing, prescribing, and dispensing their medications.

Medications can cause wonderful healing or relief from acute or chronic illness, but the public has lost trust in the way drugs are made, regulated, prescribed, and dispensed to them. This mistrust is *not* misplaced. The time has passed for tolerating unethical and uninformed behavior by individuals and companies in this process. The time has come for patients to have enforced legal rights and new responsibilities so that they can partner with those who would medicate them.

Chapter Eight

After the Harm:
Apology, Disclosure, and Trust

Cheryl Brown, DBA, RN

MY STORY

We were both medical professionals. But at that very moment, I and my about-to-be-newborn daughter were the patients and he was the obstetrician. I was full term, in active labor, and failing to progress. Time and drugs weren't working to move the delivery along, so a C-section was briefly discussed. Then epidural anesthesia was decided upon with my agreement. I was contracting, dry heaving, and quietly weeping. The nurses sat me up on the side of the bed with my legs dangling. They told me to bend forward over my full-term belly and be "still." Active labor and dry heaving are not still moments. But I concentrated on staying still, knowing that a needle was about to be directed between the two vertebrae in my spinal column. As an RN myself, I had assisted on numerous spinal procedures in the emergency department. The doctor prepared the site on my lower back.

Unsuccessful epidural attempt #1 sent instantaneous electricity down my right leg into my big toe, involuntarily causing my leg to twitch. I knew he hit my nerves. I knew what was happening and couldn't do anything about it. It was a reflex. He assertively told me not to move, as if the reflex was my fault. In between heaving and contracting, I tearfully told him, "I didn't move, you did that." He never said he was sorry nor acknowledged the pain he was causing. He also never explained anything to me or his plans to try again. Unsuccessful epidural attempt #2 was a repeat of the first, but on the other side, sending instantaneous electricity down my left leg into my big toe, again, involuntarily causing my other leg to twitch. I knew he hit my spinal nerves again. My contractions, heaving, and quiet weeping continued.

With frustration in his voice he aggressively told me to stop moving without acknowledging the pain he caused. I told him, "I didn't do that either, you did." He proceeded and prepped for the third attempt. Unsuccessful epidural attempt #3 sent rapid electricity through my perineum, causing my whole body to involuntarily jump with pain. I immediately told him to stop. He left the room in haste.

The nurses comforted me while I continued to contract, weep, and dry heave. Labor finally progressed. I was given an intravenous medication to assist with pain. The doctor returned to the room with an arrogant, nonapologizing affect. Thankfully, my daughter was born healthy, but not before I was wounded three times. During the following nine days I experienced a spinal headache from cerebral spinal fluid loss during the three failed attempts. A procedure to "patch" the area was offered, but I was too fearful to return to have that done. Through an anonymous source, I learned within the week that my doctor had paged anesthesia services to assist him with my anesthesia needs during labor. But apparently the anesthetist refused to come. I never learned the reasons behind the refusal to respond to my doctor's request for assistance.

Never having a history of headaches up to that point, I've learned to manage sixteen years of migraines induced from that harmful experience. For the first six years following that event, I felt angry toward the doctor every time I had a migraine headache. Anger and pain don't mix well, probably causing more head pain than I needed. I later learned how to manage my migraines from a neurologist who suffered from cluster headaches. I worked through the anger toward my obstetrician and learned pain management.

My thirty years of observing and working with numerous health care providers has been not only rewarding but disappointing on occasion. The rewards were usually filled with compassion and genuine caring. However, following an unanticipated medical event, I was acutely aware of provider avoidance, silence, and communication delays. Unfortunately, coupled with these events was a lack of genuine apology, disclosure, and resolution with patients and families. I now work full time in the patient safety arena not only facilitating sentinel event investigations and teaching patient safety lectures, but also advocating for health care providers' appropriate responses following harm events and/or medical mistakes.

MEDIOCRE CARE: A SHORT HISTORY

Early descriptions of the US medical system during the late 1980s reflected increasing medical-legal issues and a new focus on patient safety. Compensation for poor care was very rarely awarded. A Harvard medical practice study found that the tort system failed to compensate the majority of patients injured by their medical care. The research findings spurred the development of the patient safety movement. At the same time, the growth in medical malpractice litigation reached crisis levels in many states, with physicians unable to afford (or in some high-risk specialties even obtain) malpractice insurance. States began to address both sets of problems through tort reform laws. One reform required—that hospitals inform patients about quality problems in their medical care—also created an opportunity for improved patient safety.[1]

Fast-forward a quarter of a century. Our costs are soaring, the service is typically mediocre, and the quality is often unreliable. Every clinician has his or her own way of doing things, and the rates of failure and complication (not to mention the costs) for a given service routinely vary by a factor of two or three, even within the same hospital.[2] How shall we the health care community and we the patients become empowered to take on these challenges? Seems daunting at best, but an ever-growing medical and legal movement toward conquering this challenge is to take steps toward apology and disclosure. There is no value in withholding information or apologies, but there is valuable evidence for transparency, apology, and truth-telling/disclosure.

TRUSTING PATIENTS, SILENT PROVIDERS

Most of us are going to be touched by the health care system, and we want everything to go just right. "I am sorry" are the words we want to hear when someone has done something wrong to us—especially if (s)he has seriously hurt us. The trust factor between patients and their physicians/providers is heavily affected throughout such a relationship. To face someone who refuses to acknowledge his or her mistakes, and the harm that was caused, compounds the original wrong and undermines any future trust the patient may hope to have in that provider. Nearly two decades ago Wu et al. stated that "when mistakes are not acknowledged in a timely manner, there may be a perception of a cover-up, and public confidence in physicians may be undermined."[3] Yet when physicians and hospitals commit errors, "I'm sorry" is often the last thing that patients hear. Medical mistakes are often not even disclosed to patients, even—or especially—when those mistakes are deadly.[4]

We all know personalities, in and out of the health care arena, that are uncomfortable saying they are sorry. An apology would require acknowledging shortcomings or that they did something wrong or failed to do something. When the patient receives neither a sympathetic apology nor an appropriate, timely, responsible apology and explanation, (s)he may think, "they don't care," "they're neglectful," "I can't trust them," and so on, driving him or her to feel dismissed, hurt, alone, and later, maybe angry. Ultimately patients can't trust a person who they perceive is not committed to the truth of disclosure and apology. Persistent, repetitive incompetence, fear, and/or arrogant silence are unacceptable and predictably costly.

Patients want to and most often do approach the health care system knowing that they are entering into a relationship of trust. Even those of us who are health care professionals expect the same when we find ourselves as patients with our peers in our own health care system. There are a myriad of legal, ethical, and personal reasons why health care providers choose to or choose not to apologize and disclose unanticipated medical events. While many physicians feel ashamed and scared, others are untrained. Then, there are those who are avoiders, purposely denying any reason to render an apology. Certainly in the most recent past they were often told to stay silent by medical lawyers trying to protect against liability risk. And most aren't taught how to apologize, which isn't easy to do when the people they hurt are the people they meant to help.

Increased attention to health care quality and impending changes due to health reform are calling for health care leaders at all levels to strengthen their skills in leading quality improvement initiatives.[5] These initiatives involve training and education for providers in the appropriate delivery of bad news and/or explaining what really happened that led up to a harm event. Any type of successful health care encounter should be based on trust and open communication. So if everything doesn't go just right (an error or harm event), then we innately desire clear and timely communication about the event. This hasn't always been the case, though.

Historically, after an adverse event, the organization's actions in response to the event—particularly in the first twenty-four hours—have often determined whether or not the patient and family feel they are going to encounter truth and receive support.[6] The task of disclosing a medical error or adverse event is difficult, and the consequences of doing it badly can be severe: breakdown in relationships, failure to prevent future error, increased emotional stress, and litigation.[7] Alexander Pope once said, "To err is human, to forgive divine. . . ." To err *is* human, and because medicine is practiced by humans, medical mistakes will continue to occur every day.[8] Those mistakes and unanticipated outcomes deserve a genuine acknowledgement, an apology, an openness of explanation, and sincere regard for those harmed. Doctors and other health care workers should not second-guess themselves because they worry an apology could come back to haunt them.[9] The majority of medical professionals want to apologize; however, they are afraid of domestic terrorists known as contingency fee lawyers.[10] But most importantly, the system perpetuates medical error because the adversarial nature of litigation induces a so-called "culture of silence" in physicians eager to shield themselves from liability; this silence leads to the pointless repetition of error, as the open discussion and analysis of the root causes of medical mistakes do not take place as fully as they should.[11]

POLICIES, LAWS, AND THE BUSINESS OF APOLOGIES

Medical malpractice reforms have attracted broad attention, with current interest focusing on promoting disclosure, apology, and early compensation offers.[12] Pulling the truth out is costly at best. Litigation is an expensive and unproductive way to get to the "truth" for health care providers, hospitals, and patients.[13] Writing policy has been an effective approach to this challenge, while numerous health care systems have already developed apology policies in conjunction with mediation to avert costly litigation and promote healthy communication.[14]

Many institutions are embracing a new "full disclosure" philosophy with more open communication, honesty, and maybe even an apology when a medical error occurs, but these policies often take years to truly take hold.[15] Some hospitals have reported that as transparency about medical errors goes up and safety improves, lawsuits go down.[16] Change and a critical step forward have come to most states that now have laws that encourage medical apology by offering some form of protection for those who engage in it, usually by ensuring that the apology itself cannot be used against the physician if a suit is brought.[17]

Passing laws has been another effective approach. Likewise, many states have passed medical apology laws to prevent apologies offered in the hospital from being used as admissions of liability in the courtroom.[18] These apology laws (I'm Sorry laws or benevolent gesture laws) are now popular among thirty-eight states. Their aim is to encourage apologies from health care providers to patients and/or families who may have been adversely affected by a poor medical outcome without the apology being used against them in court as an admission of liability.[19] This has been a relief to both the medical and the legal side.

Apologies made by physicians for adverse medical events have been identified as a mitigating factor in whether patients decide to litigate. Historically, doctors have been socialized to avoid apologies because apologies admit guilt and invite lawsuits. An apology law, which specifies that a physician's apology is inadmissible in court, is written to encourage patient-physician communication. State-level apology laws could expedite the settlement process and increase the number of settlements by 15 percent within three to five years of law adoption. Apology laws have the greatest reduction in average payment size and settlement time in cases involving more severe patient outcomes. In the short run the law increases the number of resolved cases while decreasing the average settlement payment for cases with more significant and permanent injuries. While their impact on settlement payments for cases involving minor injuries is insignificant, the apology laws do reduce the total number of such cases.

Apology laws reduce the amount of time it takes to reach a settlement in what would normally be protracted lawsuits, leading to more resolved cases in the short run. In the long run, the evidence suggests there could be fewer cases overall.[20] It turns out that good apologies are also good business. Hospitals across the country that have moved from deny-and-defend stances to policies endorsing early apology and restitution have found dramatic reductions in lawsuit payouts.[21]

Several states agree that a medical apology is advantageous on several accounts. One hospital system in Michigan saw its lawsuit payoffs decrease by 60 percent after instituting a policy that mandated immediate reporting of errors, trained practitioners in communication and medical apology, and supported practitioners who did apologize.[22] Texas law clearly prohibits the admission of an expression of sympathy by a health care provider to be used as an admission of fault in a court of law.[23] Maryland has its own medical apology law stating that an apology or statement of regret by a doctor is inadmissible in a medical malpractice trial. However, in Maryland, if there is an admission of guilt in conjunction with an apology, it can be used in court. Massachusetts enacted legislation that emphasized an approach of "disclosure, apology and offer" to medical malpractice claims.[24]

A recently passed "apology law" gave Pennsylvania doctors the freedom to apologize without fear that their words could be used against them in medical malpractice suits. The law, officially called the Benevolent Gesture Act, was unanimously approved by the Senate and House and signed by Governor Corbett. It went into effect in December 2013. Pennsylvania, at that time, joined at least thirty-six other states and the District of Columbia with similar measures. Dr. Amelia Pare, president of the Allegheny County Medical Society, told Luis Fabregas, a *Pittsburgh Review* medical editor, that "this allows you to be more of a human being . . . it really keeps that doctor-patient relationship open." Mr. Fabregas also commented that the law doesn't cover statements beyond an apology or expression of care or concern. So you likely won't be hearing statements that admit negligence, such as "I wasn't thinking when I left the sponge in your husband's abdomen" or "I can't believe I removed the left foot instead of the right one."[25]

Wisconsin governor Scott Walker signed a bill in April 2014 that allows doctors and other health care providers to apologize to patients without worrying about the statements being used against them in court. The new law, pushed by Republicans, makes apologies, condolences, or expressions of sympathy inadmissible in civil proceedings and in administrative hearings concerning the health care provider's actions. Supporters argue the new law will encourage open communication between doctors and patients. Opponents, including trial attorneys, say the change will make it harder for patients to bring successful malpractice lawsuits.[26] Also, this year (2014), Rhode Island introduced a medical apology bill that would exclude expressions of benevolence but not full admissions of fault. It includes any and all statements, writing, gestures, or affirmations made by a health care provider or employee of a health care provider that express apology, sympathy, compassion, condolence, or benevolence relating to the pain, suffering, or death of a patient as a result of an unanticipated outcome of medical care that is given to the patient, the patient's family, or a friend.[27] And as of this writing (April 2014), Alaska's legislature passed an I'm Sorry bill for the same reasons as above: to make expressions of apology or compassion inadmissible as evidence in medical malpractice cases.

The I'm Sorry laws allow doctors and other health care providers to express regret without fear of the apology being used against them in a medical malpractice lawsuit. The law shields doctors so that an apology following an unwanted or unexpected medical outcome could not be used as evidence of negligence in a lawsuit. It protects any action or statement that conveys a sense of apology or explanation "emanating from humane impulses." These statutes do not protect factual statements or admissions of guilt for a medical outcome or error. Most also apply to nursing home staff and administrators. These laws are finally appearing on behalf of our hurt and harmed patients and families who deserve the utmost respect when pledging their unwavering trust to the medical community.

TALK ABOUT IT

Unforeseen or unanticipated medical outcomes ethically deserve disclosure and apology. Bioethicist Art Caplan says he is a "strong supporter" of such laws. He also goes on to say that "having an apology when an error or mistake takes place is something that patients and their families deserve. . . . Mistakes are going to happen, they do. And I think people need to hear regret. . . . [Doctors and nurses] are not going to do it if they are worried about lawsuits."[28] Caplan says that these laws do not excuse doctors for medical negligence or malpractice, but malpractice lawyers argue there is too much gray area between an apology and an admission of neglect. "It doesn't prohibit lawsuits, it just says you can talk about regret, you can talk about your feelings, without having that held against you or being the trigger to your lawsuit," Caplan says. "I think many of these apologies are absolutely sincere, absolutely not done to deflect a lawsuit. It's because people really do feel bad, and I think they really ought to get that chance. I know some lawyers are [worried], that somehow or another they're going to lose business or, if you will, bad conduct will go unpunished because of these apologies. But, I think people in health care—patients, families—they want to hear really what the doctor feels."[29] Emotional benefits are achieved through open communication between the provider and the patient, which permits the provider to apologize for the unexpected outcome without admitting to liability and allows the patient to obtain information related to the incident.

In 2001 The Joint Commission recommended, under the section entitled "Rights and Responsibilities of the Individual," that patients and their families be informed of all outcomes, whether they are positive, negative, unanticipated, preventable, or adverse events. Disclosure and apology, two separate concepts with specific skill sets, are often confused with one another. Disclosure requires many informational, factual conversations over a period of time between the provider and the patient about the outcome of care rendered. More accurately, disclosure is a serial communication of available information over sequential conversations.[30] An apology is a voluntary expression of remorse and sorrow coupled with an admission of wrongdoing. Apology is also an acknowledgement of responsibility for harm caused plus an invitation toward reconciliation.[31] Psychologists teach us that an apology is an important way of "showing respect and empathy for the wronged person." Apologies improve patient-doctor communication and reduce patient anger.[32] An apology can lead to open discussion from which the hospital may obtain information that will help avoid similar errors in the future. And a prompt apology coupled with an explanation of the event and a fair offer of compensation are critical steps in rebuilding trust between the physician and the patient.[33]

Physicians respond [to unanticipated medical events] by choosing their words carefully; mentioning the event but not that an error occurred; and failing to reveal what caused the error, how it might have been prevented, and how they may act differently in the future.[34] When a medical error or adverse event occurs, health care professionals are likely to experience powerful emotions such as shame, guilt, or failure.[35] Without time to process those reactions, they will have difficulty focusing on the needs of the patient or family, much less thinking about what they can learn from the event to improve patient safety. Physicians have expressed that they wish discussions with colleagues about medical errors or adverse events were part of hospital culture.

If senior staff members responded to news of an error by discussing their own past mistakes, such openness would be a powerful source of support for other physicians.[36] Moreover, health care providers who feel emotionally supported are more likely to feel comfortable talking to patients after an error, answering questions, and expressing their own feelings.[37] As Lucian Leape—a physician who has been at the vanguard of advocacy for disclosure and apology in medicine—has argued, a culture that precludes physicians from apologizing can be traumatizing for health care practitioners, whom he calls the "second victims" of medical error. He cites the critical repair that can come from acknowledging one's mistakes, expressing remorse, and helping to mitigate harm or offer reparations. Allowing room for true remorse, it turns out, can be healing to both sides of the medical encounter. And healing is what medicine is all about.[38]

ADMIT IT

Most of our literature reflects a decade's worth of acknowledging the struggles and multifaceted challenges of apologizing, the need for reform, and the gap in education and training. Patients want and ask for basic information about adverse events; an apology; and the prevention of future events. "What should doctors do when [they] make a mistake? . . . Of course, from a moral perspective, there is no controversy. We should do what we expect others to do. When we err, we should admit it and apologize for it."[39]

Physicians have experience in delivering bad news to patients and discussing hard choices about treatment options. Much of the expertise they have developed in that context is relevant to disclosure conversations, but there are other skills—often referred to as active listening skills, used routinely by mediators and conflict resolvers—that are less familiar to physicians and that should be a focus of training.[40]

A program run by COPIC Insurance Company, Colorado, a physician-owned medical professional liability insurer, started a postincident risk management program in 2000. The program encourages an early disclosure conversation described as open, honest, and empathic. Physicians answer patients' questions, explain what happened, and offer an apology if appropriate. COPIC pays for the patient's out-of-pocket expenses related to the injury and does not ask the patient for a waiver or general release from liability—patients are free to pursue a lawsuit if they choose. The anecdotal evidence is that few patients who have participated in the COPIC program have sued.[41]

NECESSARY TRAINING

Doctors are trained in many skills, like how to intubate a patient or how to calibrate medication dosing. But they are not trained in how to apologize. This is a problem, because if anything is certain in medicine, it is this: every doctor will make mistakes that may end up harming someone—not because they are incompetent or don't care, but because they are caring for so many.[42] Many of these mistakes come down to straight statistics. The more people you take care of, the more likely you are to make a mistake. It's not if, it's when.

Given the limited occasions when a physician will be engaged in a disclosure conversation, the goal of training health care providers should be twofold. One goal is to give hospital staff a brief introduction to the conflict resolution and communication skills used in disclosure conversations. The second is to prepare a core group of skilled and experienced staff members who can help others prepare for disclosure conversations, can participate when appropriate, and can debrief afterward. Brief introductory training for as many members of the staff as possible can make them aware of the complexity of disclosure conversations, give them elementary communication tools, and sensitize them to the value of a consultation with a process expert.[43] The following is a list of disclosure and apology recommendations and training goals for physicians and hospitals:[44]

1. Physicians and other health care professionals should develop an awareness of the communication skills most likely to be useful during disclosure conversations;
2. Hospitals should develop in-house process experts available as consultants to aid in planning, conducting, and debriefing disclosure conversations;
3. Hospitals should encourage physicians, patient safety officers, and risk managers to spend time planning before conducting disclosure conversations;
4. Physicians, hospital leaders, and other health care providers should offer an appropriate apology after an adverse event or error;
5. Hospitals and senior physicians should provide opportunities for debriefing and support for health care professionals after an error; and
6. Hospitals should use mediation as soon as practicable after an adverse event to settle potential claims.

DOING THE RIGHT THING ISN'T CHEAP

Why isn't this type of training prevalent in our medical schools, residency programs, continuing education requirements, and mandatory hospital education programs? Professional and layperson literature has made strong recommendations for these programs for decades. This call for action is indisputably relevant. Recommendations for robust patient safety and medical apology training programs should include honesty; open communication; expressions of sympathy; admission of fault; early reporting and investigation of errors; active disclosure of medical errors; learning about medical liability reform and about I'm Sorry legislation; plus learning about medical error disclosure programs. Training programs of this caliber also require committed buy-in from leadership (appointing a champion to lead, advocate, and sustain ongoing training); culture change; transparency; plus early, timely, and frequent contact/intervention with patients. Fostering ongoing outreach and educational programs for physicians also includes developing and investing time into the program, writing policies and procedures for the program, marketing the program, and lastly, considering hiring for the program.

There is a defining moment when unanticipated circumstances cause a shift and a necessity to acknowledge and apologize. Proper preparation is the key. Simple, practical points, practiced ahead of time for these defining moments, help providers to live at an accountable practicing level. Timely provider feedback gives patients a reasonable assurance that something is being done, that the truth is being researched, and that someone responsible is going to follow up with them. Some physicians, health care providers, organizations, and states have gotten on board with this culture change. Restoration of the provider-patient relationship is necessary, because pockets of resistance will only prove to be their downfall.

Chapter Nine

The Consumer Advocates Who Kicked the Hospital-Infection Nest

Lisa McGiffert, Director,
Consumers Union Safe Patient Project[1]

When Tom Vallier fell off the roof of his house in 2001, breaking a femur and fracturing vertebrae, he had no idea of the journey he was about to embark upon. He immediately had several spinal surgeries and by 2003 was the survivor of four hospital-acquired infections. He was not expected to live, and, while grateful, he discovered "that certain things in life are actually worse than death." His infections led to permanent spinal damage that causes him constant pain and the threat of recurring infections. His active, outdoor lifestyle was permanently changed to a sedentary existence. "To be frank, I was not only physically injured, but financially, emotionally, and spiritually devastated by the experience," said Tom.[2]

Several years after Tom's accident, *Consumer Reports* published an article titled "How Safe Is Your Hospital?" which included subscribers' feedback about their hospital experiences.[3] Six percent of respondents to the magazine's survey reported developing an infection during or within one week of their hospital stay. That was remarkably close to the Centers for Disease Control and Prevention (CDC) estimate at the time: five percent of US hospital patients infected each year, nearly two million people; and 88,000 of them died from the infection.[4] Later that year, *Consumer Reports*' president, Jim Guest, challenged the organization's advocacy division (Consumers Union) to identify targeted consumer issues and create nationwide campaigns, allowing for multistate advocacy. He wanted to home in on issues that would engage consumers from across the United States and would make a real difference in their lives. The need to address hospital-acquired infections was obvious. We proposed a national campaign to pass state laws that require hospitals to publish their infection rates, and Consumers Union's Stop Hospital Infections campaign[5] was born.

Consumers Union (CU) saw public transparency as a tool to stimulate change. The campaign became a catalyst to raise public awareness and to help people make more informed choices by passing laws requiring reporting of infections acquired in hospitals, breeding grounds for dangerous drug-resistant infections. Even if they had only one hospital in their community, with access to infection data, they could compare its performance with others in their state, and if that was unsatisfactory, the community could press for change—through the media, conversations among doctors, employer conversations with hospitals, and conversations between patients and their doctors. We believed patients had a right to know their hospital's record on infections.

Today most states require hospitals to report certain infections, and they post the information on publicly available websites. After more than half of the states had reporting laws, in 2011 the federal government began a public reporting program that makes infection information from the remaining states public. CDC has a sophisticated electronic reporting system that collects data from thousands of health care providers through its National Healthcare Safety Network (NHSN). The US Health and Human Services agency is in the fifth year of an action plan that sets specific targets toward eliminating health care–acquired infections (HAIs) and proposing new targets for 2020.[6] Thousands of hospitals have enrolled in local and national programs to improve their infection prevention. There is growing evidence that public reporting is having an impact on reducing these infections by motivating hospitals to improve: infections are being prevented, based on statistics from state and national reports. Lives are being saved. A 2014 CDC report on the prevalence of HAIs in 2011 indicated that one in twenty-five hospital patients was infected. That marked a 1 percent improvement since the agency's 2002 estimate.[7] Progress is being made, but we still have a long way to go.

How did all of this happen in a nation that for decades had been fairly complacent in the face of these shocking statistics? Most are unaware of the pivotal role that a network of consumer advocates played in pushing hospital-acquired infections onto the national radar, and eventually compelling prevention efforts in response. This is the story of how advocates changed the culture of medical care from one that treated infections as inevitable to one that strives for their elimination.

100,000 DEAD AND NO SENSE OF URGENCY

Ten years ago, this is what the health care landscape looked like to CU's hospital infection campaign: there was no big national push for infection control, and there was a culture of acceptance among health care providers that these infections were inevitable and that most were not preventable. The public knew very little about the scope of the problem. Virtually every infection expert we encountered thought public reporting of infections was a bad idea; some said it could not be done. We thought that hospitals were intentionally keeping their infection rates a secret, but we soon discovered that hospitals generally didn't know how many patients they were infecting because they didn't have to know—it was a "don't ask, don't tell" mentality. The prevailing attitude appeared to be that infections were of no concern as long as hospitals' annual sampling of infections put them in line with the CDC's estimate of the national average.

CU organized a totally consumer-driven campaign in this environment, which seemed incongruously complacent in the midst of an epidemic of harm. We developed a model state bill, and CU activists asked their legislators to file the bill informing the public of hospitals' track records on controlling infections. We also collected stories from patients, putting the media in touch with these very compelling narratives. Those stories led us to remarkable consumer activists who transcended their significant losses due to hospital-acquired infections to push for changes in health care policies that would ensure that no one else had to endure the kind of pain that they had to endure. Many told us that it was impossible for them not to take action—it was an important part of the way they expressed their grief. Over the next ten years they would lobby, talk to the media, testify at hearings, serve on committees to implement infection laws and committees to envision future efforts to end medical harm, educate the public, and train current and future medical professionals on what patients need to stay safe. Tom Vallier and his wife DeeDee were among the first who told us their story, and they later asked us to come to their state to pass a public reporting law in Oregon—together we finally accomplished that in 2007.

In September 2003, when CU launched its Stop Hospital Infections campaign and website, only one state, Illinois, had a law specifically requiring reports on hospital-acquired infections; the bill also required reporting of nurse staffing levels.[8] Senate Bill 59, by State Senator Barack Obama, was passed in August of that year, following a much-cited 2002 investigative report by the *Chicago Tribune*.[9] The *Tribune* series highlighted patient stories and was an inspiration to the CU campaign.

But another state, Pennsylvania, turned out to be the one to lead the way for public reporting as the state's Health Care Cost Containment Council (PHC4) initiated regulations to require hospitals to report infections occurring in their facilities.[10] CU brought public support and national attention to Pennsylvania reporting. CU was present at the news conference announcing the state's first hospital-specific report in December 2006. Illinois took almost seven years to issue its first report.

TRAILBLAZER STATES

In 2004, CU's campaign focused on four states where we felt we had the most opportunity to succeed: California, because we had an office there and were familiar with the legislative landscape; Pennsylvania, where new regulations were being proposed; and Missouri and Florida, because opportunities for local collaborations arose there. The CU-drafted model law[11] covered the infections that we thought should be reported, established advisory committees with consumer representation, protected patient privacy, and mandated that public reports would be hospital specific.

California was the first state to test this model legislation—and we passed a bill closely resembling it in 2004, pulling opposition from the state's hospital association but at least getting the state chapter of the Association for Professionals in Infection Control and Epidemiology (APIC) to negotiate with us. However, Governor Schwarzenegger vetoed the bill, putting us on notice that the hospitals were going to use their influence to maintain secrecy about how many patients they infected.

In Pennsylvania we collaborated with a dynamic PennPIRG[12] group that demonstrated to us the power of having advocates on the ground in states unfamiliar to us. It would become a model for success in other states: advocates attended meetings, worked with the media, and kept up with proposals as they moved through the legislative or regulatory process. They testified at public hearings and let us know when it was important for CU staff to show up—eventually this type of collaborative partnership would also play out in Connecticut, South Carolina, Vermont, Colorado, Rhode Island, New York, Maryland, Massachusetts, and New Jersey.

In Missouri, we had our first experience working with someone from a state who had personally been affected by infections and who asked for our help to pass legislation. Ray Wagner was a lobbyist with powerful political connections. But when his teenage son shattered his elbow in a sledding accident and got an infection from the repair surgery that led to six more surgeries in one year, Ray was incredulous that this kind of thing happened in modern US hospitals. He was outraged that no public information was available about hospitals' infection rates. Several other themes emerged in Missouri that would pan out in other states: the bill sponsor was not a powerful chair of a health committee, who often had a close relationship with hospital associations, but someone with a passion for this issue. The hospital associations would fight us and be the entities with which we had to negotiate compromises. The power of people's stories had a significant impact in rallying support. Ray's son's story ended up in a front-page article in the *Wall Street Journal*,[13] with a tagline of "Aim Is to Empower Consumers, Spur Prevention, but Critics Cite Host of Complexities, Missouri Father on a Crusade." That pushed the issue and CU's campaign onto the radar of other major media outlets like the CBS *Early Morning Show*, CNN, and *Dateline*, as well as the medical community. The article quotes Ray: "'I keep hearing that what we're trying to do can't be done,' says Mr. Wagner. He isn't buying it. 'In 10 years from now I'm hoping we can look back and say this was a very sloppy first step, but a very important first step.'"[14] Ten years later Ray still works to improve infection reporting and prevention in Missouri.[15]

After some success in 2004, we took our model bill on the road a few months before state legislatures began meeting in 2005. At that time CU had about 5,000 people signed up who had agreed to take action on various issues; today our list is a million strong. We simply e-mailed these activists to ask them to send an e-mail to their state legislators, tell them about the problem of hospital-acquired infections, ask them to follow a link to CU's model bill, and file it.

AN OUTBREAK OF LEGISLATION

In 2005, we expected five to ten legislators to respond by introducing bills and were overwhelmed when thirty states filed public reporting bills. It's rare when a legislator introduces your model bill written as is, but each bill filed contained sections identical to our model bill, so we knew they were responding to our activists. That year the New York bill was passed with the help of power hitters Art Levin, Center for Medical Consumers and former member of the Institute of Medicine committee that issued the seminal "To Err Is Human" report on medical errors, and Blair Horner, New York Public Interest Research Group (NYPIRG). These two led negotiations with legislators. CU provided technical support and grassroots actions in which we asked New Yorkers to send e-mails to their legislators urging passage of the infection-reporting bill. In New York we also connected with Reduce Infection Deaths (RID), another group focused on improving infection rates that did radio ads throughout the legislative session, which helped to raise public awareness.

New York and Virginia were the only states to adopt public reporting laws that year. But it was clear that disclosure of hospital infections resonated with policy makers and the public. It also became clear that an opportunistic strategy would be the best route for our small, three-person staff—from then on, we focused on the states where action was happening.

After 2005, the momentum for state legislation significantly picked up. New states took up the cause, and some that were unsuccessful tried again. The legislative campaign dedicated a staffer, Suzanne Henry, to track bills in every state, draft actions to follow the bills through the process, and identify people's stories that would fit with (often very specific) requests from the media. Our e-mail action strategy enabled us to follow the path of each state's bill, target members of the specific committees hearing the bills, blast the full House and Senate with e-mails when the bills came to the floor, and follow up with governors when needed. While e-mail advocacy is commonly used to get people involved today, in 2005 it was fairly new and proved to be our secret weapon. Over the course of this campaign, we would often hear from the state-based advocates that legislators were screaming about the number of e-mails!

Jean Rexford, founder of the Connecticut Center for Patient Safety, an accomplished consumer advocate on health issues and a master at getting local media coverage, predicted in 2006 that we could get the bill introduced, but it would probably take several sessions to pass. CU staff went to Connecticut, where Rexford organized a news conference, took people with personal stories to visit legislators and testify at hearings, and got supportive editorials in local papers. She enlisted other organizations to help, including a health care workers' union and the New York–based Reduce Infection Deaths. Rexford garnered support from Senator Chris Murphy and Attorney General Richard Blumenthal, building strong relationships with these two leaders who now serve in the US Senate. As was true in many states, our activists heard back from their legislators in e-mails similar to this one from Connecticut: "Thank you for your email and I echo your concern. This is a true issue and one which my own family has personal experience with the reality of this negligence."[16] Connecticut wasn't the only state where legislators came forward with their own stories—this issue really hit home for so many. At one point it looked like the bill had been so weakened by the hospital lobby that we considered walking away from it, but a compromise that retained the key components to a good public reporting law was reached, and the bill passed in one session.

Our 2006 efforts took us to Colorado, where we teamed up with a dedicated legislator, the state-based Colorado Consumer Health Initiative, and CO-PIRG to pass legislation there. CU worked mostly with the House sponsor while Kerry O'Connell, a construction engineer from Denver who survived numerous hospital-acquired infections, focused on the Senate sponsor. In 2004 Kerry fell off a ladder, dislocating his elbow and fracturing the radius bone in his forearm. The repair of these injuries resulted in a cascade of medical errors and infections and an encounter with a bad medical device.

Before his eighth surgery to repair paralyzed arm muscles, Kerry decided to take matters into his own hands. He studied medical textbooks, created a spreadsheet with all of the possible combinations of tendon surgeries done in the past hundred years, analyzing the pros and cons of each, and met with his surgeon to mutually decide how his arm would be repaired.

After helping to pass the infection reporting law, Kerry served as the chair of Colorado's hospital infection advisory committee. He has gained national recognition, speaking often at national conferences, has debated leading epidemiologists, and wrote about the patient's perspective of medical harm in the journal *Health Affairs*.[17] He is a leader in CU's patient safety network and in our circle is famous for a folksy brilliance in his observations of the absurdities routinely faced by infected patients. For example, he pegged harmed patients "Numerators" in reference to how infection rates are calculated by an impersonal health care system. He coined the term "iatrogenic bonding" because post-harm, the patient and the doctor will never forget each other's names. And "if a doctor recommends treatment, he will tell you all of the benefits but none of the risks. If a patient suggests treatment, the doctor will tell you all of the risks but none of the benefits. So if you get two opinions and tell the second doc it was your idea, you should get the full truth."[18]

Also in 2006, our collaboration with other super-advocates led to passage of infection reporting laws: Helen Haskell, the founder of Mothers Against Medical Errors in South Carolina, whose fifteen-year-old son Lewis Blackman died from medical errors that could have easily been prevented;[19] Lori Nerbonne, an RN in New Hampshire whose mother died after infections and medication errors;[20] businessman Gene Cenci; and professional health consultant Jean Keller in Vermont.[21] All were committed to improving the safety of Vermont hospitals. Michael Bennett, whose father died of multiple infections, was successful in Maryland. Even before an infection reporting bill was filed, the Maryland hospital association developed a position paper about why a bill was unnecessary and lobbied legislators to kill the bill[22] but they did not succeed.

When his father died, Michael Bennett embarked on a mission to find out what happened, gain some accountability, and change hospital care so similar horrors would not happen to others. His outrage, always visible, vocal, and appropriate, is a constant reminder to the CU activist network to avoid complacency as incremental progress is being made. A painter and paperhanger by profession, he is also a tenacious advocate with an incredible scientific mind. Mentored by two leading epidemiologists of our time—Dr. Barry Farr and Dr. William Jarvis—Michael became an expert on MRSA (methicillin-resistant *Staphylococcus aureus*) infections. He pushed for legislation in Maryland to require what is known as *active detection and isolation* (ADI), a prevention protocol based on a Society for Healthcare Epidemiology of

America (SHEA) guideline. The protocol involves actively identifying people who are colonized carriers of certain organisms like MRSA, but have no
visible symptoms, and then isolating them to prevent its spread.[23] This method to fight the spread of the MRSA superbug has had success in other
countries. Michael is a veteran of countless state and national print, TV, and
radio interviews. In his book—a loving tribute to his father's life and a frank
and honest telling of his terrible death—he summed up his patient safety
advocacy, which is so similar to others who are a part of our network:

> Over the next six years I became an activist and a patient advocate. Again and
> again I testified before legislative committees on patients' rights and safety
> issues and railed against the "tort reformers" for trying to wrest justice or fair
> and just compensation from victims of medical negligence. I met with ump-
> teen politicians and public officials on the state as well as the federal level,
> some of whom became outraged by what was happening; others simply re-
> mained complacent. Almost a week did not go by when I wasn't in a studio or
> standing on a ladder or sitting in my truck doing interviews over my cell
> phone, or rushing home to change my work clothes ahead of an arriving
> reporter and cameraman. I didn't crave the limelight; I dreaded it. And every
> interview intensified my grief. But at the same time, like other victims in
> similar circumstances, I was grateful for the opportunities, because I was fight-
> ing for my father.[24]

By the end of 2006, nine more states had passed public reporting legislation, and a total of forty-three states had considered bills. Pennsylvania had
issued the country's first public report disclosing the infection rates for each
hospital. We were on our way to changing how people thought about and
dealt with hospital-acquired infections.

PERSISTENCE PAYS OFF

After two failed attempts to require disclosure of hospital-specific infection
rates in California,[25] CU had decided it was fruitless to try again, since we
had our hands full in other states. But we were soon to meet a force of nature
in Carole Moss, who refused to take no for an answer. Her fifteen-year-old
son, Nile, had gone to a local hospital for a series of medical tests; after
returning home he began to have flu-like symptoms. As Carole put it, "within
48 hours, his life on earth came to an end."[26] She and her husband, Ty, later
learned that Nile died of an MRSA infection, something they had never heard
about and for which they had not been prepared. In an effort to raise awareness, they created Nile's Project[27] and began doing public education. Since
Ty Moss is a professional musician, they used music as a way of bringing
people together to learn about MRSA. They hold concerts during which
attendees get information about MRSA infections.

The Moss family also took their story to the state capitol. CU told Carole if she could find a sponsor to take this on, we would help. She found two sponsors and enlisted numerous dedicated local supporters and a seasoned union lobbyist to help.[28] In the end, Senator Elaine Alquist championed the passage of Nile's Law, one of the strongest infection reporting and prevention bills in the country. It requires hospitals to report infections that occur throughout the hospital as well as to screen certain patients at risk of carrying the MRSA bacteria into the hospital.

But we were not done in California. Alicia Cole, a dynamic activist who had barely survived a flesh-eating infection called necrotizing fasciitis, joined the state implementation effort, serving on the state's advisory committee with Carole. That process proved contentious, as the majority of the committee representing hospitals and the health department staff seemed to have little interest in public reporting. It was so bad that in 2010, CU issued a status report[29] on the failure of California to implement its patient safety laws, including the infection reporting laws, and testified, along with Carole, at a Senate hearing on the lack of progress.[30] This pressured the agency to actually produce reports by the legislative deadlines.

California's first report was a mess, and most didn't believe it reliably represented infections occurring in hospitals, but that has improved over time. The law required a phase-in reporting of certain infections. When reporting of surgical infections was due, the health department and hospital members of the committee agreed to require limited reporting that did not comply with the law. After mailing these instructions to all hospitals, Senator Alquist immediately demanded that the agency comply fully with the law. The health department leadership made the infection division change their directive to the hospitals. In response, the California Hospital Association sued the state. The judge's response was firm: if the hospital association didn't like the law, they should go back to the legislature to change it, but the current law clearly required reporting infections that were acquired during twenty-nine different types of surgical procedures.[31] This ruling was a huge win for consumers and ensured there would be no more stonewalling. The advisory committee was reconstituted with Carole, Alicia, and another CU activist, Rae Greulich, on board; new leadership at the health department; and hospital representatives who are serious about preventing infections.

Although it would take most states two years from passage of new laws to publication of their first reports—and a few took longer—by 2006 we had proven that it was not impossible to report infections to the public. Still, implementation of these laws required more commitments from activists. As in California, after helping to pass legislation in their states, activists served for years on state-created advisory committees formed to help guide the process of public reporting. We were always outnumbered—typically committees had one or two consumer representatives, but some states had more.

Meetings were often held at state hospital association offices, sometimes placing another layer of intimidation over those of us who passionately wanted the public to see infection rates. Some state health department employees who were given the task to head up these efforts demonstrated a strong commitment and vision for implementation—of note, Rachel Stricof in New York and Pat Jones in Vermont. But we met with resistance in more states. Often it was subtle, a delay here or there to give the hospitals more time to get used to the idea or get organized—often delivered with jargon empathetic to patients but that didn't quite feel authentic.

Texas was perhaps the worst example of delays, where every turn was met with another barrier. The first bill, introduced in 2005, turned into a study—a common delay tactic. Since Texas holds biennial legislative sessions, every delay translated into a two-year wait. The study committee, including CU staff and activist Raquel Sanchez,[32] whose father had died of an infection in a Houston hospital, recommended reporting infections to the public. In 2007 a public reporting bill was finally passed, but there was another delay because the legislature had not appropriated funds to do the work. Then in late 2009, funding was allocated, but then the health department decided there was a problem with some language in the original law that would have to be fixed to allow sharing information with CDC. That amendment was passed in 2011. By the time the state finally issued its first report in 2013, the federal Hospital Compare website had beat them to it, publishing Texas hospital reports in the first national posting of infection information. Texas is a good illustration of the tenacity required by consumer advocates to get these laws passed and implemented.

THE EXPERTS TAKE NOTE

We began drawing the attention of frontline infection control professionals. On the national level, they were not always as stridently opposed to our efforts as hospitals but were not proactively advocating for reporting either. While fending off local opposition by the epidemiology community (most of whom worked for hospitals) in most states, one national organization representing these professionals reached out to us.

In 2004, national APIC staff approached CU to work as allies in support of public reporting. The national organization realized that public reporting offered an opportunity to improve the work environment for infection control professionals (now called infection preventionists) and raise the status of this problem so hospitals might provide the resources desperately needed for infection control. CU was invited to speak at the 2005 APIC convention in Atlanta, where the general audience of state-based professionals was less than friendly, but there were some who saw the benefits of reporting. CU maintains an ongoing collaborative relationship with APIC. That audience was a breeze compared to the hundreds of openly hostile physician epidemiologists who confronted me when I spoke of the need for public reporting at the 2005 SHEA convention in Los Angeles. They were not happy with the hornets' nest we had stirred up. In 2006, SHEA, the Infectious Diseases Society of America (IDSA), and APIC put out their model bill that closely followed our consumer initiative.[33]

Early in our campaign, CDC staff contacted us to discuss what we were doing and informally provided us with some guidance on the wording of our model bill. CU staff started to regularly attend meetings of the CDC's national infection advisory committee, known as the Healthcare Infection Control Practices Advisory Committee (HICPAC),[34] with an eye toward getting the agency's support for public reporting. After all, CDC was the federal agency with responsibility to monitor, control, and prevent infections, and these committee members were national experts, so surely they would be interested in an effort to identify where these infections were happening. But there certainly didn't seem to be much urgency around a problem that, according to them at the time, affected two million people and killed nearly 100,000 every year.[35]

Following legislative debates in their states, HICPAC members from California and Pennsylvania proposed that the committee issue an official "guidance" to state legislatures regarding the best way to publish infection rates. Most of the HICPAC members thought they should simply tell legislators it was a bad idea but were finally convinced that the issue was not going away. CU advised the committee that our Stop Hospital Infection campaign was just picking up steam, and others pointed to the explosion of bills supporting this popular idea. In February 2005,[36] the committee reluctantly drafted the guidance to the states on public reporting.[37] CDC sought CU's input regarding the best way to word the guidance for legislators. Having this official document in hand improved our ability to pass legislation. However, the guidance carefully included a statement of ambivalence on the part of the agency and committee:

> Advocates of mandatory public reporting of HAIs believe that making such information publicly available will enable consumers to make more informed choices about their health care and improve overall health care quality by reducing HAIs. Further, they believe that patients have a right to know this information. However, others have expressed concern that the reliability of public reporting systems may be compromised by institutional variability in the definitions used for HAIs, or in the methods and resources used to identify HAIs. Presently, there is insufficient evidence on the merits and limitations of an HAI public reporting system. Therefore, the Healthcare Infection Control Practices Advisory Committee (HICPAC) has not recommended for or against mandatory public reporting of HAI rates.[38]

As we were advocating for these new laws, we often encountered similar arguments against public reporting from experts: there was no evidence that public reporting prevented infections, so, as scientists, they could not endorse the idea. For consumer advocates, it seemed like an obvious first step—how can you possibly *know* that infection rates are declining if you are not documenting infections? And we were incredulous that they didn't agree that awareness of which hospitals had the biggest problems was a necessary step toward preventing infections from happening. To us, it was a no-brainer. To them, it was unscientific.

CDC finally publicly embraced disclosure of infection rates in 2010,[39] to coincide with the first release of hospital ratings on infections by *Consumer Reports*.[40] Staff from the two entities had conferred frequently as *Consumer Reports* developed these ratings. At last, CDC concluded that it was "scientific": ". . . public reporting of healthcare-associated infections (HAIs) is an important component of national HAI elimination efforts. Research shows that when healthcare facilities are aware of their infection issues and implement concrete strategies to prevent them, rates of certain hospital infections can be decreased by more than 70 percent." Since then, the agency has become an active supporter of public disclosure.

In 2007, the National Quality Forum (NQF)[41] established a committee to endorse hospital-acquired infection measures for public reporting and quality assessment purposes. CU staff represented consumers on the committee. It proved to be an eye-opener as to how far we still had to go. There was active resistance by providers who made up a majority on the committee and subcommittees. Few of these members supported the concept of publicly reporting infection rates, and their discussions revealed weaknesses in hospital infection surveillance. For example, discussions revealed that few hospitals tracked catheter-associated urinary tract infections (CAUTIs), one of the most common types of hospital-acquired infections, and most had no systematic methods to track which patients had urinary catheters in place. One physician relayed that in order to do a study on CAUTIs, she had to literally go from bed to bed and lift the sheets to determine how many patients were even catheterized, much less infected. This was a shocking validation of our assessment of hospitals' "don't ask, don't tell" mentality, since the primary way to prevent CAUTIs is to avoid using catheters in the first place or remove them ASAP. In the end, the committee endorsed measures that were already being reported by twenty states. It seemed at the time a wasted opportunity to push beyond what was already being done, but in the long run it broke through some long-standing resistance and eased the way for the Centers for Medicare and Medicaid Services (CMS) to later require hospitals to report these infection measures in exchange for payment incentives. When CMS put CAUTIs on their hospital-acquired conditions list[42] —preventable harmful events for which CMS stopped paying hospitals—hospitals had to quickly develop strategies for tracking which patients had urinary catheters.[43]

Key to implementation of state laws was the evolution of CDC's NHSN, a secure, Internet-based surveillance system through which hospitals can report infections. It replaced an outdated system that for thirty years had been collecting infection data from 300 hospitals that voluntarily participated.[44] This upgrade coincided with CU passing infection-reporting laws across the country. It provided states with strapped budgets the tools they needed to comply with the new laws. NHSN was available at no cost to the states, but the real task was convincing local infection control professionals that it would work for them. With state laws mandating hospital participation, CDC saw the opportunity to expand its ability to tap into more comprehensive data about infections. CDC staff spent countless hours speaking to state advisory committees and assisting state health departments with training staff in thousands of hospitals on identification of infections. CDC held regular meetings with state health departments that provided feedback on how to improve NHSN. By the time CMS proposed to link a Medicare payment program to infection reporting, NHSN was the national standard for reporting, and the transition was fairly easy—at least for hospitals in those states that had passed legislation.

At a 2008 congressional hearing Don Wright, in a new administrator position at US Health and Human Services (HHS), was raked over the coals about the federal agency's lack of response to hospital-acquired infections. CU activist Ed Lawton testified about his devastating encounter with multiple deadly hospital infections that left him unable to stand, walk, or engage in other normal activities.[45] A US General Accounting Office (GAO) report[46] released a month earlier was presented to the committee, calling on HHS to prioritize the problem of hospital infections and improve coordination among federal agencies to assess the problem and prevention strategies. Later the GAO published an overview of state initiatives on infections.[47] The GAO interviewed CU staff for these reports.

In response, Wright initiated the development of a national action plan to eliminate infections. CU and activists in our network attended meetings on the plan's development and every annual gathering to assess progress. Throughout the process, in an effort to increase consumer input, HHS staff reached out to CU to recruit advocates. It was crucial to have consumers in the room pushing for more reporting, because the other participants were often complaining about having to report on the few types of infections that were required or were busy praising each other for how much they were doing to prevent infections. Meanwhile, millions of patients continued to be infected each year. New York activist Mary Brennan Taylor was a featured speaker at several HHS meetings, where she presented an articulate timeline of all that went wrong with her mother's care that led to her death. There was progress, but not enough.

In 2009 CDC finally updated their estimate of the annual cost of hospital-acquired infections from $6 billion to $45 billion,[48] an astounding increase that only included the cost of hospital-related care. To this day, there are no good estimates of the other costs that infected patients incur for services like medications, wound care, doctor visits, and physical therapy. That same year, the federal government provided a measly $40 million in American Recovery and Reinvestment Act (ARRA)[49] grants to be distributed to states that applied for funding of local action plans. Even so, this modest funding helped many states hire staff at health departments to run their infection programs and to validate what hospitals were reporting. Consumer advocates had identified validation as a great concern because we knew infections were being underreported. Our model bill required the states to ensure accuracy of the data, and we felt it should be a key component to every state program. In the end, ARRA funds used for validation served the dual purpose of training hospital staff on how to do basic surveillance—something hospitals should have already been doing.

PATIENT STORIES MAKE IT REAL

Consumers Union's entry into the patient safety arena as a strong, recognizable national voice of consumers and patients added the critical element of public "buzz" needed to jolt a passive health care system into action. Media on the national, state, and local levels covered our work and the legislative activity in nearly every state. We knew that the media was key to getting the word out about the devastating infection statistics. It provided added pressure on hospitals and elected officials considering legislation. The campaign was featured in hundreds of news stories around the country and connected journalists with hundreds of patients and family members to interview about the devastation of hospital infections. Putting a human face on these statistics was instrumental to our media strategy, led by CU's Michael McCauley. McCauley strategically sent out news releases and op-eds in the states to bolster the work of legislative sponsors and CU. He built a national list of reporters covering hospital infection issues and sent them media alerts whenever bills were moving or something was happening in their state. Several times a year he sent national updates so they could see that their states were part of a national movement to end secrecy around hospital infections.

We began collecting stories as soon as we launched our campaign, and by the time Daniela Nuñez joined our campaign staff in 2008, we had thousands of them. For the first years of the campaign, Suzanne Henry had been a jack-of-all-trades, including developing patient stories. With Daniela on board we had someone whose primary job was to gather patients' infection stories, match them up with reporters looking to write about infections, and cultivate relationships with those who wanted to become full-blown activists. She also brought strong social media skills to the campaign, giving us a constant online presence. By tweeting regularly about patient safety issues from the consumer perspective she expanded the number of people who follow our work. At this writing, CU's patient safety campaign has collected over 6,000 stories from across the United States—a good portion of them are infection stories, but they also include experiences with other types of medical harm.

In 2009, the Stop Hospital Infections campaign became the Safe Patient Project (SPP), expanding our work to include medical errors, doctor account-ability, and medical device safety. Through outreach, media, social network-ing, and mining of stories patients shared with the campaign, SPP's thriving network of advocates continued to grow and serve as a vital hub for the patient safety movement. We first began to work with those activists who were harmed or had family members who were harmed by preventable medi-cal errors as victims of the system. But over time, they became empowered consumer advocates and experts on patient safety. Many now serve as consu-mer members on state and federal advisory committees and are invited to speak before medical societies, medical schools, and patient safety groups. Some have established local nonprofit organizations that work year-round on patient safety issues. SPP provides technical support and networking tools, such as a listserv, and opportunities for working together, multiplying their impact and ours. Once a year, we bring these activists together to strategize on future collaborations and strengthen relationships.

A CHANGING TIDE

Attitudes toward infection reporting have changed over the years at the CDC and other federal agencies, often due to the commitment of numerous federal employees to fully engage consumers in efforts to eliminate infections. At CDC, positive change happened when Abbigail Tumpey was hired as the communications director for the division doing infection-related work. She organized regular conference calls with consumer advocates to advise and seek their input concerning "hot" issues and upcoming reports—similar to calls that had been going on for years with hospitals, epidemiologists, and infection control professionals. CDC hosted two "consumer days" where consumer advocates met with CDC scientists at their Atlanta headquarters. CU and individual activists have developed working relationships with CDC experts, collaborating on various projects. In 2008 CU was invited to serve as the first consumer liaison to the CDC HICPAC committee,[50] giving us a regular platform to raise issues important to patients.

The landscape has changed dramatically in the past ten years. While we were building an army of grassroots activists, other organizations became active, and new government programs made infections a bit more difficult for hospitals to ignore. The Surgical Care Improvement Project (SCIP)[51] was an early effort to systematically educate hospitals about best practices to prevent infections and to document and track their use by hospitals. In 2002 participation was low until reporting was connected to an annual 2 percent inflation increase in Medicare payments in 2006; then participation shot up immediately. By 2009, on average, hospitals were using these best practices close to 100 percent of the time. In 2005, the Institute for Healthcare Improvement (IHI) launched a campaign[52] that guided hospitals to adopt evidence-based protocols for preventing errors and infections and other similar efforts followed at IHI and other organizations. Also, the 2010 Accountable Care Act created financial incentives for hospitals to reduce infections—this is anticipated for FY 2015.[53]

After ten years, it is clear that a three-part strategy is important: accountability through public disclosure, training and education at the hospital level, and getting hospital leadership's attention by tying money to safety measures.

The sheer scope of the hospital-acquired infection problem demands urgent action, but that is clearly not what is happening—722,000 hospital-acquired infections occur each year, causing 75,000 deaths according to CDC's most recent estimates.[54] The numbers alone should have sounded alarms years ago—but for some reason, this national problem has not risen to the level of urgency that its statistics should demand. Researchers' estimates are fairly consistent, reflecting a huge problem. One in five patients is infected while in the hospital getting treatment for something else. But often reporters and others become fixated on why the numbers don't add up or whether all infections have been captured. A CU activist from Texas, John James, put it nicely in his 2013 estimate of the number of people who die from preventable medical errors, including infections:[55]

> There was much debate after the IOM report about the accuracy of its estimates. In a sense, it does not matter whether the deaths of 100,000, 200,000 or 400,000 Americans each year are associated with PAEs [preventable adverse events] in hospitals. Any of the estimates demands assertive action on the part of providers, legislators, and people who will one day become patients. Yet, the action and progress on patient safety is frustratingly slow; however, one must hope that the present, evidence-based estimate of 400,000+ deaths per year will foster an outcry for overdue changes and increased vigilance in medical care to address the problem of harm to patients who come to a hospital seeking only to be healed.

We have the knowledge and the research that tells us what needs to be done to prevent infections. We have the momentum. But those of us in the thick of it often wonder if the momentum is strong enough to sustain work that needs to be done over the long haul. The business of preventing infections never ends—it requires constant vigilance. The stories continue to come in from infected patients, hospitals continue to resist accounting for more of the harm they cause, improvements are still lacking. Consumers, the public, must sustain our outrage to keep hospitals from turning their attention away from preventing infections for some future demand. Every day hospitals make decisions on how to spend their money. They too often fail to prioritize the things that keep patients safe. More nurses, more infection-control monitoring, and more education are needed.

We are clearly on a path of slow progress. It is evident in many state reports, each year demonstrating decreases on specific infection measures, and in the latest national infection prevalence report showing a 1 percent decline. However, reporting is still quite limited, and widespread validation of what the hospitals report still doesn't exist. Many remain skeptical that hospitals are reporting all of the infections they cause, so it is difficult to assess whether significant change has happened. In the beginning, some told us we should change the name of our Stop Hospital Infections campaign because infections simply could not be completely stopped. But we believe that is the wrong emphasis in light of the huge numbers of patients being infected. If hospitals don't hold zero as the goal, they have an excuse to stop trying to prevent every infection. Today many hospitals, nurses, and doctors are aiming for zero—and that alone is progress. These tragic deaths and injuries are a disgrace to our country, and their elimination should be a national priority.

IN CONCLUSION—LESSONS LEARNED FOR AN EFFECTIVE CAMPAIGN

- Create a model law. This can be drafted from scratch, a copy of an existing law, or a combination of sections from multiple existing laws. It helps to have some components of related existing laws to counter skepticism.
- Identify passionate, committed people living in the targeted state and enlist them as full partners. Regular people with compelling stories can have a strong influence with state legislators and can help to keep tabs on bills as they are moving through the process.
- Be persistent and expect pushback from entrenched parties who benefit from the status quo.
- Identify key legislators. Sometimes these will be legislators who are knowledgeable on health issues, but legislators who "get it" because of

some personal experience or association with someone with a personal experience are often the best advocates on an issue. Whomever you work with, work to become a resource to them—if you don't know the answers to their questions when asked, find them and follow up with the legislator with the information.

- Identify ally organizations and ask them to endorse the model law. Even if health care providers are opposed to what you are trying, maintain a working relationship with them. Don't give up, but don't burn bridges; at some point you may have to negotiate with them.
- Mount a public awareness campaign through the media. This can include very effective social media blitzes. Develop relationships with reporters who cover the particular issue.
- Follow up to ensure that the law is implemented once it passes.

Chapter Ten

Medical Guidelines and Informed Consent—Routes to Safer Medical Care

Denise Lasater, DBA, RN; Cheryl Brown, DBA, RN; and John T. James, PhD

WHY DO MEDICAL GUIDELINES AND INFORMED CONSENT MATTER?

Medicine, like most other institutions, is not only changing at a rapid rate but is being challenged on every level. Long recognized as a subtle admixture of science and art, medicine has moved notably in the direction of a science as new tools and techniques have been developed to help practitioners of "the healing" understand better what works in the treatment of patients; plus this dramatic expansion of medical knowledge (and technology), and of the ways by which medical knowledge is advanced, is changing the face of medical practice.[1] Practicing an acceptable standard of care is an expectation of every patient when they enter into a medical environment.

American medicine has long sought to control the standard of care that physicians are expected to provide to their patients; so, one effort to insulate the standard of care from external interference, called a "safe harbors" approach, would enable physicians to avoid liability for malpractice if they adhered to medical practice guidelines.[2] The idea is to eliminate the "battle of experts" and reduce defensive medicine by requiring judges and juries to accept guidelines as conclusive evidence of the standard of care; current efforts to improve the guideline development process, including the use of evidence-based guidelines, are unlikely to be able to overcome the shortcomings that led safe harbors initiatives to fail in the early 1990s.[3]

Patients find more satisfaction and better outcomes in the delivery of health care when their providers use evidence-based practices that apply

155

medical guidelines based on research findings to deliver safe, patient-centered, and collaborative health care. To remain abreast of the latest medical knowledge in a specialty, a provider, left without the help of medical guidelines, would have to review research and practice recommendations for more than seventeen hours a day to be able to apply the latest findings to his clinical practice.[4] This is not going to happen when clinicians and other health care practitioners spend more than eight hours a day providing health care to patients.

Medical guidelines, now numbering about 2,500, are formulated by expert groups to guide clinicians in the practice of medicine with a goal of optimizing outcomes for each patient. In other words, guidelines are intended to foster evidence-driven use of medical services, reduce the overuse of unnecessary medical services, and increase utilization of necessary medical services. The goal is to provide safe and affordable care to all patients. It has not turned out that way.

Doctors are frustratingly slow to adopt clinical practices consistent with evidence-based guidelines, especially if adoption of those guidelines may reduce the need for their services. To confound matters, some guidelines were written by "experts" with potential bias and were not thoroughly peer-reviewed by outside experts. The Institute of Medicine (IOM), the medical branch of the US National Academy of Sciences, assembled an expert committee and published a book outlining ways to improve the trustworthiness of clinical practice guidelines. In 2006 the IOM declared that by 2020 clinical decisions should be supported by accurate, timely, and current clinical information 90 percent of the time, reflecting the best evidence available to optimize outcomes for patients.[5] Poor-quality care harms patients and increases medical care costs. The Centers for Disease Control and Prevention ranks preventable harm as the third leading cause of patient death and suggests preventable harm to patients costs an estimated $9,000 per household each year.[6]

Involving patients in their own plan of care is essential to grow partnerships between patients and clinicians. Patients who are informed about clinical decision making are more likely to actively participate in their care. Care must be consistent with patients' values, goals, and capabilities. They should expect their doctors to be cognizant of current medical guidelines and inform them when, and for what reason, they intend to deviate from guidelines.[7] Physicians may recommend a deviation from medical guidelines for a specific patient; however, if they make that recommendation, the patient must be fully informed of the rationale for the deviation.

MEDICAL GUIDELINES INCLUDE TRANSPARENT
INFORMED CONSENT

A necessary component of the partnership between provider and patient includes informed consent. The provider is accountable to communicate sufficient information so the patient can make an informed decision about the need for procedures and the potential consequences. The relationship between a provider and patient is based on consent, which requires voluntary agreement for the provider to perform an invasive treatment or procedure on a patient.[8] The provider is ethically and legally obligated to personally explain a procedure and describe potential risks, benefits, and alternatives to the chosen medical recommendation, including doing nothing, so the patient can make an informed decision.[9] An informed and cautious patient will ask many questions and seek a second, *independent* opinion if necessary. A trustworthy clinician will have no hesitation in allowing the patient to seek a second opinion.

What happens when a provider doesn't disclose the risks involved in a medical treatment or procedure? Generally nothing, because the patient does not know she has been denied sufficient information to make an informed decision. However, in a legal case from twenty years ago a surgeon did not divulge all of the risks to the patient. The patient experienced one of the known risks that had not been disclosed to him prior to the surgery. As a result, he acquired a permanent surgical complication. The case was not warranted as malpractice because the surgeon's behavior did not violate standard of care.[10] Lack of informed consent cases are considered hard to win because the burden of proof that the consent was not informed lay with the patient.[11] Thus, it becomes imperative that the patient and provider develop a style of communication based on understanding and *genuine informed* consent.[12] The reliability of evidence-based practice in reducing harm lies on providers sharing information, patients developing partnerships with providers, and providers committing to informed consent.

Providers are often tied to traditional practices that are comfortable for them. This is nowhere more apparent than with the problem of implementing guidelines designed to curtail the overuse of antibiotics in patients with acute respiratory infections. Overuse of antibiotics is a long-term health risk because it potentially fosters an emergence of antibiotic-resistant strains that are difficult to treat and can be highly invasive (discussed in chapter 5). A team of investigators examined whether a simple intervention might foster better compliance with guidelines. Clinicians were asked to display a poster-size correspondence letter with their photograph in each patient examination room. The letter declared their commitment to discontinuing the overprescribing of antibiotics. The posters were likely to generate conversations between clinician and patients about the need for antibiotics. The inappropriate use of antibiotics dropped from 43 percent to 34 percent—not a rousing improvement, but at least a nudge in the right direction.[13] This result had important, high-value implications. It was a challenge to convince clinicians to stop doing something that had become traditional, even in the face of evidence that it caused more harm than good. The challenges of phasing out or rejecting low-value care are much greater than the challenges of adopting new, high-value care. This imbalance in adopting change includes loss of income from an abandoned procedure, entrenched beliefs about the value of the procedure that should be abandoned, and a biased view of risks and benefits from procedures in general.[14] It seems that providing no or diminished payment for low-value services would quickly overcome these psychological biases. The informed patient must ask how a proposed procedure will affect their care.

Sometimes clinicians omit information that seems trivial to them but will be very important to the patient. A young woman was about to start a teaching internship in the fall and had decided to have Lasik procedure on her eyes in the summer before her internship. Her ophthalmologist failed to tell her that after the procedure she would have to put eyedrops in her eyes every ten minutes for one month while she was awake. Not knowing this, and given other activities of the summer, she decided to have the procedure performed a few days before her internship started. She was livid when she learned, immediately *after* the procedure, that as she tried to teach fifth-graders and was being evaluated by her mentors, she was going to have to pause every ten minutes to put in eyedrops.

Another scenario that plays out far too many times in health care began with a surgical team that often functioned together with their favorite surgeon performing non-urgent gallbladder removals. Prior to a surgical procedure, a count of instruments, sponges, needles, and sharps is required; however, this particular team had become confident in their skills and chose to use their judgment to routinely *not* count surgical items prior to surgery. So all goes well for years, and then the day comes when they must open the patient in order to respond to complicating surgical events. Beyond anyone's imagination, the instrument room technician miscounted the small clamps used to stop bleeding. When the surgery converted to an open operation, everyone *assumed* they knew what to expect for the final count. This was habitual risky behavior. The error compounded when the staff told the surgeon that the postoperative count was correct.

How does this end? The patient had multiple postoperative complications that resulted in additional care and extended the patient's hospital stay. The surgeon ordered an X-ray within hours after the surgery due to the unexpected patient responses during the recovery period. There was the problem: a four-inch-long clamp! The patient returned to surgery. The clamp was removed. The patient filed a lawsuit and won a monetary settlement. The surgeon was reported to the National Practitioner Data Bank (discussed in chapter 2). This harm could have been prevented. The staff knew they were habitually ignoring the standards and did not hold each other accountable. Unintended, retained foreign objects after surgery account for increased medical and liability costs in 95 percent of the reported occurrences.[15]

BARRIERS TO THE USE OF MEDICAL GUIDELINES AND INFORMED CONSENT

In 1999, leaders of the IOM focused on patient safety.[16] The landmark report *To Err Is Human* claimed that up to 98,000 lives were lost each year due to medical errors in hospitals, costing $29 billion annually. The IOM's estimate was based on data taken from medical records of patient care in New York State in 1984, a year in which evidence-based guidelines were in their infancy. Research following the release of the IOM report of 1999, a blueprint for quality improvement, has examined the importance and scope of adverse events. However, a study published in 2013, based on a more thorough analysis of medical errors, including errors of omission due to failure to follow guidelines, resulted in an estimate of 440,000 premature deaths as a result of hospital-associated infections and medical errors in hospitals.[17]

Researchers looked into the recurring theme of poor communication among providers and between providers and patients.[18] This pattern of poor communication was detrimental to quality care, informed consent, and risk management. In 2012 another group of researchers found that fifty-seven private health care facilities and thirty-four academic centers had delayed diagnoses and treatments, resulting from an organizational culture that tolerated a lack of documentation on admission assessments and diminished compliance with national standards of care.[19] How can these patterns that create risk to the patient be mitigated? Wise patients and their advocates will ensure that providers are listening to them and communicating well with each other.

PATIENTS AND PROVIDERS PARTNER

Hospitals must share information with other hospitals and continuously improve ways to share it.[20] Another point is that patients' experiences must be systematically solicited. This means hospitals can identify instances where patients have experienced adverse events (things that did not go as well as expected) and the patients can disclose whether they were given sufficient information to make informed decisions about their care. Obviously, if the patient is rendered unstable or dead, then the patient's advocate must serve this role.[21]

An example of conflicting priorities between patient and provider is as follows. A twenty-nine-year-old woman is delighted to be experiencing her first pregnancy but finds disappointment in the lackluster approach her respected obstetrician is taking. She repeatedly tries to engage her provider in developing a birth plan only to hear words of discouragement, delay, and dismissal. The well-educated woman has read much on the standard of care for delivery for those who are having their first baby. All the indicators point to allowing nature to take its course with vaginal delivery, the desired clinical path as long as the mother and baby are doing well. However, the obstetrician continues to advocate for induction or cesarean delivery. The expectant mother has read advice presented by the American Congress of Obstetricians and Gynecologists.[22] As a professional society, the stated goal for obstetricians managing a pregnant and laboring woman is to be patient-centered and optimize safety for mother and baby. This means allowing a vaginal delivery. So if the goal of the provider is to give kindness, acceptance, and respect to the maternal experience, why does the provider continue to promote induction or scheduled cesarean section? The truth is he had a vacation planned at the time of her due date.

RECOMMENDATIONS TO PATIENTS

Application of medical guidelines and *transparent* informed consent reside at the core of patient-centered medical care. Care that fails to follow guidelines without informing the patient (or their advocate) of the need to deviate from guidelines is not giving the patient sufficient information to give their informed consent to the provider. Patients must be aware of the following:

- Medical guidelines exist for diagnosis and treatment of most conditions. Ask your clinician which guideline he is following for your care.
- If your doctor says that your care needs to deviate from guidelines, ask questions until you understand if this means you will be at greater risk for an adverse outcome.
- Recent guidelines factor in patient preferences (e.g., serious aversion to any surgery); therefore, you should be certain that your doctor understands your preferences.
- Never let yourself be intimidated by the informed-consent forms that you will be presented with as a hospital patient.
- Know the basics of informed consent and document whether each of these has been addressed for you before you give any consent.

One of the great challenges facing patients and their advocates is remaining cautious, yet empowered, in the complex and busy environment characteristic of most hospitals. Each must ask questions until they understand every step and reason for treatment and what to expect as an outcome.

Chapter Eleven

Medical Imaging: Does It Help?

Kiran Sagar, MD, FAHA, FACC

INTRODUCTION

We live in the age of rapidly evolving technology. We rarely find a person without a cell phone that is able to display images. Facebook and Twitter are integral parts of our life, especially within the younger generation. In clinical medicine we use imaging procedures such as computed axial tomography (CAT)[1] and magnetic resonance imaging (MRI)[2] to diagnose diseases, which would have required high-risk, invasive testing twenty years ago. A good example is detection of brain or spinal cord tumors. In past decades, we would have used air encephalogram and myelography (X-ray visualization of structures after injection of air and a dye). We would have to inject air and a dye to delineate the masses—a somewhat risky process. Patients would suffer from severe headache and neck stiffness and would have to be hospitalized. Without these tests we would likely miss the diagnosis.

I know about missed diagnoses from personal experience. In 1994 my husband was diagnosed with a spinal cord tumor at age fifty. The tumor had been growing slowly. Doctors had mistakenly attributed his symptoms of ten years to vertebral disc disease. Had an MRI been done years earlier, paralysis of his legs could have been prevented. He was left with weakness, rigidity of legs, numbness, pain in his lower body, and inadequate control of bladder and bowel function. He loved to hike and ski, but now he can barely walk. I would have loved to have had the fictitious tricorder from the television series *Star Trek: The Next Generation*. The tricorder diagnosed a disease at macro- and microcellular level.

I am the first to admit that there are cracks in the clinical application of current imaging procedures for diagnosis of diseases. Inappropriate use of imaging, lack of quality control of imaging sites, substandard training of physicians that read the images, and overuse of procedures as cash cows for doctors and hospitals often undermine the inherent value of imaging. In the ensuing chapter I will highlight problems associated with medical imaging and suggest guidelines for patients, doctors, and professional societies. Together we may be able to cut costs and improve the quality of medical imaging.

A LOSS OF CRITICAL THINKING

We doctors have given up critical thinking or forming differential diagnoses based on the history and physical examination of a patient. In the past we ordered tests after forming a provisional clinical diagnosis. These days we order tests before taking a thorough history or comprehensively examining a patient. Then we fit the diagnosis to the test results, seldom using patient history and physical examination as a basis for diagnosis. Virtually all patients coming to the emergency room with chest pain, irrespective of their risk factors or quality of pain, undergo a battery of tests such as imaging stress testing, echocardiogram, and in some emergency rooms, a cardiac CAT coronary angiogram. A young menstruating woman without risk factors for coronary artery disease does not require these tests. A middle-aged man with chest pain, diabetes mellitus, history of smoking, and increased blood cholesterol should have an imaging stress test,[3] as he is likely to have coronary artery disease.

ACCURACY OF IMAGING

In clinical medicine there is no iron-clad, bright line between normal and abnormal test results. Typically the "normal" band of a numerical test will include 95 percent of results of a given population with the remaining, extreme 5 percent deemed "abnormal." A good test may be normal in people with disease (false negative) and be positive in people without disease (false positive). False positive tests, such as often occur in mammography screening for breast cancer, have consequences. They may lead to further tests, painful biopsies, more MRIs, increased costs, and even erroneous attempts at surgery when no abnormalities exist. Screening tests yield best results when there is a reasonable likelihood of disease. A screening test such as mammography is best when applied to people who are at high risk of disease. Bleyer and Welch reported that screening mammography only marginally reduced the rate at which women presented with advanced breast cancer.[4] They also noted that there was a sustained overdiagnosing of breast cancer. Their observations resulted in an argument regarding benefits of a routine screening mammography in relationship to new guidelines for mammography screening. Experts modeled the costs associated with following the guidelines, which specify biennial screening of women from fifty to seventy-four unless the woman is at higher risk of breast cancer, or continuing to screen women annually from the ages of forty to eighty-four. Assuming that 85 percent of eligible women seek screening, they estimated that following the guidelines rather than following current practices would save about $7.6 billion each year.[5] Similar studies raised questions about routine MRI in patients with low back pain.[6] MRI of the spine should be done if back pain is associated with neurological deficit. This applies to diagnosis of ovarian cancer and use of ultrasound.[7]

Transvaginal ultrasound is an imaging technique sometimes used to screen for ovarian cancer; however, this and other screening tests for ovarian cancer are not recommended for women without symptoms possibly associated with this cancer. What makes this cancer worrisome is that its five-year survival rate is only 25 percent, but it is also a rare cancer. Unnecessary surgeries, resulting in removal of normal ovaries after this screening, are common when the screening yields what turns out to be a false positive.[8]

Perceived risks of being sued cause defensive medical practice by doctors. They order more tests, many of them imaging tests, to protect themselves from accusations of negligence. Defensive medicine increases health care costs without improving health outcomes, although the added costs of defensive medicine is not large compared to the other wastes. For example, curtailing malpractice awards and gains from not doing defensive medicine was estimated to save about $11 billion annually, whereas a substantial reduction in insurance company profits would save $12 billion, eliminating inpatient harms would save $13 billion, and reducing avoidable outpatient complications by 50 percent would save $200 billion.[9]

MAKING MONEY AND MAINTAINING SKILLS

Many patients find that their doctor has ordered a variety of tests, but they do not have a clue as to why. Patients must ask, "Are these tests necessary to diagnose or monitor my condition?" Sometimes they are ordered for financial gain for doctors and hospitals as opposed to defensive medicine purposes.[10] There are two ways money affects the number of tests ordered. First, doctors are often paid according to revenues generated. The more money they bring in, the better their compensation. Reimbursement of imaging and its interpretation is significantly higher than that of seeing a patient. More and more doctors are performing imaging procedures in their offices. These days imaging stress tests, echocardiograms, CAT, and MRI are often performed in physician offices. Patients generally do not directly pay for tests nor understand the need. They are afraid to question the doctor, so they comply. As more doctors, many unqualified to read images, perform more imaging procedures, costs go up and the quality of test results goes down.

Many factors can affect the quality of imaging results: quality of equipment, training of technicians, frequency of procedures performed, and physician training and experience. Office-based imaging is usually inferior to that performed in large, dedicated imaging centers. There are no regulations for equipment or image quality. Federal guidelines require a physician to read 480 mammograms per year (two or three per week). Several years ago a radiologist at Kaiser Permanente pored over doctors' records of mammography reports, decided to keep score of missed cancers, and printed their data in bar/pie graphs. He discovered that nearly half of the physicians reading mammograms did not meet federal qualifications. In contrast to dedicated experts who read 1,400 mammograms per year, these physicians read fewer than 480 per year.[11] It seemed that reading more than 480 mammograms per year was not sufficient to ensure optimal quality of the readings. Smith-Bindman and her colleagues[12] asked what the rate of false-positive readings was when physicians read 481 to 750 screening mammograms per year compared to the false-positive rate of those reading 2,500 to 4,000 screening mammograms per year. The physicians in the high-reading group had 50 percent fewer false positives than those in the moderate-reading group (481 to 750).

Similar problems are present in other specialties. In most community hospitals all cardiologists perform and interpret echocardiograms, both transthoracic (TTE) and transesophageal (TEE). These doctors often do not have appropriate training and read fewer echocardiograms than a dedicated echocardiographer. In 2009, Thompson and colleagues reported an error rate of 29 percent in interpretation of TTEs and TEEs in a community hospital.[13] Here are two examples of the types of errors and their consequences. First was a forty-four-year-old, morbidly obese woman who was sent to surgery for a double heart valve replacement. The diagnosis of two leaky valves had been made from TTE and TEE performed and interpreted by her cardiologist. She was in the operating room, intubated and anesthetized. The surgeon requested preoperative TEE before opening the woman's chest. Pre- and intraoperative TEEs are routinely performed to monitor the progress of valve surgery. The cardiologist performing the TTE was a specialist in echocardiography and did not find evidence of leaky valves requiring surgery. She discovered that the patient had hypertrophic cardiomyopathy (enlargement of heart muscles), which did not need surgery. Anesthesia was reversed and the patient was extubated and sent home that evening. A second patient who was a victim of misread images was taken to the operating room for repair of an acute aortic dissection, diagnosed with TEE by the patient's general cardiologist. The surgeon opened the chest and did not find any abnormality of the aorta. He closed the chest without performing any intervention. I was asked to review the patient's TTE and TEE the next morning. The physician originally reading the patient's TEE had mistaken an artifact for aortic dissection. In both cases of misread images the physicians lacked training and experience.

TOWARD SAFER IMAGING

Professional societies should develop and enforce training/quality guidelines based on evidence that specific guidelines lead to better outcomes and that wasteful imaging is not practiced. The insurance companies and the government (Medicare and Medicaid) could base reimbursement on whether the physician has adequate training. Freestanding, for-profit imaging centers frequently send flyers to our homes advertising inexpensive screening for carotid artery disease, abdominal aortic aneurysm, and calcium scores for heart disease. The patient must keep in mind that to date there are no data showing that screening of asymptomatic people is beneficial.

What can be done to improve quality and accuracy and cut down the overuse of medical imaging? Collaborative efforts between patients, physicians, and professional-medical societies are needed. The General Accounting Office of the Department of Health and Human Services proposed that the Centers for Medicare and Medicaid Services establish minimum standards for diagnostic imaging centers.[14] To reduce waste nine professional societies were asked to propose five potentially wasteful tests in their medical discipline. Of the forty-five tests put forth, twenty-four of them were imaging tests.[15] Patients should be educated and should learn to ask questions about the necessity of an imaging test and how it will change their therapy. Sometimes a watch-and-wait attitude makes more sense than extra tests. At times one needs to say no. A simple "no" may save your life.[16]

Physicians must take an active role to reduce misuse of imaging procedures. A critical thought process should be developed to form a clinical diagnosis before ordering multiple and maybe unnecessary tests. There should be no fear involved in asking a colleague what she or he thinks about interpretation of an image. Only experts in the field should be allowed to interpret imaging studies. Experts must continually hone their skills through collaboration and feedback on the outcomes of images they have interpreted. Challenging images must at times be shared among experts to improve interpretations. Financial incentives should not be part of a perverse incentive for unnecessary imaging.

A recent collaborative study by Swedish and New York City researchers proposed an easy approach to curb inappropriate imaging: "a gentle shaming" of doctors who do not follow guidelines. The researchers determined that gentle shaming reduced rates of imaging among Swedish men with a low risk of prostate cancer from 43 percent to 3 percent. [17] Patients must not count on their physicians to give them all the information they need when being screened with an MRI for either prostate cancer or breast cancer. A study of more than three hundred men and women between the ages of fifty and sixty-nine found that only thirty of the patients reported that their physician informed them of the potential harm from overdiagnosis and overtreatment. Indeed, one study found that the majority of doctors involved in screening cannot provide a correct estimate of potential harm in prostate and breast cancer screening. [18]

CONCLUSIONS

Medical imaging provides an early diagnosis often alleviating the need for invasive procedures while early diagnosis often allows for a second opinion if an invasive procedure is necessary. The wise patient will ask about the alternatives to invasive testing, to include a "watchful waiting" approach. A cautious patient will ask about the credentials of the physician reading the images and the pedigree of the instrumentation used to create the images. It's also a good idea to ask about the accreditation status of an imaging center. Properly obtained and read images can save your life, but misread images may subject you to substantial harm from invasive procedures. Do not expect regulatory agencies to protect you. They won't.

Epilogue

We brought together a group of people that had stories to tell and insights to share. Our reserved passion poured into these pages, stemming from first-hand experiences and a sense that the time for a new beginning is at hand. Costs are out of control; too many caregivers are burned out; access to care is unjustly distributed; and too many patients have needlessly suffered and died.

We recall words spoken by Abraham Lincoln 150 years ago: "that we here highly resolve that these dead shall not have died in vain; that this nation shall have a new birth of freedom, and that government of the people, by the people, for the people, shall not perish from the earth."

We desire that anyone seeking health care can trust the system and their caregivers, but we acknowledge that they must be careful, because the checks and balances that would otherwise protect patients fail too often. Our governments, both state and national, have for far too long listened to the message of profit-driven special interests. It is time for the voice of the people to be heard and action to be taken, lest we perish as a nation of free people. As Dr. Martin Luther King Jr. observed, "Injustice anywhere is a threat to justice everywhere."

Notes

INTRODUCTION

1. D. L. Light, J. Lexchin, and J. J. Darrow, "Institutional Corruption of Pharmaceuticals and the Myth of Safe and Effective Drugs," *Journal of Law, Medicine and Ethics* 14 (2013): 590–600, accessed March 22, 2014, http://ssrn.com/abstract=2282014.

2. D. Drake, "How Being a Doctor Became the Most Miserable Profession," *Daily Beast*, accessed April 24, 2014, http://www.thedailybeast.com/articles/2014/04/14/how-being-a-doctor-became-the-most-miserable-profession.html.

3. J. T. James, "A New Evidence-Based Estimate of Patient Harms Associated with Hospital Care," *Journal of Patient Safety* 9 (2013): 122–128.

4. L. Hines, "Retail Clinics Challenging Pediatricians for Business," *Houston Chronicle*, April 13, 2014, D5.

5. "Accountable Care Organizations," Centers for Medicare and Medicaid Services, US Department of Health and Human Services, accessed April 10, 2014, http://www.cms.gov/Medicare/Medicare-Fee-for-Service-Payment/ACO/.

6. "An Accountable Care Organization," Kelsey-Seybold Clinic, accessed April 10, 2014, http://www.kelsey-seybold.com/kelseycare/pages/what-is-an-accountable-care-organization.aspx.

7. Ask.com, "How Many Hospitals Are in the USA? Most Current Hospital Data According to the U.S. Census Bureau," accessed April 24, 2014, http://answers.ask.com/Education/Schools/how_many_hospitals_are_there_in_the_usa?ad=semD&an=google_s&am=broad&o=2731.

8. M. Makary, *Unaccountable: What Hospitals Won't Tell You and How Transparency Can Revolutionize Health Care* (New York: Bloomsbury Press, 2012), 147.

9. R. Healy, "(Non) Profit Hospitals: Charity Pays," 100 Reporters—New Journalism for a New Age, accessed April 14, 2014, http://100r.org/2014/04/nonprofit-hospitals-charity-pays/.

10. K. E. Joynt, E. L. Orav, and A. K. Jha, "Mortality Rates for Medicare Beneficiaries Admitted to Critical Access and Non-Critical Access Hospitals, 2002-2010," *JAMA* 309 (2013): 1379–1387.

11. O. W. Brawley, *How We Do Harm: A Doctor Breaks Ranks about Being Sick in America* (New York: St. Martin's Griffin, 2011), 3–6.

12. "Adverse Events in Skilled Nursing Facilities: National Incidence among Medicare Beneficiaries," Office of Inspector General, accessed April 13, 2013, https://oig.hhs.gov/oei/reports/oei-06-11-00370.pdf.

13. N. Daneman, A. Gruneir, S. E. Bronskill, et al., "Prolonged Antibiotic Treatment in Long-Term Care," *JAMA Internal Medicine* 173 (2013): 673–682.

14. B. A. Briesacher, J. Tjia, T. Field, et al., "Antipsychotic Use among Nursing Home Residents," *JAMA* 309 (2013): 440–442.

15. B. Tonsing, *Stand in the Way: Patient Advocates Speak Out.* (Lulu Publishing Services, Lulu.com, 2014), xi–xiii.

16. V. Combs, "Activist Group Targets J&J and Its Transvaginal Mesh Lawsuits with Social Media Attack," Medcity News, accessed April 14, 2014, http://medcitynews.com/2014/04/activist-group-targets-jj-transvaginal-mesh-social-media-attack/?utm_source=MedCity+News+Subscribers&utm_campaign=2c710c8608-RSS_EMAIL_CAMPAIGN&utm_medium=email&utm_term=0_c05cce483a-2c710c8608-67014761.

17. T. Tamkins, "Medical Bills Prompt More Than 60 Percent of U.S. Bankruptcies," CNN Health, accessed April 14, 2014, http://www.cnn.com/2009/HEALTH/06/05/bankruptcy.medical.bills/.

18. "Problems Paying Medical Bills: Early Release of Estimates From the National Health Interview Survey, January 2011–June 2012," Centers for Disease Control and Prevention, accessed April 14, 2014, http://tinyurl.com/ky27w8q.

19. "Why Intuitive Issued a Recall for da Vinci Surgical System," accessed April 14, 2014, http://www.advisory.com/daily-briefing/2013/12/06/intuitive-says-da-vinci-surgical-system-can-stall-issues-recall.

20. Anonymous, "A Randomized Trial of Propranolol in Patients with Acute Myocardial Infarction: I. Mortality Results," *JAMA* 247 (1982): 1707–1714, accessed April 24, 2014, http://www.ncbi.nlm.nih.gov/pubmed/7038157.

21. T. H. Lee, "Eulogy for a Quality Measure," *New England Journal of Medicine* 357 (2007): 1175–1177.

22. Patient Centered Outcome Research Institute, accessed April 14, 2014, http://www.pcori.org/.

23. Association of American Medical Colleges, accessed April 24, 2014, https://www.aamc.org/newsroom/newsreleases/358410/20131024.html.

24. J. J. Norcini, J. R. Boulet, W. D. Dauphinee, et al., "Evaluating the Quality of Care Provided by Graduates of International Medical Schools," *Health Affairs* 8 (2010): 1461–1468.

25. V. R. Fuchs. "Major Trends in the US Health Economy Since 1950," *New England Journal of Medicine* 366 (2012): 973–977.

26. T. J. Caverly, B. P. Combs, C. Moriates, et al., "Too Much Medicine Happens Too Often," *JAMA Internal Medicine* 174 (2014): 8–9.

27. A. Carroll, "Too Few Generalist Physicians Doesn't Necessarily Mean Too Many Specialists," June 26, 2013, accessed April 24, 2014, http://newsatjama.jama.com/2013/06/26/too-few-generalist-physicians-doesnt-necessarily-mean-too-many-specialists/.

28. S. Kliff, "How Much Does an Appendectomy Cost? Somewhere between $1,529 and $186,955," *Washington Post*, April 24, 2012, accessed April 25, 2014, http://www.washingtonpost.com/blogs/wonkblog/post/how-much-does-an-appendectomy-cost-somewhere-between-1529-and-186955/2012/04/24/gIQAMeKMeT_blog.html.

29. T. R. Reid, *The Healing of America: A Global Quest for Better, Cheaper, and Fairer Health Care* (New York: Penguin Press, 2009), 171.

30. President Clinton: Patient Bill of Rights, February 20, 1998, accessed April 14, 2014, http://archive.ahrq.gov/hcqual/press/pbor.html.

31. J. T. James, *A Sea of Broken Hearts: Patient Rights in a Dangerous, Profit-Driven Health Care System* (Bloomington, IN: Authorhouse, 2007), 143–145.

1. THE FAILURE OF STATE MEDICAL BOARDS TO PROTECT THE PUBLIC

1. L. Brunton, J. Lazo, and Keith Parker, *Goodman & Gilman's The Pharmacological Basis of Therapeutics*, 11th ed. (New York: McGraw-Hill, 2005).

2. Lexi-Corp, Acetazolamide: Drug information, *UpToDate*, 1978–2006.

3. Ibid.

4. R. J. Mason, et al., *Murray and Nadel's Textbook of Respiratory Medicine*, 4th ed. (Philadelphia, PA: Elsevier Saunders, 2005).

5. P. Jones and M. Greenstone, "Carbonic Anhydrase Inhibitors for Hypercapnic Ventilatory Failure in Chronic Obstructive Pulmonary Disease," *Cochrane Database of Systematic Reviews* (2001): doi: 10.1002/14651858.CD002881.

6. D. C. Johnson and H. Kazemi, "Disorders of Ventilatory Control," *UpToDate*, 2007.

7. A. M. Luks and E. R. Swenson, "Medication and Dosage Considerations in the Prophylaxis and Treatment of High-Altitude Illness," *Chest* 133 (2008): 744–755.

8. Thomas Similowski, William Whitelaw, and Jean-Philippe Derenne (eds.), *Clinical Management of Chronic Obstructive Pulmonary Disease, Lung Biology in Health and Disease*, vol. 165 (New York: Marcel Dekker, 2002).

9. C. F. Ameringer, *State Medical Boards and the Politics of Public Protection* (Baltimore, MD: John Hopkins University Press, 1999).

10. R. L. Hollings and Christal Pike-Nase, *Professional and Occupational Licensure in the United States* (Westport, CT: Greenwood Press, 1997).

11. Federation of State Medical Boards, "2009 State of States' Physician Regulation," accessed March 6, 2014, http://www.fsmb.org/pdf/2009_state_of_states.pdf.

12. US Department of Health and Human Services (DHHS), Office of Inspector General, "Federal Initiatives to Improve State Medical Boards' Performance," oei-01-93-00020, February 1993.

13. N. Sawicki, "Character, Competence, and the Principles of Medical Discipline," *Journal of Health Care Law and Policy* 13 (2010): 285–323.

14. US Department of Health and Human Services (DHHS), "State Discipline of Physicians: Assessing State Medical Boards through Case Studies," by Randall R. Bovbjerg, Pablo Aliaga, and Josephine Gittler. Contract #HHS-100-03-0011 (Washington, DC: 2006).

15. Federation of State Medical Boards, "What Is a State Medical Board? Answers to Your Questions about the Role of State Medical Boards in Health Care," accessed March 6, 2014, http://www.fsmb.org/what_is_a_smb.html.

16. Ameringer, 2.

17. R. C. Derbyshire, "How Effective Is Medical Self-Regulation?" *Law and Human Behavior* 7 (1983): 193–202.

18. Ameringer, 3.

19. A. Stein, "Doctors Who Get Away with Killing and Maiming Must Be Stopped," February 2, 1986, accessed April 16, 2014, http://www.nytimes.com/1986/02/02/opinion/doctors-who-get-away-with-killing-and-maiming-must-be-stopped.html .

20. "State Medical Boards' Disciplinary Actions," Public Citizen, accessed March 20, 2014, http://www.citizen.org/statemedicalboardsdisciplinaryactions.

21. National Conference of State Legislatures, "Ensuring the Public Trust 2012, Program Policy Evaluation's Role in Serving State Legislatures," accessed March 11, 2014, http://www.ncsl.org/legislators-staff/legislative-staff/program-evaluation/survey-ensuring-the-public-trust.aspx.

22. US Department of Health and Human Services (DHHS), Office of Inspector General, Office of Analysis and Inspections, *Medical Licensure and Discipline: An Overview*, Control Number: P-01-86-00064 (Boston, MA: 1986).

23. US Department of Health and Human Services (DHHS), Office of Inspector General, *Performance Indicators, Annual Reports, and State Medical Discipline: A State-by-State Review*, oei-01-89-00563, July 1991.

24. US Department of Health and Human Services (DHHS), Office of Inspector General, *Federal Initiatives to Improve State Medical Boards' Performance*, oei-01-93-00020, February 1993.

25. *Seattle Times*, "License to Harm," April 25, 2006, accessed March 20, 2014, http://seattletimes.com/news/local/licensetoharm/index.html.

26. W. Heisel, "State Medical Boards Leave Patients in Danger and in Dark," *Reporting on Health*, December 29, 2010, accessed March 21, 2014, http://www.reportingonhealth.org/node/10331.

27. M. Twohey, "Dr. Ricardo Arze and Sex Abuse Cases Shows Disconnect between Law Enforcement, State Regulators of Doctors," *Chicago Tribune*, July 29, 2010, accessed March 21, 2014, http://www.chicagotribune.com/health/ct-met-doctor-sex-charges-20100729,0,5520049.story.

28. J. Kohler, "Missouri Secretive, Lax on Doctor Discipline," *St. Louis Post-Dispatch*, December 12, 2010, accessed March 21, 2014, http://www.stltoday.com/lifestyles/health-med-fit/fitness/article_5cc342ba-dd6c-5428-b25e-99f8faeca638.html.

29. C. Crowley, "Medical Board Soft on Doctors," *Times Union*, August 20, 2012, accessed March 12, 2014, http://www.timesunion.com/local/article/Medical-board-softer-on-doctors-3798607.php.

30. R. Meryhew and G. Howatt, "Minimum Standards Mean Less Discipline," *Star Tribune*, February 6, 2012, accessed March 12, 2014, http://www.startribune.com/local/138692919.html?page=all&prepage=1&c=y#continue.

31. D. Wahlberg, "Wisconsin Doctors Who Make Mistakes Often Don't Face Serious Consequences," *Wisconsin State Journal*, January 26, 2013, accessed March 20, 2014, http://host.madison.com/news/local/health_med_fit/wisconsin-doctors-who-make-mistakes-often-don-t-face-serious/article_3c6f0602-673d-11e2-a66c-001a4bcf887a.html.

32. S. Elbein, "Anatomy of a Tragedy," *Texas Observer*, August 28, 2013, accessed March 20, 2014, http://www.texasobserver.org/anatomy-tragedy/.

33. Institute of Medicine, *To Err Is Human: Building a Safer Health System* (Washington, DC: National Academies Press, 2000), accessed March 30, 2014, .

34. B. Starfield, "Is US Health Really the Best in the World?" *JAMA* 284 (2000): 483–485.

35. J. T. James, "A New, Evidence-Based Estimate of Patient Harms Associated with Hospital Care," *Journal of Patient Safety* 9 (2013): 122–128. doi: 10.1097/PTS.0b013e3182948a69.

36. P. Levitt, "Still Unsafe: Why the American Medical Establishment Cannot Reduce Medical Errors," *Skeptic Magazine* 18 (2013): 44–48.

37. A. Levine, R. Oshel, and S. Wolfe, "State Medical Boards Fail to Discipline Doctors with Hospital Actions against Them," accessed March 20, 2014, http://www.citizen.org/hrg1937.

38. P. Eisler and B. Hansen, "Thousands of Doctors Practicing Despite Error, Misconduct," *USA Today*, August 20, 2013, accessed March 20, 2014, http://www.usatoday.com/story/news/nation/2013/08/20/doctors-licenses-medical-boards/2655513/.

39. Derbyshire, 1983.

40. American Board of Internal Medicine, "Why Maintenance of Certification Matters," accessed March 12, 2014,http://www.abim.org/pdf/publications/why-MOC-matters.pdf.

41. M. J. Mehlman, "Professional Power and the Standard of Care in Medicine," *Arizona State Law Journal* 44 (2012): 1165–1235.

42. D. M. Eddy, "Evidence-Based Medicine: A Unified Approach," Health Affairs 24 (2005): 9–17. doi: 10.1377/hlthaff.24.1.9.

43. O. W. Brawley, *How We Do Harm—A Doctor Breaks Ranks about Being Sick in America* (New York: St. Martin's Press, 2012), 243.

44. Ibid., 243.

45. D. T. Chen, M. K. Wynia, R. M. Moloney, and G. C. Alexander, "U.S. Physician Knowledge of the FDA-Approved Indications and Evidence Base for Commonly Prescribed Drugs: Results of a National Survey," *Pharmacoepidemiology Drug Safety* 18 (2009): 1094–1100. doi: 10.1002/pds.1825.

46. J. Carey, "Medical Guesswork," *Business Week*, May 28, 2006, accessed April 1, 2014, http://www.businessweek.com/stories/2006-05-28/medical-guesswork.

47. D. A. Davis, P. E. Mazmanian, and M. Fordis, "Accuracy of Physician Self-Assessment Compared with Observed Measures of Competence: A Systematic Review," *JAMA* 296 (2006): 1094–1102. doi: 10.1001/jama.296.9.1094.

48. Anne-Marie J. Audet, M. M. Doty, J. Shamsudin, and S. C. Schoenbaum, "Measure, Learn, and Improve: Physicians' Involvement In Quality Improvement," *Health Affairs* 24 (2005): 843–853. doi: 10.1377/hlthaff.24.3.843.

49. S. H. Miller, "American Board of Medical Specialties and Repositioning for Excellence in Lifelong Learning: Maintenance of Certification," *Journal of Continuing Education in the Health Professions* 25 (2005): 151–156.

50. Brawley, 193.

51. G. Regehr and K. Eva, "Self-Assessment, Self-Direction, and the Self-Regulating Professional," *Clinical Orthopaedics and Related Research* 449 (2006): 34–38.

52. J. Kruger and D. Dunning, "Unskilled and Unaware of It: How Difficulties in Recognizing One's Own Incompetence Lead to Inflated Self-Assessments," *Journal of Personality and Social Psychology* 77 (1999): 1121–1134. doi: 10.1037/0022-3514.77.6.1121.

53. Glenn Regehr and Kevin Eva, 34–38.

54. T. A. Brennan, R. I Horwits, F. D. Duffy, et al., " The Role of Physician Specialty Board Certification Status in the Quality Movement," *JAMA* 292 (2004): 1038–1043. doi: 10.1001/jama.292.9.1038-1043.

55. Idrees v. American University of the Caribbean, No. 80 CIV 6629 (DNE), 546 F Supp. 1342, 1982.

56. J. T. James, *A Sea of Broken Hearts, Patient Rights in a Dangerous, Profit-Driven Health Care System* (Bloomington, IN: AuthorHouse, 2007), 107–115.

57. American Medical Association, "Continuing Medical Education for Licensure Reregistration," accessed March 14, 2014, http://www.ama-assn.org/resources/doc/med-ed-products/continuing-medical-education-licensure.pdf.

58. Institute of Medicine, *Conflict of Interest in Medical Research, Education, and Practice* (Washington, DC: National Academies Press, 2009),http://www.ncbi.nlm.nih.gov/books/NBK22942/.

59. M. A. Rodwin, "Drug Advertising, Continuing Medical Education, and Physician Prescribing: A Historical Review and Reform Proposal," *Journal of Law, Medicine & Ethics* 38 (2010): 807–815. doi: 10.1111/j.1748-720X.2010.00534.x.

60. L. Morris and J. K. Taitsman, " The Agenda for Continuing Medical Education—Limiting Industry's Influence," *New England Journal of Medicine* 361 (2009): 2478–2482.

61. M. A. Bowman and D. L. Pearle, "Changes in Drug Prescribing Patterns Related to Commercial Company Funding of Continuing Medical Education," *Journal of Continuing Education Health Professions* 8 (1988): 13–20. doi: 10.1002/chp.4750080104.

62. Travel Medical Seminars, "Earn CME Credits on Your Own Time, Take the Vacation You Want and Get the Education You Need," accessed March 25, 2014, http://www.travelmedicalseminars.com/index.php .

63. American Medical Association, "Reporting Impaired, Incompetent or Unethical Colleagues," accessed March 14, 2014, http://www.ama-assn.org//ama/pub/physician-resources/medical-ethics/code-medical-ethics/opinion9031.page.

64. M. Makary, *Unaccountable: What Hospitals Won't Tell You and How Transparency Can Revolutionize Health Care* (New York: Bloomsbury Press, 2012).

65. C. M. DesRoches, S. R. Rao, and J. A. Fromson, et al., "Physicians' Perceptions, Preparedness for Reporting, and Experiences Related to Impaired and Incompetent Colleagues," *JAMA* 304 (2010): 187–193. doi: 10.1001/jama.2010.921.

66. K. H. Berge, M. D. Seppala, and A. M. Schipper, "Chemical Dependency and the Physician," *Mayo Clinic Proceedings* 84 (2009): 625–631.

67. R. Horowitz, *In the Public Interest, Medical Licensing and the Disciplinary Process* (New Brunswick, NJ: Rutgers University Press, 2013).

68. D. Grant and K. C. Alfred, "Sanctions and Recidivism: An Evaluation of Physician Discipline by State Medical Boards," *Journal of Health Politics Policy Law* 32 (2007): 867–885.

69. W. Heisel, "Off the Record: Legislators Try to Put Doctor Discipline behind the Curtain," *Reporting on Health,* accessed March 10, 2014, http://www.reportingonhealth.org/2014/02/28/record-legislators-try-put-doctor-discipline-behind-curtain .

70. B. Cullen, "Commission Case Reports," *Washington State Medical Quality Assurance Commission Update,* 3 Winter 2013, accessed April 16, 2014, http://www.doh.wa.gov/Portals/1/Documents/3000/658002%28December2013%29.pdf.

71. US Department of Health and Human Services (DHHS), Office of Inspector General, *State Medical Boards and Medical Discipline.* oei-01-89-00560, August 1990.

72. Sawicki, 303–306.

73. Bradford Winters, J. Custer, S. M. Galvagno Jr., et al., "Diagnostic Errors in the Intensive Care Unit: A Systematic Review of Autopsy Studies," *BMJ Quality and Safety* 21 (2012): 894–902. doi: 10.1136/bmjqs-2012-000803.

74. M. L. Graber, "The Incidence of Diagnostic Error in Medicine," *BMJ Quality and Safety* 22 (2013): ii21–ii27. doi: 10.1136/bmjqs-2012-001615.

75. O. W. MacDonald, "Physician Perspectives on Preventing Diagnostic Errors," Group Publisher, QuantiaMD, 2011, accessed March 16, 2014, http://quantiamd.com/qqcp/QuantiaMD_PreventingDiagnosticErrors_Whitepaper_1.pdf?cid=1540.

76. H. Singh, A. N. D. Mayer, and E. J. Thomas, "The Frequency of Diagnostic Errors in Outpatient Care: Estimations from Three Large Observational Studies Involving US Adult Populations," *BMJ Quality and Safety* (2014). doi: 10.1136/bmjqs-2013-002627.

77. S. Boodman, "Rarely Mentioned Medical Mistake: Patients Harmed by High Rates of Misdiagnosis," The California Report, State of Health, accessed April 16, 2014, http://blogs.kqed.org/stateofhealth/2013/05/07/doctors-mistakes-in-diagnosis-rarely-mentioned-harm-patients/ .

78. G. D. Schiff, O. Hasen, S. Kim, et al., "Diagnostic Error in Medicine, Analysis of 583 Physician-Reported Errors," *Archives of Internal Medicine* 169 (2009): 1881–1887.

79. M. Graber, "Diagnostic Errors in Medicine: A Case of Neglect," *Joint Commission Journal on Quality and Patient Safety* 31 (2005): 106–113.

80. P. Groskerry, "From Mindless to Mindful Practice—Cognitive Bias and Clinical Decision Making," *New England Journal of Medicine* 368 (2013): 2445–2448. doi: 10.1056/NEJMp1303712.

81. Brawley, 282.

82. J. Banja, "The Normalization of Deviance in Healthcare Delivery," *Business Horizons* 53 (2010): 139. doi: 10.1016/j.bushor.2009.10.006.

83. D. Johnson and L. Talmage, "The Evolution of Medical Discipline in 20th Century America, " Federation of State Medical Boards, accessed March 15, 2014, http://www.iamra.com/pdf/IAMRA%20Conference%20%20October%203/Workshops/Evolution%20of%20Medical%20Discipline%20in%2020th%20Century%20America.pdf.

84. Oregon State Medical Board, "Anatomy of a Complaint," accessed April 16, 2014, http://www.oregon.gov/omb/Investigations/Documents/anatomy-of-complaint.pdf.

85. Kansas Statutes, Chapter 65: Public Health, Article 28: Healing Arts, accessed April 16, 2014, http://kansasstatutes.lesterama.org/Chapter_65/Article_28/#65-2838a.

86. Colorado of Department Regulatory Agencies, Division of Registrations, "What Happens When You File a Complaint," accessed April 16, 2014, http://www.dora.state.co.us/reg_investigations/file_complaint.htm.

87. Texas Statutes, Occupations Code, Title 3, Health Professions, Subtitle B. Physicians, Chapter 164. Disciplinary Actions and Procedures, accessed April 16, 2014, http://www.statutes.legis.state.tx.us/Docs/OC/htm/OC.164.htm.

88. Federation of State Medical Boards, "Physician Profile Information—Board-by-Board Overview," accessed March 22, 2014, http://www.fsmb.org/pdf/GRPOL_Physician_Profiling.pdf .

89. Federation of State Medical Boards, "U.S. Medical Regulatory Trends and Actions," March 2014.

90. C. M. Ostrom, "Legislative Measure Seeks Medical-Board Transparency," *Seattle Times*, March 16, 2011, accessed March 22, 2014, http://seattletimes.com/html/localnews/2014517578_doctorcomplaints17m.html.

91. Horowitz, 177.

92. Federation of State Medical Boards, " *The Exchange*, vol. 1: Licensing Boards, Structure and Disciplinary Functions" (Euless, TX: FSMB, looseleaf compilation), 2003.

93. S. Wolf to Secretary Kathleen Sebelius, Department of Health and Human Services, March 15, 2011, accessed March 1, 2014, http://www.citizen.org/documents/1937A.pdf .

94. Federation of State Medical Boards, "Summary of 2010 Board Actions," accessed April 16, 2014, http://www.fsmb.org/pdf/2010-summary-of-board-actions.pdf.

95. C. F. Ameringer, "State Medical Boards and the Problem of Unnecessary Care and Treatment," *Journal of Medical Regulation* 99 (2013): 25–32.

96. J. S. Weissman, E. C. Schneider, S. N. Weingart, et al., "Comparing Patient-Reported Hospital Adverse Events with Medical Record Review: Do Patients Know Something That Hospitals Do Not?" *Annals of Internal Medicine* 149 (2008): 100–108. doi: 10.7326/0003-4819-149-2-200807150-00006.

2. SECRETS OF THE NATIONAL PRACTITIONER DATA BANK AND THE FAILURE OF MEDICAL LICENSING BOARDS, HOSPITALS, AND THE LEGAL SYSTEM TO PROTECT THE PUBLIC FROM DANGEROUS PHYSICIANS

1. The Data Bank was subsequently supplemented by the Healthcare Integrity and Protection Data Bank (HIPDB). The HIPDB was established by the Health Insurance Portability and Accountability Act of 1996 (HIPPA) to include licensure information on nonphysicians and nondentists as well as some criminal convictions as well as similar sanctions information on health care entities. Most HIPDB information was added to the Data Bank on March 1, 2010. Remaining HIPDB information was added to the Data Bank on May 6, 2013, when the HIPDB was closed to eliminate duplicative reporting, as mandated by the Patient Protection and Affordable Care Act of 2010.

2. M. Makary, *Unaccountable: What Hospitals Won't Tell You and How Transparency Can Revolutionize Health Care* (New York, Bloomsbury Press, 2012), 74.

3. 99th Congress, 2d. Session House of Representatives, Rpt 99-903. Report to Accompany HR 5540 [by the Committee on Energy and Commerce], p. 2.

4. National Practitioner Data Bank, http://www.npdb-hipdb.hrsa.gov/hcorg/register.jsp .

5. 42 USC 11101, *et seq* accessed April 28, 2014, http://www.npdb.hrsa.gov/resources/titleIv.jsp . For the secrecy provision, see 42 USC 11137(b).

6. 42 USC 11135, accessed April 28, 2014, http://www.law.cornell.edu/uscode/text/42/11135 .

7. National Practitioner Data Bank 2010 Annual Report, available at http://www.npdb-hipdb.hrsa.gov/resources/reports/2010NPDBAnnualReport.pdf , table 6. The 2010 Annual Report is the latest report available as of November 10, 2012.

8. National Practitioner Data Bank, accessed April 28, 2014, http://www.npdb-hipdb.hrsa.gov/hcorg/billingAndFees.jsp . Users may also enroll practitioners in the Data Bank's continuous query service, which provides immediate copies of all new reports on enrolled practitioners. This service costs $3.00 per year per name enrolled.

9. National Practitioner Data Bank 2002 Annual Report, page 11, http://www.npdb-hipdb.hrsa.gov/resources/reports/2002NPDBAnnualReport.pdf .

10. Physicians include allopathic physicians (MDs), osteopathic physicians (DOs), and their respective interns and residents.

11. The following statistics were calculated by the author based on analysis of the National Practitioner Data Bank's Public Use Data File of December 31, 2013, as downloaded from

http://www.npdb-hipdb.hrsa.gov/resources/publicData.jsp. The Public Use Data File is updated quarterly.

12. Physicians with dozens of reports typically had them for various types of malpractice. In contrast, those with hundreds of reports typically repeated the same mistake over and over, such as prescribing tetracycline to young children, which caused permanent discoloration of their permanent teeth and could cause growth problems.

13. Author's analysis of the Data Bank Public Use File of December 31, 2013.

14. Author's analysis of the Data Bank Public Use File of December 31, 2013.

15. The author of this chapter was the Data Bank's associate director for research and disputes prior to retirement. In this capacity the author read hundreds, if not thousands, of reports to the Data Bank.

16. "The AMA believes that medical liability claims data is a poor indicator of quality," http://www.ama-assn.org/ama/pub/physician-resources/legal-topics/business-management-topics/national-practitioner-data-bank.page .

17. Author's analysis of the Data Bank Public Use File of June 30, 2012.

18. Author's analysis of the Data Bank Public Use File of June 30, 2012.

19. It would be illegal for the author to confirm or deny that this case was reported to the Data Bank.

20. "Doctor Sued for Inserting Screwdriver into Patient's Back," *Good Morning America*, February 17, 2006, http://abcnews.go.com/GMA/story?id=1630844 .

21. Data provided by the Division of Practitioner Data Banks, US Department of Health and Human Services, in private communication to Public Citizen, September 2012.

22. Public Citizen compared state medical board websites in 2006. "Report of Doctor Disciplinary Information on State Web Sites: A Survey and Ranking of State Medical and Osteopathic Board Web Sites in 2006," http://www.citizen.org/Page.aspx?pid=700 . Although some board websites may have been improved or changed since that time, the sites still vary greatly in the amount of information they provide.

23. A. Young, A. J. Chaudhry, and J. V. Thomas et al., "A Census of Actively Licensed Physicians in the United States, 2010," *Journal of Medical Regulation* 96 (2011), table 1.

24. The AMA has adopted various resolutions (1) opposing making Data Bank information public, (2) proposing to severely restrict the information in the Data Bank so that it would be a less comprehensive listing of a physician's past malpractice and medical disciplinary history and could not serve to identify patterns of problem behavior or incompetence, and (3) even opposing the very existence of the Data Bank.

- H-355.985: "Our AMA: (1) opposes all efforts to open the National Practitioner Data Bank to public access; (2) strongly opposes public access to medical malpractice payment information in the National Practitioner Data Bank; and (3) opposes the implementation by the National Practitioner Data Bank of a self-query user fee. (Res. 824, I-93; Reaffirmed: BOT Rep. 31, I-00; Reaffirmation & Reaffirmed: Res. 216, A-01; Reaffirmed: CME Rep. 2, A-11)."

- AMA Resolution H-355.987: "Our AMA affirms its support for the Federation of State Medical Boards Action Data Bank and calls for the dissolution of the National Practitioner Data Bank. (Sub. Res. 814, A-93; Reaffirmed by Sub. Res. 807, I-95; Reaffirmed by CME Rep. 3, A-96; Reaffirmed by Ref. Cmt. H, A-96; Reaffirmed by Rules & Credentials Cmt., A-96; Reaffirmed: BOT Rep. 31, I-00; Reaffirmed: CMS Rep. 6, A-10)."

- AMA Resolution H-355.991: "It is the policy of the AMA to seek to abolish the National Practitioner Data Bank. (Res. 828, I-91; Reaffirmed by Ref. Cmt. H, A-96; Reaffirmed: Sub. Res. 812, I-97; Reaffirmed: BOT Rep. 31, I-00; Reaffirmed: CMS Rep. 6, A-10)."

- H-355.999: "Our AMA believes that (1) the National Practitioner Data Bank requirements should be modified so that settlements and judgments of less than $30,000 are not reported or recorded; (2) reports, other than licensure revocation, in the Data Bank should be purged after five years; (3) proctoring of physicians for the purpose of investigation should not be reportable. . . ."

- H-355.995: "It is the policy of the AMA to (1) work with HHS to establish a mechanism to inform physicians when an inquiry to the Data Bank has been made; (2) reaffirm its policy that reports, other than licensure revocation, in the Data Bank should be purged after five years. . . ."

- H-450.950: "Our AMA: (1) communicates to legislators the fundamental unfairness of the civil judicial system as it now exists, whereby a jury, rather than a forum of similarly educated peers, determines if a physician has violated the standards of care and such results are communicated to the National Practitioner Data Bank; and (2) impresses on our national legislators that only when a physician has been disciplined by his/her state licensing agency should his/her name appear on the National Practitioner Data Bank. (Res. 809, I-99; Reaffirmed: BOT Rep. 31, I-00; Reaffirmation & Reaffirmed: Res. 216, A-01; Reaffirmed: CME Rep. 2, A-11)."
- H-175.976: "Our AMA will take all necessary actions to oppose and rescind the Health Care Integrity and Protection Data Bank [which has been merged into the NPDB Data Bank]. If not possible to repeal the establishment of the data bank, the AMA should take steps to protect the legal due process rights of practitioners. (Sub. Res. 803, A-99; Reaffirmation I-07)."

25. M. Makary, video trailer promoting book *Unaccountable* (at 1:56), http://www.youtube.com/watch?v=d9Pi8F-lWuA&feature=em-share_video_use , accessed November 21, 2012.

26. A. R. Localio, A. G. Lawthers, and T. A. Brennan, et al., "Relation between Malpractice Claims and Adverse Events Due to Negligence: Results of the Harvard Medical Practice Study III," *New England Journal of Medicine* 325 (1991): 245–251. The authors state the ratio of adverse events caused by negligence to malpractice claims is 7.6 to 1 [13 percent]. They go on to say, "This relative frequency overstates the chances that a negligent adverse event will produce a claim, however, because most of the events for which claims were made in the sample did not meet our definition of adverse events due to negligence."

27. A. B. Jena, S. Seabury, and D. Lakdawalla, et al., "Malpractice Risk According to Physician Specialty," *New England Journal of Medicine* 365 (2011): 629–636.

28. The total number of physicians losing privileges and those not losing privileges is greater than the total number of physicians reported because some had both kinds of actions taken in different facilities or even in the same facility.

29. Data provided by the Division of Practitioner Data Banks, US Department of Health and Human Services, in private communication to Public Citizen, September 2012.

30. 42 USC Sec. 11111, accessed April 28, 2014, http://www.law.cornell.edu/uscode/text/42/11111 .

31. All the following examples are from Gerald N. Rogan, MD, et al., "How Peer Review Failed at Redding Medical Center, and Why It Is Failing across the Country and What Can Be Done About It—Disaster Analysis Redding Medical Center Congressional Report," June 1, 2008.

32. J. Kohler, "Sole Layman on Healing Arts Board is Attorney for Doctors," *St. Louis Post-Dispatch*, December 14, 2010,.

33. Licensing board query volume data provided by the Division of Practitioner Data Banks in response to a data request from Consumers Advancing Patient Safety, September 2012. It should be noted that licensing boards obtain information on licensure actions by other state boards from the Federation of State Medical Boards (FSMB), but the FSMB does not supply licensing boards with malpractice payment, clinical privileges action, or other types of information supplied by the Data Bank. Licensing boards typically say they do not query because they do not have the budget to pay for queries and they get information from the FSMB. It is also likely that they do not have adequate staffing to make use of the information if they got it. Data on the number of physicians and licenses used to calculate the ratio of queries to physicians and licensees is from A. Young, A. J. Chaudhry, and J. V. Thomas, et al., "A Census of Actively Licensed Physicians in the United States, 2010," *Journal of Medical Regulation* 96, no. 4 (2011): table 1.

34. Public Citizen, "State Medical Boards Fail to Discipline Doctors with Hospital Actions against Them," March 2011, http://www.citizen.org/documents/1937.pdf .

35. Ibid., table 1, p. 5.

36. Ibid., p. 6.

37. Ibid., table 2, p. 7.

38. B. Joseph, "Flaws Found in State Consumer Protection Enforcement," *Orange County Register*, October 26, 2012, http://www.ocregister.com/articles/boards-375814-board-cases.html .

39. Author's analysis of the National Practitioner Data Bank Public Use File of June 30, 2010.

40. ⁴⁰ Author's analysis of the National Practitioner Data Bank Public Use File of December 31, 2013.

41. Institute of Medicine, *To Err Is Human: Building a Safer Health System*, 1999, 1, http://www.nap.edu/catalog/9728.html .

42. D. Wilson, "Mistakes Chronicled on Medicare Patients," *New York Times*, November 15, 2010, http://www.nytimes.com/2010/11/16/business/16medicare.html?_r=0 .

43. Office of Inspector General, Department of Health and Human Services, "Adverse Events in Hospitals: National Incidence among Medicare Beneficiaries," November 2010, OEI-06-09-00090, pg. ii, http://oig.hhs.gov/oei/reports/oei-06-09-00090.pdf .

44. J. T. James, "A New, Evidence-Based Estimate of Patient Harms Associated with Hospital Care," *Journal of Patient Safety* 9 (2013): 122–128.

45. Public Citizen suggests that "boards are likely to do a better job disciplining physicians if most, if not all, of the following conditions exist:

- They receive adequate funding (all money from license fees going to fund board activities instead of going into the state treasury for general purposes). In an era of especially tight state budgets, money allocated to board revenue from doctors' licensing fees frequently has been transferred to fund other parts of state executive branch functions;
- They have adequate staffing;
- They engage in proactive investigations, rather than only reacting to complaints;
- They use all available/reliable data from other sources such as Medicare and Medicaid sanctions, hospital sanctions and malpractice payouts;
- They have excellent leadership;
- They have independence from state medical societies;
- They are independent from other parts of the state government; and
- A reasonable legal framework exists for disciplining doctors (the "preponderance of the evidence" rather than "beyond reasonable doubt" or "clear and convincing evidence" as the legal standard for discipline)."

S. M. Wolfe, C. Williams, and A. Zaslow, "Public Citizen's Health Research Group Ranking of the Rate of State Medical Boards' Serious Disciplinary Actions, 2009–2011," May 17, 2012, http://www.citizen.org/documents/2034.pdf .

46. Use of electronic meetings and virtual peer review, as has been done by rural hospitals in Texas, would facilitate use of randomly assigned outside peer reviewers. See J. R. Williams, K. M. Mechler, and R. B. Akins, et al., "The Rural Physician Peer Review Model©: A Virtual Solution," http://www.ahrq.gov/downloads/pub/advances2/vol2/Advances-Williams_115.pdf .

3. FAILURES AND SUCCESSES OF PHYSICIAN PEER AND PERFORMANCE REVIEW

1. The National Practitioner Data Bank, HHS, accessed April 28, 2014, http://www.npdb.hrsa.gov/.

2. Centers for Medicare and Medicaid Services, accessed April 28, 2014, http://www.gpo.gov/fdsys/pkg/CFR-2011-title42-vol5/pdf/CFR-2011-title42-vol5-sec482-21.pdf.

3. California Department of Public Health, accessed April 28, 2014, http://www.cdph.ca.gov/programs/LnC/Pages/lnc.aspx.

4. OIG News, December 11, 2003, accessed April 28, 2014, https://oig.hhs.gov/publications/docs/press/2003/121103release.pdf.

5. Martin Luther King, Jr., Hospital History, accessed April 28, 2014, http://www.mlkcommunityhospital.org/our-story.

6. D. Meldi, F. Rhoades, and A. Gippe, "The Big Three: A Side by Side Matrix Comparing Hospital Accrediting Agencies," January/February 2009, accessed April 28, 2014, http://cms.ipressroom.com.s3.amazonaws.com/107/files/20125/Comparing_Accreditation_Programs_Synergy_.pdf.

7. M. W. Scott letter to the U. S. Department of Justice, November 15, 2005, accessed May 1, 2014.

8. G. N. Rogan, F. Sebat, and I. Grady, *How Peer Review Failed at Redding Medical Center, Why It Is Failing Across the Country and What Can be Done About It*, June 1, 2008, accessed April 28, 2014.

9. S. Klaidman, *Coronary: A True Story of Medical Care Gone Awry* (New York: Scribner, 2008).

10. Asiana Flight 214 crash, July 6, 2013 at San Francisco International Airport, accessed May 1, 2014, http://en.wikipedia.org/wiki/Asiana_Airlines_Flight_214.

11. J. Battard-Menendez, "The Impetus for Legislation Revoking the Joint Commission's Deemed Status as a Medicare Accrediting Agency," *JONA's Healthcare Law, Ethics, and Regulation* 12 (2010): 69–76, accessed April 28, 2010, http://www.ncbi.nlm.nih.gov/pubmed/20733410.

12. B. Blackmond, "Hospital Accreditation—Alternatives to the Joint Commission," accessed April 28, 2014, http://www.healthlawyers.org/Events/Programs/Materials/Documents/HHS09/blackmond.pdf.

13. Public Citizen, "Physician Accountability," accessed May, 1, 2014, http://www.citizen.org/Page.aspx?pid=1248.

14. Food and Drug Administration, "The Mammography Quality Standards Act Final Regulations: Modifications and Additions to Policy Guidance Help System #9," April 19, 2006, accessed May 2014, http://www.fda.gov/RadiationEmittingProducts/MammographyQualityStandardsActandProgram/DocumentArchives/ucm114207.htm.

15. American Society of Cytopathology, "Quality Control and Quality Assurance Practices," November 10, 2000, accessed May 1, 2014, http://www.cytopathology.org/quality-control-and-quality-assurance-practices/.

16. E. G. Brown, Attorney General of the State of California, Case Number 02-2002-139527, accessed April 28, 2014, http://www2.mbc.ca.gov/BreezePDL/document.aspx?path=%5cDIDOCS%5c20070508%5cDMRAAABI16%5c&did=AAABI070508224526093.DID&licenseType=A&licenseNumber=32120#page=1.

17. State of California, accessed April 28, 2014, https://www.breeze.ca.gov/datamart/detailsCADCA.do?selector=false&selectorType=&selectorReturnUrl=&anchor=b727bcb.0.0.

18. Medicare, Hospital Compare, accessed April 28, 2014, http://www.medicare.gov/hospitalcompare/search.html?AspxAutoDetectCookieSupport=1.

19. Institute of Medicine, *Toward Quality Measures for Population Health and the Leading Health Indicators* (Washington DC, National Academies Press, 2013), accessed April 29, 2014, http://www.iom.edu/Reports/2013/Toward-Quality-Measures-for-Population-Health-and-the-Leading-Health-Indicators.aspx.

20. T. Bishop, *Baltimore Sun*, "Cardiologist's License Revoked over Accusations of Placing Unneeded Stents," accessed April 28, 2014, http://articles.baltimoresun.com/2011-07-13/health/ms-md-midei-license-revoked-20110713_1_midei-unneeded-stents-stent-business.

21. License sanctions by the State of Maryland, July 2011, accessed April 28, 2014, http://www.mbp.state.md.us/forms/jul11sanctions.pdf.

22. Staff Report on Cardiac Stent Usage at St. Joseph Medical Center, December 2010, accessed April 29, 2014, http://www.finance.senate.gov/newsroom/chairman/release/?id=ce0c5525-b352-474f-9970-96f5afc140bb.

23. Government Accountability Office, VA Healthcare, December 2013, accessed April 28, 2014, http://www.gao.gov/assets/660/659378.pdf.

24. E. Kenniston. "The Joint Commission and Patient Safety Outcomes: Have Accreditor Policies Improved Patient Safety?" 2011, accessed April 28, 2014, http://hlaw.ucsd.edu/prospectivestudents/documents/Kenniston_HavePoliciesImprovedPatientSafety.pdf.

25. D. Drake, *Daily Beast*, accessed April 23, 2014, http://www.thedailybeast.com/articles/2014/04/14/how-being-a-doctor-became-the-most-miserable-profession.html.

26. D. A. Davis, P. E. Mazmanian, M. Fordis, et al., "Accuracy of Physician Self-Assessment Compared with Observed Measures of Competence—A Systematic Review," *JAMA* 296 (2006): 1094–1102.

27. W. Hall, C. Violato, R. Lewkonia, et al., "Assessment of Physicians Performance in Alberta: The Physician Achievement Review," *Canadian Medical Association Journal* 161 (1999): 52–57.

28. I. Dubinsky, K. Jennings, M. Greengarten, and A. Brans, "360-Degree Physician Performance Assessment," *Healthcare Quarterly* 13 (2009): 71–76.

29. K. Overeem, H. C. Wollersheim, O. A. Arah, et al., "Evaluation of Physicians' Professional Performance: An Iterative Development and Validation Study of Multisource Feedback Instruments," *BMC Health Services Research* 12 (2012): 8, accessed April 24, 2014, http://www.biomedcentral.com/1472-6963/12/80.

30. T. Donnon, A. Al Ansari, S. Al Alawi, and C. Violato, "The Reliability, Validity, and Feasibility of Multisource Feedback Physician Assessment: A Systematic Review," *Academic Medicine* 89 (2014): 1–6.

4. DANGEROUS MEDICAL DEVICES

1. D. M. Zuckerman, P. Brown, and S. E. Nissen, "Medical Device Recalls and the FDA Approval Process," *Archives of Internal Medicine* 171 (2011):1006–1007.

2. US Government Accountability Office, "FDA Should Take Steps to Ensure That High-Risk Device Types Are Approved through the Most Stringent Pre-market Review Processes," GAO-09-190: January 2009, http://gao.gov/new.items/d09190.pdf, accessed February 26, 2014.

3. Institute of Medicine (IOM), *Medical Devices and the Public's Health: The FDA 501(k) Clearance Process at 35 Years* (Washington: National Academies Press, 2011), 1–12.

4. R. Sutton, J. D. Fisher, C. Linde, and D. G. Benditt, "History of Electrical Therapy for the Heart," *European Heart Journal* 9 (Supplement 1) (2007): 3-4.

5. Ibid., 5–8.

6. D. Walter, *Collateral Damage—A Patient, a New Procedure and the Learning Curve* (privately published in Charleston, SC, 2011), 1–182.

7. M. Mansour, T. Mela, J. Ruskin, and D. Keane, "Successful Release of Entrapped Circumferential Mapping Catheters in Patients Undergoing Pulmonary Vein Isolation for Atrial Fibrillation," *Heart Rhythm* 1 (2004): 558–561.

8. Zuckerman, 1007–10.

9. U.S. Government Accountability Office.

10. S. Sarosiek, M. Crowther, and J. M. Sloan, "Indications, Complications, and Management of Inferior Vena Cava Filters," *JAMA Internal Medicine* 173 (2013): 513–517.

11. V. Prasad, J. Rho, and A. Cifu, "The Inferior Vena Cava Filter," *JAMA Internal Medicine* 173 (2013): 493–495.

12. American Academy of Orthopaedic Surgeons, "Current Concerns with Metal-on-Metal Hip Arthroplasty," December 2012, http://www.aaos.org/about/papers/advistmt/1035.asp, accessed February 27, 2014.

13. S. R. Knight, R. Aujla, and S. P. Biswas, "Total Hip Arthroplasty—Over 100 Years of Operative History," *Orthopedic Reviews 2011*, http://www.pagepress.org/journals/index.php/or/article/view/or.2011.e16/3190, accessed February 27, 2014.

14. American Academy of Orthopaedic Surgeons.

15. K. T. Mäkelä, T. Visuri, P. Pulkkinen, et al., "Risk of Cancer with Metal-on-Metal Hip Replacements: Population Based Study," *BMJ* 345 (2012): e4646, http://www.bmj.com/content/345/bmj.e4646, accessed February 27, 2014.

16. Food and Drug Administration, "Information for Patients Who Have Metal-on-Metal Hip Implants," January 17, 2013, http://www.fda.gov/MedicalDevices/ProductsandMedicalProcedures/ImplantsandProsthetics/MetalonMetalHipImplants/ucm241766.htm, accessed February 27, 2014.

17. Food and Drug Administration, "Information for Patients Considering a Metal-on-Metal Hip Implant System," January 17, 2013, http://www.fda.gov/MedicalDevices/ProductsandMedicalProcedures/ImplantsandProsthetics/MetalonMetalHipImplants/ucm241767.htm, accessed February 27, 2014.

18. A. K. Skipor, P. A. Campbell, L. M. Patterson, et al., "Serum and Urine Metal Levels in Patients with Metal-on-metal Surface Arthroplasty," *Journal of Materials Science Materials in Medicine* 13 (2002): 1227–1234.

19. S. S. Tower, "Arthroprosthetic Cobaltism: Neurological and Cardiac Manifestations in Two Patients with Metal-on-Metal Arthroplasty: A Case Report," *Journal of Bone and Joint Surgery, American Volume* 92 (2010): 2847–2851.

20. J. J. Jacobs, "Commentary on an Article by Stephen S. Tower, MD: 'Arthroprosthetic Cobaltism: Neurological and Cardiac Manifestations in Two Patients with Metal-on-Metal Arthroplasty. A Case Report,'" *Journal of Bone and Joint Surgery, American Volume* 92 (2010): e35.

21. T. Kelly, S. Bauer, and S. Tower, "Power, Credibility and Expertise in a Colonized Medical Discourse," PhilSci Archive, 3rd Annual Values in Medicine, Science, and Technology Conference, Dallas, TX, May 22–24, 2013, accessed 29 May 2014, http://philsci-archive.pitt.edu/9777/.

22. J. G. Sotos and S. S. Tower, "Systemic Disease after Hip Replacement: Aeromedical Implications of Arthroprosthetic Cobaltism," *Aviation, Space, and Environmental Medicine* 84 (2013): 242–245.

23. M. P. Estey, E. P. Diamandis, C. Van Der Straeten, et al., "Cobalt and Chromium Measurement in Patients with Metal Hip Protheses," *Clinical Chemistry* 59 (2013): 880–886.

24. S. S. Tower, "Arthroprosthetic Cobaltism Associated with Metal on Metal Hip Implants," *BMJ* 344 (2012): e430.

25. S. Tower, "Arthroprosthetic Cobaltism: Identification of the At-Risk Patient," *Alaska Medicine* 52 (2010): 28–32.

26. Y-M Kwon, A. V. Lombardi, J. J. Jacobs, et al., "Risk Stratification Algorithm for Management of Patients with Metal-on-Metal Hip Arthroplasty," *Journal of Bone and Joint Surgery, American Volume* 96 (2014): e4(1–6).

27. MEDICINEWISE N., "Monitoring for Potential Toxicity in Patients with Metal-on-Metal Hip Protheses: Advice for Health Professionals," 2013.

28. X. Mao, A. A. Wong, and R. W. Crawford, "Cobalt Toxicity—An Emerging Clinical Problem in Patients with Metal-on-Metal Hip Protheses?" *Medical Journal of Australia* 194 (2011): 649–651.

29. C. Machado, A. Appelbe, and R. Wood, "Arthroprosthetic Cobaltism and Cardiomyopathy," *Heart, Lung and Circulation* 21 (2012): 759–760.

30. S. E. Graves, A. Rothwell, K. Tucker, et al., "A Multinational Assessment of Metal-on-metal Bearings in Hip Replacement," *Journal of Bone and Joint Surgery, American Volume* 93 Supplement 3 (2011): 43–47.

31. S. E. Graves, "What Is Happening with Hip Replacement?" *Medical Journal of Australia* 194 (2011): 620–621.

32. L. A. Allen, A. V. Ambardekar, K. M. Devaraj, et al., "Clinical Problem-Solving: Missing Elements of the History," *New England Journal of Medicine* 370 (2014): 5595–5596.

33. K. Dahms, Y. Sharkova, P. Heitlan, et al., "Cobalt Intoxication Diagnosed with the Help of Dr. House," *Lancet* 383 (2014): 573–574.

34. S. Tower, "Dr. Tower Writes to Senator re Concerns about the Regulatory Malfeasance at the FDA—Metal-on-Metal Hip Replacement," accessed April 29, 2014, http://earlsview.

com/2013/01/10/dr-tower-writes-to-senator-re-concerns-about-the-regulatory-malfeasance-at-the-fda-metal-on-metal-hip-replacement-debacle/.

35. B. Meier, "Johnson & Johnson in Deal to Settle Hip Implant Lawsuits," November 19, 2013, http://www.nytimes.com/2013/11/20/business/johnson-johnson-to-offer-2-5-billion-hip-device-settlement.html?_r=0, accessed February 27, 2014.

5. A CONTEMPORARY REVIEW OF HEALTH CARE-ASSOCIATED INFECTIONS

1. A. Gawande, "The Disturbing Truth about Doctors and Your Medical Safety," May 18, 2007, accessed January 15, 2014, http://www.truth-out.org/archive/item/70678:atul-gawande--the-disturbing-truth-about-doctors-and-your-medical-safety.

2. T. N. Raju, "Ignac Semmelweis and the Etiology of Fetal and Neonatal Sepsis," *Journal of Perinatology* 19 (1999): 307–310.

3. Nulond, S. *The Doctor's Plague: Germans, Childbed Fever, and the Strange Story of Ignac Semmelweis.* New York: W. W. Norton, 2004.

4. R. M. Klevens, J. R. Edwards, C. L. Richards, Jr., et al., "Estimating Health Care-Associated Infections and Deaths in U.S. Hospitals," *Public Health Reports* 122 (2007): 160–166.

5. A. Srinivasan, M. Craig, and D. Cardo, "The Power of Policy Change, Federal Collaboration, and State Coordination in Healthcare-Associated Infection Prevention," *Clinical Infectious Diseases* 55 (2012): 426–431.

6. Centers for Disease Control and Prevention (CDC), "Healthcare Facility HAI Reporting Requirements to CMS via NHSN—Current Requirements 2013," accessed April 28, 2014, http://www.cdc.gov/nhsn/PDFs/CMS/CMS-Reporting-Requirements-Deadlines.pdf.

7. P. Pronovost, D. Needham, S. Berenholtz, et al., "An Intervention to Decrease Catheter-Related Bloodstream Infections in the ICU," *New England Journal of Medicine* 355 (2006): 2725–2732.

8. C. L. Bosk, M. Dixon-Woods, C. A. Goeschel, et al., "Reality Check for Checklists," *Lancet* 374 (2009): 444–445.

9. D. M. Saman, K. T. Kavanagh, B. Johnson, et al., "Can Inpatient Hospital Experiences Predict Central Line-Associated Bloodstream Infections?" *Plos One* 8 (2013): e61097.

10. N. Arora, K. Patel, C. A. Engell, et al., "The Effect of Interdisciplinary Team Rounds on Urinary Catheter and Central Venous Catheter Days and Rates of Infection," *American Journal of Medical Quality*, September 4, 2013.

11. N. Freixas, F. Bella, E. Limon, et al., "Impact of a Multimodal Intervention to Reduce Bloodstream Infections Related to Vascular Catheters in Non-ICU Wards: A Multicentre Study," *Clinical Microbiology and Infection* 19 (2013): 838–844.

12. C. Lindberg, G. Downham, P. Buscell, et al., "Embracing Collaboration: A Novel Strategy for Reducing Bloodstream Infections in Outpatient Hemodialysis Centers," *American Journal of Infection Control* 41 (2013): 513–519.

13. A. Marigliano, P. Barbadoro, L. Pennacchietti, et al., "Active Training and Surveillance: 2 Good Friends to Reduce Urinary Catheterization Rate," *American Journal of Infection Control* 40 (2012): 692–695.

14. Gawande, "The Disturbing Truth about Doctors and Your Medical Safety."

15. *WHO Guidelines on Hand Hygiene in Health Care: First Global Patient Safety Challenge Clean Care Is Safer Care* (Geneva: World Health Organization, 2009), accessed April 28, 2014, http://whqlibdoc.who.int/publications/2009/9789241597906_eng.pdf.

16. D. Pittet, S. Hugonnet, S. Harbarth, et al., "Effectiveness of a Hospital-Wide Programme to Improve Compliance with Hand Hygiene: Infection Control Programme," *Lancet* 356 (2000): 1307–1312.

17. C. M. White, A. M. Statile, P. H. Conway, et al., "Utilizing Improvement Science Methods to Improve Physician Compliance with Proper Hand Hygiene," *Pediatrics* 129 (2012): e1042–1050.

18. A. Hartocollis, "With Money at Risk, Hospitals Push Staff to Wash Hands," 2013, accessed January 18, 2014, http://www.nytimes.com/2013/05/29/nyregion/hospitals-struggle-to-get-workers-to-wash-their-hands.html?_r=0.

19. M. McGuckin, J. Storr, Y. Longtin, et al., "Patient Empowerment and Multimodal Hand Hygiene Promotion: A Win-Win Strategy," *American Journal of Medical Quality* 26 (2011): 10–17.

20. Y. Longtin, H. Sax, B. Allegranzi, et al., "Patients' Beliefs and Perceptions of Their Participation to Increase Healthcare Worker Compliance with Hand Hygiene," *Infection Control and Hospital Epidemiology* 30 (2009): 830–839.

21. Gawande, "The Distrurbing Truth about Doctors and Your Medical Safety,"

22. M. Day, "Doctors Are Told to Ditch 'Disease Spreading' Neckties," *BMJ* 332 (2006): 442.

23. R. J. Brilli, R. E. McClead Jr., W. V. Crandall, et al., "A Comprehensive Patient Safety Program Can Significantly Reduce Preventable Harm, Associated Costs, and Hospital Mortality," *Journal of Pediatrics* 163 (2013): 1638–1645.

24. K. L. Rich, S. M. Reese, K. A. Bol, et al., "Assessment of the Quality of Publicly Reported Central Line-Associated Bloodstream Infection Data in Colorado, 2010," *American Journal of Infection Control* 41 (2013): 874–879.

25. D. L. Thompson, M. Makvandi, and J. Baumbach, "Validation of Central Line-Associated Bloodstream Infection Data in a Voluntary Reporting State: New Mexico," *American Journal of Infection Control* 41 (2013): 122–125.

26. D. M. Saman and K. T. Kavanagh, "A Tale of Two Cows: Why We Have a Cow Map and Not a Healthcare Acquired Infection Map," *Epidemonomics* blog, March 13, 2012, accessed April 28, 2014, http://www.cddep.org/blog/posts/tale_two_cows_why_we_have_cow_map_and_not_health care_acquired_infection_map.

27. D. M. Roddy and D. Malloy, "John Murtha Dies at 77," *Pittsburgh Post-Gazette*, February 9, 2010, accessed March 1, 2014, http://www.post-gazette.com/nation/2010/02/08/Rep-John-Murtha-dies-at-77/stories/201002080195 .

28. D. M. Saman, K. T. Kavanagh, and S. K. Abusalem, "Redefining the Standardized Infection Ratio to Aid in Consumer Value Purchasing," *Journal of Patient Safety* 9 (2013): 55–58.

29. L. Landro, "Why Hospitals Want Patients to Ask Doctors, 'Have You Washed Your Hands?'" *Wall Street Journal*, September 30, 2013, accessed October 1, 2013, http://online.wsj.com/news/articles/SB10001424052702303918804579107202360565642.

30. A. Ottum, A. K. Sethi, E. A. Jacobs, et al., "Do Patients Feel Comfortable Asking Healthcare Workers to Wash Their Hands?" *Infection Control and Hospital Epidemiology* 33 (2012): 1282–1284.

31. D. M. Hacek, S. M. Paule, R. B. Thomson Jr., et al., "Implementation of a Universal Admission Surveillance and Decolonization Program for Methicillin-Resistant Staphylococcus aureus (MRSA) Reduces the Number of MRSA and Total Number of S. aureus Isolates Reported by the Clinical Laboratory," *Journal of Clinical Microbiology* 47 (2009): 3749–3752.

32. F. J. McIntyre and R. McCloy, "Shaving Patients before Operation: A Dangerous Myth?" *Annals of the Royal College of Surgeons of England* 76 (1994): 3–4.

33. A. O. Adisa, O. O. Lawal, and O. Adejuyigbe, "Evaluation of Two Methods of Preoperative Hair Removal and Their Relationship to Postoperative Wound Infection," *Journal of Infection in Developing Countries* 5 (2011): 717–722.

34. B. R. Swenson, T. L. Hedrick, R. Metzger, et al., "Effects of Preoperative Skin Preparation on Postoperative Wound Infection Rates: A Prospective Study of 3 Skin Preparation Protocols," *Infection Control and Hospital Epidemiology* 30 (2009): 964–971.

35. M. J. Kuehnert, D. Kruszon-Moran, H. A. Hill, et al., "Prevalence of Staphylococcus aureus Nasal Colonization in the United States, 2001–2002," *Journal of Infectious Diseases* 193 (2006): 172–179.

36. R. J. Gorwitz, D. Kruszon-Moran, S. K. McAllister, et al., "Changes in the Prevalence of Nasal Colonization with Staphylococcus aureus in the United States, 2001-2004," *Journal of Infectious Diseases* 197 (2008): 1226–1234.

37. Centers for Disease Control and Prevention (CDC), "Clostridium difficile Infection," 2013, accessed January 16, 2014, http://www.cdc.gov/HAI/organisms/cdiff/Cdiff_infect.html .

38. G. Patel, S. Huprikan, S. H. Factor, et al., "Outcomes of Carbapenem-Resistant Klebsiella pneumoniae Infection and the Impact of Antimicrobial and Adjunctive Therapies," *Infection Control and Hospital Epidemiology* 29 (2008): 1099–1106.

39. Centers for Disease Control and Prevention (CDC), "Making Health Care Safer: Stop Infections from Lethal CRE Germs," *CDC Vital Signs*, March 2013, accessed April 28, 2014, http://www.cdc.gov/vitalsigns/hai/cre/.

40. D. M. Sievert, P. Ricks, J. R. Edwards, et al., "Antimicrobial-Resistant Pathogens Associated with Healthcare-Associated Infections: Summary of Data Reported to the National Healthcare Safety Network at the Centers for Disease Control and Prevention, 2009–2010," *Infection Control and Hospital Epidemiology* 34 (2013): 1–14.

41. D. P. Nicolau, "Carbapenems: A Potent Class of Antibiotics," *Expert Opinion on Pharmacotherapy* 9 (2008): 23–37.

42. K. A. Hazlewood, S. D. Brouse, W. D. Pitcher, et al., "Vancomycin-Associated Nephrotoxicity: Grave Concern or Death by Character Assassination?" *American Journal of Medicine* 123 (2010): e181–187.

43. H. W. Boucher, G. H. Talbot, D. K. Benjamin, et al., "10 × '20 Progress—Development of New Drugs Active against Gram-Negative Bacilli: An Update From the Infectious Diseases Society of America," *Clinical Infectious Diseases*, April 17, 2013, accessed April 28, 2014, http://cid.oxfordjournals.org/content/early/2013/04/16/cid.cit152.full.pdf.

44. Society for Healthcare Epidemiology of America, Infectious Diseases Society of America, and Society PID, "Policy Statement on Antimicrobial Stewardship by the Society for Healthcare Epidemiology of America (SHEA), the Infectious Diseases Society of America (IDSA), and the Pediatric Infectious Diseases Society (PIDS)," *Infection Control and Hospital Epidemiology* 33 (2012): 322–327.

45. A. C. Nyquist, R. Gonzales, J. F. Steiner, et al., "Antibiotic Prescribing for Children with Colds, Upper Respiratory Tract Infections, and Bronchitis," *JAMA* 279 (1998): 875–877.

46. Centers for Disease Control and Prevention (CDC), "Office-Related Antibiotic Prescribing for Persons Aged </= 14 years—United States, 1993–1994 to 2007–2008," *MMWR: Morbidity and Mortality Weekly Report* 60, no. 34 (September 2, 2011): 1153–1156, accessed April 28, 2014, http://www.cdc.gov/mmwr/preview/mmwrhtml/mm6034a1.htm.

47. L. A. Hicks, T. H. Taylor, and R. J. Hunkler, "U.S. Outpatient Antibiotic Prescribing, 2010," *New England Journal of Medicine* 368 (2013): 1461–1462.

48. D. Gould, "Survey Reveals Growing Consumer Demand For Antibiotic-Free Meat," 2012, *Forbes*, accessed March 2, 2014, http://www.forbes.com/sites/daniellegould/2012/06/26/survey-reveals-growing-consumer-demand-for-antibiotic-free-meat/.

49. J. Halloran, "The Overuse of Antibiotics in Food Animals Threatens Public Health: Consumers Union," 2012, accessed March 2, 2014, http://consumersunion.org/news/the-overuse-of-antibiotics-in-food-animals-threatens-public-health-2/.

50. T. N. Palmore, D. K. Henderson, M. J. Bonten, et al., "Enhancing Patient Safety by Reducing Healthcare-Associated Infections: The Role of Discovery and Dissemination," *Infection Control and Hospital Epidemiology* 31 (2010): 118–123.

51. S. R. Deeny, B. S. Cooper, B. Cookson, et al., "Targeted versus Universal Screening and Decolonization to Reduce Healthcare-Associated Methicillin-Resistant Staphylococcus aureus Infection," *Journal of Hospital Infection* 85 (2013): 33–44.

52. Klevens et al., "Estimating Heath Care-Associated Infections and Deaths in U.S. Hospitals."

53. Centers for Medicaid and Medicare Services and Medicare.gov, "Healthcare Associated Infections," 2013, accessed April 28, 2014, https://data.medicare.gov/Hospital-Compare/Healthcare-Associated-Infections/ihvx-zkyp.

54. Saman et al. "Can Impatient Hospital Experiences Predict Central Line-Associated Bloodstream Infections?"

55. Klevens et al., "Estimating Health Care-Associated Infects and Deaths in U.S. Hospitals."

6. OVERSIGHT OF PHYSICIAN OFFICES: DR. WELBY OR DR. APPLEBEE?

1. A. Hahn, "Would You Go under Anesthesia If Your Doctor's Only Backup Plan Was to Call 911?" *Online Metroland,* October 21, 2004, http://metroland.net/back_issues/vol_27_no43/features.html.

2. "Office-Based Surgery (OBS) Frequently Asked Questions (FAQ's) for Practitioners," New York State Department of Health, http://www.health.ny.gov/professionals/office-based_surgery/obs_faq.htm.

3. R. Urman and F. Shapiro, "Improving Patient Safety in the Office: The Institute for Safety in Office-Based Surgery," Spring-Summer 2011, Anesthesia Patient Safety Foundation, http://www.apsf.org/newsletters/html/2011/spring/02_officesafety.htm.

4. American Social History Productions, Inc., "Upton Sinclair Hits His Readers in the Stomach," *History Matters: The US Survey Course on the Web*, http://historymatters.gmu.edu/d/5727/.

5. "Restaurant Inspections in Your Area," *Food Safety News*, http://www.foodsafetynews.com/restaurant-inspections-in-your-area/#.UlRyKRbAXfg.

6. A. Gawande, "Big Med," *New Yorker,* August 13, 2012, http://www.newyorker.com/reporting/2012/08/13/120813fa_fact_gawande?currentPage=all.

7. S. L. Chen and T. R. Morgan, "The Natural History of Hepatitis C Virus (HCV) Infection," *International Journal of Medical Sciences* 3, no. 2 (2006): 47–52.

8. E. V. McKnight and T. T. Bennington, *A Never Event: Exposing the Largest Outbreak of Hepatitis C in American Healthcare History*, History Examined, 2010.

9. M. Mailliard, personal communication with the author, December 15, 2010.

10. A. Macedo de Oliveira, K. L. White, D. P. Leschinsky, et al., "An Outbreak of Hepatitis C Virus Infections among Outpatients at a Hematology/Oncology Clinic," *Annals of Internal Medicine* 142 (2005): 901.

11. A. Y. Guy, N. D. Thompson, M. K. Schaefer, et al., "Patient Notification for Bloodborne Pathogen Testing due to Unsafe Injection Practices in the US Health Care Settings, 2001-2011," *Medical Care* 50 (2012): 786.

12. "About Dr. Roberts," Perlmutter Health Center, www.perlhealth.com/about-dr-roberts/.

13. "WFP Health Talk: The Benefits of Integrative Medicine with Dr Carol Roberts, MD," Wiseman Family Practice, http://www.wisemanfamilypractice.com/wfp-healthtalk-the-benefits-of-integrative-medicine-with-dr-carol-roberts-md/.

14. R. Sanderson, "Outbreak of Hepatitis C in an Outpatient Alternative Medicine Clinic," Association for Professionals in Infection Control, 2010 Annual Conference and Educational Meeting, July 11–15, New Orleans, LA.

15. E. V. McKnight and L. Lollini, "There Isn't Anything I Can't Do—Melisa French's Story," Hepatitis Outbreaks National Organization for Reform, March 17, 2014, http://www.honoreform.org/blog/?cat=2.

16. C. Gentry, "Alternative-Medicine Doctor Reprimanded, Fined in Hepatitis C Outbreak," WUSF News, October 12, 2014, http://wusfnews.wusf.usf.edu/post/alternative-medicine-doctor-reprimanded-fined-hepatitis-c-outbreak.

17. "About Dr. Roberts," Perlmutter Health Center, http://www.perlhealth.com/about-dr-roberts/.

18. L. Landro, "Taming the Wild West of Outpatient Surgery—Doctors' Offices," *Wall Street Journal*, October 26, 2010, http://blogs.wsj.com/health.

19. H, Vila Jr., R. Soto, A. B. Cantor, et al., "Comparative Outcomes Analysis of Procedures Performed in Physician Offices and Ambulatory Surgery Centers," *Archives of Surgery* 138 (2003): 994.

20. "OSHA Fact Sheet: OSHA Inspections," Occupational Safety and Health Administration, https://www.osha.gov/OshDoc/data_General_Facts/factsheet-inspections.pdf.

21. "Clinical Laboratory Improvement Amendments (CLIA)," Centers for Medicare and Medicaid Services, http://www.cms.gov/Regulations-and-Guidance/Legislation/CLIA/index.html?redirect=/clia/.

22. "Health Information Privacy," US Department of Health and Human Services, http://www.hhs.gov/ocr/privacy/.

23. "Medicaid Fraud Control Units—MFCUs Office of Inspector General," Office of Inspector General US Department of Health and Human Services, https://www.oig.hhs.gov/fraud/medicaid-fraud-control-units-mfcu/index.asp.

24. "Recovery Audit Program," Centers for Medicare and Medicaid Services, http://www.cms.gov/Research-Statistics-Data-and-Systems/Monitoring-Programs/Medicare-FFS-Compliance-Programs/Recovery-Audit-Program/?redirect=/recovery-audit-program/.

25. "HEDIS and Quality Compass," National Committee for Quality Accreditation, http://www.ncqa.org/HEDISQualityMeasurement/WhatisHEDIS.aspx.

26. "Rating List Information," Douglas County Health Department, http://www.douglascountyhealth.com/food-a-drink/food-facility-ratings/rating-list-information.

27. "Viral Hepatitis Outbreaks: Viral Hepatitis Statistics and Surveillance, Healthcare-Associated Hepatitis B and C Outbreaks Reported to the Centers for Disease Control and Prevention (CDC) in 2008-2012," Centers for Disease Control and Prevention, http://www.cdc.gov/hepatitis/Outbreaks/HealthcareHepOutbreakTable.htm.

28. E. V. McKnight and L. Lollini, "Service above Self—Johnny Robertson's Story," Hepatitis Outbreaks National Organization for Reform, October 28, 2013, http://www.honoreform.org/blog/?p=141#more-141.

29. "What to Ask Healthcare Providers," One and Only Campaign, http://oneandonlycampaign.org/content/what-ask-healthcare-providers.

30. "Questions to Ask Your Doctor," Agency for Healthcare Research and Quality, http://www.ahrq.gov/patients-consumers/patient-involvement/ask-your-doctor/index.html.

31. H. Haskell, "Many Medical Errors Don't Happen in the Hospital but in Doctors' Offices," *TEDMED Great Challenges 2012* (unpublished).

32. T. Torrey, "How to Find a Doctor's Medical Malpractice Track Record," About.com, http://patients.about.com/od/doctorinformationwebsites/a/malpracticeinfo.htm.

33. R. Lieber, "Your Money: The Web Is Awash in Reviews, but Not for Doctors. Here's Why," *New York Times,* March 9, 2012, http://www.nytimes.com/2012/03/10/your-money/why-the-web-lacks-authoritative-reviews-of-doctors.html?pagewanted=all.

34. "How to Choose a Doctor," ConsumerReports.org, March 2013, http://www.consumerreports.org/cro/2012/12/how-to-choose-a-doctor/index.htm.

35. "About FDA: What Does FDA Do?" US Food and Drug Administration, http://www.fda.gov/aboutfda/transparency/basics/ucm194877.htm.

36. "Fast Facts on US Hospitals," American Hospital Association, http://www.aha.org/research/rc/stat-studies/fast-facts.shtml.

37. A. Young, H. Chaudhry, J. Thomas, et al., "A Census of Actively Licensed Physicians in the United States," 2010. *Journal of Medical Regulation* 96 (2011):11.

38. M. Beck, "U.S. News: More Doctors Steer Clear of Medicare," *Wall Street Journal,* July 29, 2013, http://online.wsj.com/news/articles/SB10001424127887323971204578626151017241898.

39. "Legislative Reference," American Association for Accreditation of Ambulatory Surgery Facilities, Inc., http://www.aaaasf.org/pub/OPT_Legislative_Reference.pdf.

40. "Clinic Outcry Grows," *Las Vegas Review Journal,* February 29, 2008, http://www.reviewjournal.com/news/clinic-outcry-grows.

41. M. Glabman, "Lobbyists That the Founders Just Never Dreamed Of," *Managed Care Magazine,* August 2002, http://www.managedcaremag.com/archives/0208/0208.lobbying.html.

42. K. Johnson, "Denver Woman Sentenced in Hepatitis Infection Case," *New York Times,* February 24, 2010, http://www.nytimes.com/2010/02/25/us/25hepatitis.html?_r=0.

43. M. Guillermo, "Dipak Desai Gets Life in Prison in Hep C Outbreak Case," KVVU Broadcasting Corporation, January 2, 2014, http://www.fox5vegas.com/story/23780441/dipak-desai-gets-life-in-prison-in-hep-c-outbreak-case.

44. M. R. Yessian and M. B. Kvaal, "Quality Assurance Activities of Medical Licensure Authorities in the United States and Canada," US Department of Health and Human Services Office of Inspector General, http://oig.hhs.gov/oei/reports/oei-01-89-00561.pdf .

45. "CertiFacts Online Frequently Asked Questions," American Board of Medical Specialties, http://www.certifacts.org/faq.html#14.

46. "HHS Has Taken Steps to Address Unsafe Injection Practices, but More Action Is Needed," US Government Accountability Office, July 2012, GAO-12-712.

47. T. Gandhi and T. Lee, "Patient Safety beyond the Hospital," *New England Journal of Medicine* 363 (2010): 1003.

48. "Choosing a Patient Safety Organization: Tips for Hospitals and Health Care Providers," Agency for Healthcare Research and Quality, http://www.pso.ahrq.gov/sites/default/files/Choosing%20a%20PSO.pdf.

49. D. M. Berwick, "A Transatlantic Review of the NHS at 60," Physicians for a National Health Program, July 1, 2008, http://www.pnhp.org/news/2010/may/a-transatlantic-review-of-the-nhs-at-60.

7. PRESCRIPTION DRUGS—TO HEAL AND TO HARM

1. L. Beletsky, J. D. Rich, and A. Y. Walley, "Prevention of Fatal Opioid Overdose," *JAMA* 308 (2012): 1863–1864.

2. J. Whalen, D. Barrett, and P. Loftus, "Glaxo in $3 Billion Settlement," *Wall Street Journal,* July 3, 2012.

3. A. Van Zee, "The Promotion and Marketing of OxyContin: Commercial Triumph, Public Health Tragedy," *American Journal of Public Health* 99 (2009): 221–227.

4. K. Outterson, "Punishing Health Care Fraud—Is the GSK Settlement Sufficient?" *New England Journal of Medicine* 367 (2012): 1082–1085.

5. A. C. Logan, V. Yank, and R. S. Stafford, "Off-Label Use of Recombinant Factor VIIa in U.S. Hospitals: Analysis of Hospital Records," *Annals of Internal Medicine* 154 (2011): 516–522.

6. R. S. Stafford, "Regulating Off-Label Drug Use—Rethinking the Role of the FDA," *New England Journal of Medicine* 358 (2008): 1427–1429.

7. J. M. Davis, E. M. Connor, and A. J. J. Wood, "The Need for Rigorous Evidence on Medication Use in Preterm Infants—Is It Time for a Neonatal Rule?" *JAMA* 308 (2012): 1435–1436.

8. Public Citizen, accessed February 11, 2014, http://www.worstpills.org/includes/page.cfm?op_id=552.

9. W. A. Ray, K. T. Murray, K. Hall, et al., "Azithromycin and the Risk of Cardiovascular Death," *New England Journal of Medicine* 366 (2012): 1881–1890.

10. M. Mitka, "Drug for Severe Sepsis Is Withdrawn from Market, Fails to Reduce Mortality," *JAMA* 306 (2011): 2439–2440.

11. K. Fain, M. Daubreese, and G. C. Alexander, "The Food and Drug Administration Amendments Act and Postmarketing Commitments," *JAMA* 310 (2013): 202–203.

12. Institute of Medicine, *Ethical and Scientific Issues in Studying the Safety of Approved Drugs* (Washington, DC: National Academies Press, 2012), accessed March 24, 2014, http://tinyurl.com/cxovshm.

13. Food and Drug Administration, Patients and physicians may report drug side effects here, accessed March 24, 2014.

14. A. Slomski, "Falls from Taking Multiple Medications May Be a Risk for Both Young and Old," *JAMA* 307 (2012): 1127–1128.

15. C. Feudtner, D. Dai, K. R. Hexem, et al., "Prevalence of Polypharmacy among Hospitalized Children in the United States," *Archives of Pediatric and Adolescent Medicine* 166 (2011): 9–16.

16. D. Garfinkel and D. Mangin, "Feasibility Study of a Systematic Approach for Discontinuation of Multiple Medications in Older Adults," *Archives of Internal Medicine* 170 (2010): 1648–1654.

17. ProPublica. This is a public interest journalism group. To learn about doctor prescribing practices under Medicare Part D in 2011, visit http://projects.propublica.org/checkup/, accessed March 24, 2014.

18. M. Gheorghaide, W. A. Gattis, and C. M. O'Conner, "Treatment Gaps in the Pharmacologic Management of Heart Failure," *Reviews in Cardiovascular Medicine* 3 (2002): S11–S19.

19. A. Goyal and W. A. Borenstein, "Health System-Wide Quality Programs to Improve Blood Pressure Control," *JAMA* 310 (2013): 695–696.

20. R. R. Khanna, R. G. Victor, K. Bibbins-Domingo, et al., "Missed Opportunities for Treatment of Uncontrolled Hypertension at Physician Office Visits in the United States, 2005 through 2009," *Archives of Internal Medicine* 172 (2012): 1344–1345.

21. J. T. James, *A Sea of Broken Hearts—Patient Rights in a Dangerous, Profit-Driven Health Care System* (Bloomington, IN: Author-House, 2007).

22. J. N. Cohn, P. R. Kowey, P. K. Whelton, and M. Prisant, "New Guidelines for Potassium Replacement in Clinical Practice," *Archives of Internal Medicine* 160 (2000): 2429–2436.

23. W. B. Borden, R. F. Redberg, A. I. Mushlin, et al., "Patterns and Intensity of Medical Therapy in Patients Undergoing Percutaneous Coronary Intervention," *JAMA* 305 (2011): 1882–1889.

24. C. M. Bell, S. S. Brener, N. Gunraj, et al., "Association of ICU or Hospital Admission with Unintentional Discontinuation of Medications for Chronic Diseases," *JAMA* 306 (2011): 840–847.

25. J. M. Kahn and D. C. Angus, "Going Home on the Right Medications—Prescription Errors and Transitions of Care," *JAMA* 306 (2011): 878–879.

26. Open Notes. This is a project by which doctors' notes about the care of a patient can be easily viewed by the patient. To learn more visit http://www.myopennotes.org/, accessed March 24, 2014.

27. A. Ahmad, G. Nijpels, J. M. Dekker, et al., "Effect of a Pharmacist Medication Review in Elderly Patients Discharged From the Hospital," *Archives of Internal Medicine* 172 (2012): 1346–1347.

28. H. D. Nelson, B. Smith, J. C. Griffin, and R. Fu, "Use of Medications to Reduce Risk for Primary Breast Cancer: A Systematic Review for the U.S. Preventive Services Task Force," *Annals of Internal Medicine* 158 (2013): 604–614.

29. Mayo Clinic: accessed March 24, 2014, http://www.mayoclinic.com/health/breast-cancer-prevention/WO00091.

30. E. Basch, "Toward Patient-Centered Drug Development in Oncology," *New England Journal of Medicine* 369 (2013): 397–400.

31. J. C. Weeks, P. J. Catalano, A. Cronin, et al., "Patients' Expectations about Effects of Chemotherapy for Advanced Cancer," *New England Journal of Medicine* 367 (2012): 1616–1625.

32. J. E. Bekelman, M. Kim, and E. J. Emanuel, "Toward Accountable Cancer Care," *JAMA Internal Medicine* 173 (2013): 958–959.

33. P. B. Bach, "Reforming the Payment System for Medical Oncology," *JAMA* 310 (2013): 261–262.

34. T. J. Smith and B. E. Hillner, "Bending the Cost Curve in Cancer Care," *New England Journal of Medicine* 364 (2011): 2065.

35. M. Mitka, "Nursing Home Antipsychotics," *JAMA* 307 (2012): 134. The testimony can be found at https://oig.hhs.gov/testimony/docs/2011/levinson_testimony_11302011.pdf, accessed March 24, 2014.

36. Center for Medicare and Medicaid Services, Press Release: http://www.cms.gov/Newsroom/MediaReleaseDatabase/Press-Releases/2013-Press-Releases-Items/2013-08-27.html, accessed March 24, 2014.

37. American Board of Internal Medicine Foundation, Choosing Wisely may be found at http://www.choosingwisely.org/doctor-patient-lists/american-geriatrics-society/, accessed March 24, 2014.

38. C. M. Hughes and M. M. Tunney, "Improving Prescribing of Antibiotics in Long-Term Care," *JAMA Internal Medicine* 173 (2013): 682–683.

39. K. Outterson, "Regulating Compounding Pharmacies after NECC," *New England Journal of Medicine* 367 (2012): 1969–1972.

40. Centers for Disease Control, accessed March 24, 2014, http://www.cdc.gov/hai/outbreaks/meningitis-map-large.html.

41. K. Outterson, "Regulating Compounding Pharmacies after NECC."

42. Ibid.

43. K. Outterson, "The Drug Quality and Security Act—Mind the Gaps," *New England Journal of Medicine* 370 (2014): 97–99.

44. Institute of Medicine, *Preventing Medication Errors Ethical* (Washington, DC: National Academies Press, 2007), 4.

45. Food and Drug Administration. Compare the intentions of the FDA and the slow progress by visiting these sites, the first from a lanned hearing in getting information to the public in 2010 and the second from 2013: http://ww.fda.gov/drugs/newsevents/ucm219716.html, accessed March 24, 2014, and three years later there is finally a working site: http://www.fda.gov/Drugs/ResourcesForYou/Consumers/default.htm, accessed March 24, 2014.

46. Institute of Medicine, *Ethical and Scientific Issues in Studying the Safety of Approved Drugs* (Washington, DC: National Academies Press, 2012), 14.

47. Consumers Reports Best Buy Drugs, http://www.consumerreports.org/health/best-buy-drugs/index.html, accessed March 24, 2014.

48. R. D. Strand, *Death by Prescription—The Shocking Truth Behind an Overmedicated Nation* (Nashville, TN: Thomas Nelson Publishers, 2003).

49. M. Angell, *The Truth about the Drug Companies—How They Deceive Us and What to Do About It* (New York: Random House, 2004).

50. B. Goldacre, *Bad Pharma—How Drug Companies Mislead Doctors and Harm Patients* (New York: Faber and Faber, 2012).

51. D. Healy, *Pharmageddon* (Berkeley: University of California Press, 2012).

52. P. Gotzsche, *Deadly Medicines and Organised Crime—How Big Pharma Has Corrupted Healthcare* (London: Ratcliffe Publishing, 2013 A. Linsky, "Reversing Gears—Discontinuing Medication Therapy to Prevent Adverse Events," *JAMA Internal Medicine* 173 (2013): 524–525.

53. N. E. Morden, L. M. Schwartz, E. S. Fisher, et al., "Accountable Prescribing," *New England Journal of Medicine* 369 (2013): 299–302 and *Deadly Medicines and Organised Crime—How Big Pharma Has Corrupted Healthcare* (2013).

54. A. Linsky, "Reversing Gears—Discontinuing Medication Therapy to Prevent Adverse Events," *JAMA Intewrnal Medicine* 173 (2013): 524–525.

55. H. Hamilton, P. Gallagher, C. Ryan, et al., "Potentially Inappropriate Medications Defined by STOPP Criteria and the Risk of Adverse Drug Events in Older Hospitalized Patients," *Archives of Internal Medicine* 171 (2011): 1013–1019.

56. D. R. Levinson, "Prescribers with Questionable Patterns in Medicare Part D," Office of Inspector General of the Department of Health and Human Services, 2013, accessed March 24, 2014, http://oig.hhs.gov/oei/reports/oei-02-09-00603.pdf.

8. AFTER THE HARM:
APOLOGY, DISCLOSURE, AND TRUST

1. Carol B. Liebman and Chris Stern Hyman, "A Mediation Skills Model to Manage Disclosure of Errors and Adverse Events to Patients," *Health Affairs* 23, no. 4 (2004): 22, accessed August 23, 2013. doi: 10.1377/hlthaff.23.4.22.

2. Atul Gawande, "Big Med: Restaurant Chains Have Managed to Combine Quality Control, Cost Control, and Innovation. Can Health Care?" *New Yorker,* August 13, 2012, accessed September 19, 2013, http://www.newyorker.com/reporting/2012/08/13/120813fa_fact_gawande.html.

3. Albert W. Wu, Thomas A. Cavanaugh, Stephen J. McPhee, Bernard Lo, and Guy P. Micco, "To Tell the Truth: Ethical and Practical Issues in Disclosing Medical Mistakes to Patients," *Journal of General Internal Medicine,* 12 (1997), accessed August 20, 2013. doi: 10.1046/j.1525-1497.1997.07163.

4. Maggie Little, "Engaging Bioethics: A Field without Apology," *The Hoya: Georgetown University's Newspaper,* September 24, 2013, accessed December 5, 2013, http://www.thehoya.com/engaging-bioethics-an-approach-to-ethics-rooted-in-architecture.html. More than that, many doctors work in hospitals or clinical settings that are woefully underequipped in basic quality control. As Atul Gawande, a physician who has long advocated admitting to errors in medicine, has pointed out, quality control systems common to other industries, from aviation to the restaurant industry, have evaded the medical profession. Whatever the root causes of medical error, though, apology needs to become a critical part of its aftermath. But the real change has to be a cultural one. Apology needs to be seen as a sign of caring, not a sign of weakness. If airlines can apologize when a flight has been delayed, doctors should be able to apologize when a surgery goes awry.

5. Andrew Garman and Linda Scribner, "Leading for Quality in Healthcare: Development and Validation of a Competency Model," *Journal of Healthcare Management,* November 1, 2011, accessed July 7, 2013, http://www.biomedsearch.com/article/Leading-quality-in-healthcare-development/274519826.html.

6. Doug Wojcieszak, James W. Saxton, and Maggie M. Finkelstein, *Sorry Works! Disclosure, Apology, and Relationships Prevent Medical Malpractice Claims* (Indiana: AuthorHouse, 2010), accessed July 17, 2013, http://books.google.com/books.

7. Liebman and Hyman, "A Mediation Skills Model to Manage Disclosure of Errors and Adverse Events to Patients," 25.

8. Denise Atwood, "Impact of Medical Apology Statutes and Policies," *Journal of Nursing Law* 12, no. 1 (2008): 44.

9. Luis Fabregas, "New PA Law Allows Doctors to Be Human," *TribLive,* December 7, 2013, accessed December 10, 2013, http://triblive.com/opinion/luisfabregas/4614305-74.

10. Paul Carpenter, "Benevolent Gesture Law Means Medical People Can Display Human Impulses," *Morning Call,* October 30, 2013, accessed November 5, 2013, http://articles.mcall.com/2013-10-30/news/mc-pc-benevolent-gesture-legislation-20131029.

11. Duncan MacCourt and Joseph Bernstein, "Medical Error Reduction and Tort Reform through Private, Contractually Based Quality Medicine Societies," *American Journal of Law and Medicine* 35, no. 4 (2009): 505.

12. Allen Kachalia and Michelle M. Mello, "New Directions in Medical Liability Reform," *New England Journal of Medicine* 364, no. 16 (2011), accessed January 11, 2014, doi/full/10.1056/NEJMhpr1012821.

13. Atwood, "Impact of Medical Apology Statutes and Policies," 44. Health care systems with established medical apology policies and programs have increased efficacy in resolving disputes without litigation and show a demonstrated cost savings as a result. A medical apology program in conjunction with mediation is a much more efficient and effective way to find the truth, resolution, and forgiveness.

14. Ibid.

15. Rachel Zimmerman, "Delicate Doctoring Moments: A Medical Error by Another Physician," *Common Health Reform and Reality*, November 1, 2013, accessed February 20, 2014, http://commonhealth.wbur.org.

16. Kate Davidson, "How Much Is an Apology Worth?" *Marketplace Economy*, November 12, 2013, accessed January 3, 2014, http://www.marketplace.org.

17. Little, "Engaging Bioethics: A Field without Apology."

18. Ibid.

19. Tanya Albert, "Preventing Lawsuits: Coalition Pushes Apologies and Cash Up-Front," *American Medical Association News*, February 7, 2005, accessed October 20, 2013, http://www.amednews.com/article/20050207/profession/302079966/2/.

20. Benjamin Ho and Elaine Liu, "Does Sorry Work? The Impact of Apology Laws on Medical Malpractice" (Job Market Paper: Cornell University and University of Houston, 2010), accessed September 14, 2013, http://irving.vassar.edu/faculty/bh/Ho-Liu-Apologies-and-Malpractice-nov15.pdf.

21. Sheri J. Welch, "Quality Matters: Deny and Defend: Apologizing Hampered by Physician Culture Risk Management," *Emergency Medicine News*, March 2011, accessed June 30, 2014, http://journals.lww.com/em-news/Fulltext/2011/03000/Quality_Matters__Deny_and_Defend__Apologizing.12.aspx

22. Little, "Engaging Bioethics: A Field without Apology."

23. Atwood, "Impact of Medical Apology Statutes and Policies," 44.

24. Alan J. Belsky, "PA Medical Apology Law Soon to Take Effect, JHU Study Shows Lack of Courtesy among Young Doctors," Maryland Malpractice Lawyer (blog), December 6, 2013 (5:00 a.m.), http://www.marylandmalpracticelawyers.com/2013/12/pa-medical-apology-law-soon-to-take-effect-jhu-study-shows-lack-of-courtesy-among-young-doctors.html.

25. Fabregas, "New PA Law Allows Doctors to Be Human."

26. Associated Press, "Governor Signs Web Privacy, DNA Collection, Medical Apology Bills," Channel3000, April 8, 2014, http://www.channel3000.com/news/politics/governor-signs-web-privacy-dna-collection-medical-apology-bills/25383378?item=1.

27. Rhode Island General Assembly, "An Act Related to Courts and Civil Procedure: Admissibility of Health Care Providers' Reports of Medical and Health Care Errors," January 2014, accessed February 28, http://lawprofessors.typepad.com/tortsprof/2014/01/ri-medical-apology-bill-introduced.html and http://lawprofessors.typepad.com/tortsprof/2014/01/ri-medical-apology-bill-introduced.html.

28. Art Caplan, interviewed by Robin Young, *Here and Now*, "Penn Joins States with I'm Sorry Law," 90.9WBUR FM, October 25, 2013.

29. Ibid.

30. Lee Taft, "Disclosing Unanticipated Outcomes: A Challenge to Providers and Their Lawyers," *Taft Solutions, AHLA Essay* (2008), 13.

31. Ibid., 14.

32. Marilyn M. Singleton, "I'm Sorry for Your Loss," *AAPS A Voice for Private Physicians*, November 11, 2013, accessed February 8, 2014, http://www.aapsonline.org/index.php/site/article/im_sorry_for_your_loss/.

33. Liebman and Hyman, "A Mediation Skills Model to Manage Disclosure of Errors and Adverse Events to Patients," 27.

34. Ibid., 24.

35. Dan Shapiro, "Beyond the Blame: A No-Fault Approach to Malpractice," *New York Times*, September 23, 2003, accessed November 17, 2013, http://www.nytimes.com/2003/09/23/health/essay-beyond-the-blame-a-no-fault-approach-to-malpractice.html.

36. Charles Vincent, "Understanding and Responding to Adverse Events," *New England Journal of Medicine* 348, no. 11 (2003): 1055.

37. Liebman and Hyman, "A Mediation Skills Model to Manage Disclosure of Errors and Adverse Events to Patients," 28.

38. Maggie Little, "Engaging Bioethics: A Field without Apology."

39. Michael Kirsch, "How Should a Physician Apologize after a Medical Error?" *KevinMD*, December 18, 2013, http://www.kevinmd.com/blog/2013/12/physician-apologize-medical-error.html.

40. Liebman and Hyman, "A Mediation Skills Model to Manage Disclosure of Errors and Adverse Events to Patients," 24.

41. Ibid., 29.

42. Maggie Little, "Engaging Bioethics: A Field without Apology."

43. Liebman and Hyman, "A Mediation Skills Model to Manage Disclosure of Errors and Adverse Events to Patients," 25.

44. Ibid., 24.

9. THE CONSUMER ADVOCATES WHO KICKED THE HOSPITAL-INFECTION NEST

1. Consumers Union is the policy and advocacy division of *Consumer Reports*.

2. Tom Vallier, e-mail to author, October 27, 2003.

3. *Consumer Reports*, "How Safe Is Your Hospital?" January 2003, p. 16.

4. MMWR Weekly, February 25, 2000, "Fourth Decennial International Conference on Nosocomial and Healthcare-Associated Infections," accessed April 27, 2014, http://www.cdc.gov/mmwr/preview/mmwrhtml/mm4907a4.htm.

5. The Stop Hospital Infections campaign was expanded in 2009, adding work on medical errors, medical implant safety, and accountability for physicians to our advocacy to eliminate health care–acquired infections. The campaign is now called the Safe Patient Project.

6. HHS, updated April 27, 2014, accessed April 27, 2014, http://www.health.gov/hai/prevent_hai.asp.

7. R. M. Klevens, J. R. Edwards, C. L. Richards, et al., "Estimating Health Care-Associated Infections and Deaths in U.S. Hospitals, 2002," *Public Health Reports* 122 (2007): 160–166.

8. Illinois General Assembly, accessed April 27, 2014, http://www.ilga.gov/legislation/BillStatus.asp?GA=93&DocTypeID=SB&DocNum=59&GAID=3&SessionID=3&LegID=491.

9. M. J. Berens, "Investigation: Unhealthy Hospitals—Infection Epidemic Carves Deadly Path," *Chicago Tribune*, July 21, 2002, accessed April 27, 2014, http://www.chicagotribune.com/news/chi-0207210272jul21,0,2177158.story.

10. *Pittsburgh Post-Gazette*, accessed April 24, 2014, http://old.post-gazette.com/pg/04040/270958.stm; http://old.post-gazette.com/pg/04065/281295.stm; the hospital-acquired infection reports are now issued by the Pennsylvania health department rather than PHC4, but PHC4 continues to include infections in its analyses of hospital quality and costs.

11. Consumers Union Safe Patient Project, posted January 4, 2010, accessed April 27, 2014, http://safepatientproject.org/document/model_hospital_infections_disclosure_act.

12. PennPIRG, accessed April 27, 2014, http://www.pennpirg.org/.

13. R. Rundle, "Some Push to Make Hospitals Disclose Rates of Infection," *Wall Street Journal*, February 1, 2005, http://online.wsj.com/news/articles/SB110722521039541957.

14. Ibid.

15. Ray Wagner e-mail to author about improving Missouri law, February 4, 2014.

16. Lisa Freeman e-mail to author, forwarding e-mail from Connecticut State Representative John Stripp, April 11, 2006.

17. K. O'Connell, "Two Arms, Two Choices: If Only I'd Known Then What I Know Now," *Health Affairs* 31, no.8 (2012):1895–1899. doi: 10.1377/hlthaff.2011.1158.

18. Ibid.

19. K. Jewell and L. McGiffert, "To Err Is Human, to Delay Is Deadly," May 2009, 4, http://safepatientproject.org/safepatientproject.org/pdf/safepatientproject.org-ToDelayIsDeadly.pdf, accessed May 12, 2014.

20. *Consumer Reports*, "Hospitals Will Have to Pay for Their Mistakes," September 2008, http://www.consumerreports.org/cro/aboutus/mission/viewpoint/hospitals-will-have-to-pay-for-their-mistakes/overview/hospitals-paying-for-their-mistakes-ov.htm, accessed May 8, 2014.

21. Gene Cenci and Jeanne Keller e-mails to author, May 2005.

22. Maryland Hospital Association Council on Legislative and Regulatory Policy, minutes, January 14, 2005.

23. C. A. Muto, J. A. Jernigan, B. E. Ostrowsky, et al., "SHEA Guideline for Preventing Nosocomial Transmission of Multidrug-Resistant Strains of Staphylococcus aureus and Enterococcus," *Infection Control and Hospital Epidemiology* 24 (2003): 362–386.

24. M. Bennett, *My Father: An American Story of Courage, Shattered Dreams, and Enduring Love* (privately published, 2011), accessed April 24, 2014, http://www.amazon.com/My-Father-American-Shattered-Enduring/dp/0615553052/ref=sr_1_sc_1?ie=UTF8&qid=1329709796&sr=8-1-spell.

25. A dedicated advocate, State Senator Jackie Speier passed a bill in 2006, but it ended badly with a weakened compromise that mostly put into place some infection control requirements for hospitals. In hindsight, probably the most significant provision was to require every hospital to develop an antibiotic stewardship program.

26. Nile's Project, accessed April 27, 2014, http://www.nilesproject.com/.

27. Ibid.

28. Senators Elaine Alquist and Dean Florez both sponsored legislation; Alquist's was the one that eventually required public reporting. Beth Capell, who was representing Service Employees International Union, helped tremendously with her lobbying expertise.

29. Consumers Union Safe Patient Project, "Preventable Harm: California Fails to Follow through with Patient Safety Laws," March 2010, accessed April 27, 2014, http://safepatientproject.org/CAPatientSafetyReportFinal_2.pdf.

30. Consumers Union Safe Patient Project, accessed April 27, 2014, http://safepatientproject.org/document/cu_testifies_at_senate_hearing_about_californias_lax_enforcement_of_patient_safety_laws; http://safepatientproject.org/document/testimony_of_advocate_carole_moss_before_ca_senate_health_committee.

31. California Healthline, "Judge Upholds Requirements on Reporting of Hospital Infections," June 23, 2011, accessed April 27, 2014, http://www.californiahealthline.org/articles/2011/6/23/judge-upholds-requirements-on-reporting-of-hospital-infections.

32. Texas Department of State Health Services, "Recommendations and Key Findings Advisory Panel on Health Care-Associated Infections Submitted to Meet the Reporting Requirements of SB 872, 79th Legislature, Regular Session," 2006, 3.

33. "Model Legislation on Public Reporting of Healthcare-Associated Infections," Association for Professionals in Infection Control and Epidemiology, Infectious Diseases Society of America, and the Society for Healthcare Epidemiology of America, January 17, 2006. In 2005, CU worked with the National Conference of Insurance Legislators (NCOI) as it adopted a model hospital infection reporting law that closely followed the one we helped to pass in New York. NCOI Letter: "Lawmakers Unanimously Adopt Patient Safety Model Law, Support Medical Error Reporting," December 2005, 3, accessed April 27, 2014, http://www.ncoil.org/news/2005_NewsLetters/December2005.pdf.

34. Centers for Disease Control and Prevention, Healthcare Infection Control Practices Advisory Committee, accessed April 27, 2014, http://www.cdc.gov/hicpac/.

35. Ibid. Klevens, "Estimating Health Care-Associated Infections and Deaths in U.S. Hospitals, 2002," 160.

36. The guidance was released to coincide with the APIC national convention in February 2005 but was published in a peer-reviewed journal in May 2005.

37. L. McKibben, T. Horan, J. I. Tokars, et al., "Guidance on Public Reporting of Healthcare-Associated Infections: Recommendations of the Healthcare Infection Control Practices Advisory Committee," *American Journal of Infection Control* 33 (2005): 217–226.

38. Ibid., 217.

39. CDC media statement, "CDC Statement: Public Reporting of Healthcare Associated Infections," February 2, 2010, accessed April 27, 2014, http://www.cdc.gov/media/pressrel/2010/s100202.htm.

40. *Consumer Reports*, accessed April 27, 2014, http://www.consumerreports.org/cro/magazine-archive/2010/march/health/hospital-infections/ratings/hospital-infections-ratings.htm.

41. National Quality Forum, accessed April 27, 2014, http://www.qualityforum.org/Home.aspx.

42. Centers for Medicare and Medicaid Services, accessed April 27, 2014, http://www.cms.gov/Medicare/Medicare-Fee-for-Service-Payment/HospitalAcqCond/Hospital-Acquired_Conditions.html.

43. H. Wald, A. Richard, V. V. Dickson, and E. Capezuti, "Chief Nursing Officers' Perspectives on Medicare's Hospital-Acquired Conditions Non-Payment Policy: Implications for Policy Design and Implementation," *Implementation Science* 7 (2012): 78, accessed April 27, 2014, http://www.implementationscience.com/content/7/1/78.

44. The National Nosocomial Infection Surveillance System (NNIS) began in 1970. "Monitoring Hospital-Acquired Infections to Promote Patient Safety—United States, 1990-1999," *MMWR Weekly* 49 (2000): 149–153.

45. Testimony of Ed Lawton, House Committee on Oversight and Government Reform, April 16, 2008, accessed April 27, 2014, http://oversight-archive.waxman.house.gov/documents/20080416112456.pdf.

46. United States Government Accountability Office, "Health-Care-Associated Infections in Hospitals: Leadership Needed from HHS to Prioritize Prevention Practices and Improve Data on These Infections," testimony before the Committee on Oversight and Government Reform, House of Representatives, April 16, 2008, accessed April 27, 2014, http://www.gao.gov/new.items/d08673t.pdf.

47. United States Government Accountability Office, "Report to the Chairman, Committee on Oversight and Government Reform, House of Representatives: An Overview of State Reporting Programs and Individual Hospital Initiatives to Reduce Certain Infections," September 2008, accessed April 27, 2014, http://www.gao.gov/new.items/d08808.pdf.

48. R. D. Scott, "March 2009. The Direct Medical Costs of Healthcare Associated Infections in US Hospitals and the Benefits of Prevention," accessed April 27, 2014, http://www.cdc.gov/hai/pdfs/hai/scott_costpaper.pdf.

49. American Recovery and Reinvestment Act of 2009, P.L. 111-5.

50. Centers for Disease Control, accessed April 27, 2014, http://www.cdc.gov/hicpac/roster.html.

51. The Joint Commission, August 15, 2012, accessed April 27, 2014, http://www.jointcommission.org/surgical_care_improvement_project/.

52. 100,000 Lives Campaign, accessed April 27, 2014, http://www.ihi.org/Engage/Initiatives/Completed/5MillionLivesCampaign/Documents/Overview%20of%20the%20100K%20Campaign.pdf.

53. Centers for Medicare and Medicaid Services, accessed April 27, 2014, http://www.cms.gov/Medicare/Quality-Initiatives-Patient-Assessment-Instruments/hospital-value-based-purchasing/index.html?redirect=/hospital-value-based-purchasing/.

54. S. S. Magill, J. R. Edwards, W. Bamberg, et al., "Multistate Point-Prevalence Survey of Health Care–Associated Infections," *New England Journal of Medicine* 370 (2014): 1198–1208.

55. J. T. James, "A New, Evidence-Based Estimate of Patient Harms Associated with Hospital Care," *Journal of Patient Safety* 9 (2013):122–128.

10. MEDICAL GUIDELINES AND INFORMED CONSENT – ROUTES TO SAFER MEDICAL CARE

1. A. J. Rosoff, "Evidence-Based Medicine and the Law," *AHRQ: Research Findings and Reports*, http://www.ahrq.gov/research/findings/evidence-based-reports, accessed 10 May 2014.

2. M. J. Mehlman, "Medical Practice Guidelines as Malpractice Safe Harbors: Illusion or Deceit?" *Journal of Law, Medicine and Ethics* 40, no. 2 (Summer 2012): 286–300.

3. Mehlman, 286.

4. N. Brennan et al., "The Map of Medicine: A Review of Evidence for Its Impact on Healthcare," *Health Information and Libraries Journal* 28 (2011): 94.

5. IOM, Institute of Medicine (2011), "Clinical Practice Guidelines We Can Trust," http://tinyurl.com/3t9hj8t, accessed April 11, 2014.

6. P. J. Pronovost, "Enhancing Physicians' Use of Clinical Guidelines," *JAMA* 310 (2013): 2501.

7. R. M. Epstein, B. S. Alper, and T. E. Quill, "Communicating Evidence for Participatory Decision Making," *JAMA* 291 (2004): 2359–2366.

8. Roberta Carroll and Peggy L. B. Nakamura, eds., *Risk Management Handbook for Healthcare Organizations: Volume 1: The Essentials* (San Francisco, CA: John Wiley and Sons, 2011).

9. "Opinion 8.08—Informed Consent," American Medical Association, accessed April 26, 2014, .

10. Aceto v. Dougherty, 415 Mass. 654 (1993).

11. "Gross Negligence and Lack of Informed Consent," *Legal Info*, accessed April 26, 2014, www.legalinfo.com/content/medical-malpractice/gross-negligence-and-lack-of -informed-consent.html.

12. J. C. Schwartz, "A Dose of Reality for Medical Malpractice Reform," Advance online publication, *New York Law Review,* http://ssrn.com/abstract=2104964.

13. D. Meeker, T. K. Knight, M. W. Friedberg, et al., "Nudging Guideline-Concordant Antibiotic Prescribing—A Randomized Clinical Trial," *JAMA Internal Medicine* 174 (2014): 425–431.

14. B. R. Roman and D. A. Asch, "Faded Promises: The Challenge of Deadopting Low-Value Care," *Annals of Internal Medicine*, published online April 29, 2014, http://www.ncbi.nlm.nih.gov/pubmed/24781317.

15. "The Joint Commission Sentinel Event Alert: Issue 51," The Joint Commission, accessed April 26, 2014, http://www.jointcommission.org/sea_issue_51.

16. R. Bunting, "Healthcare Innovation Barriers: Results of a Survey of Certified Professional Healthcare Risk Managers," *Journal of Healthcare Risk Management* 31 (2012): 3–16.

17. J. T. James, "A New, Evidence-Based Estimate of Patient Harms Associated with Hospital Care," *Journal of Patient Safety* 9 (2013): 122–128.

18. G. Sharma, S. Awashi, A. Dixit, and G. Sharma, "Patient Safety Risk Assessment and Risk Management: A Review on Indian Hospitals," *Chronicles of Young Scientists* 2 (2011): 186–191.

19. P. Zrelak, G. Utter, S. Banafseh, et al., "Using the Agency for Healthcare Research and Quality Patient Safety Indicators for Targeting Nursing," *Journal of Nursing Care Quality* 27 (2012): 99–108.

20. L. Zipperer, and G. Amori, "Knowledge Management: An Innovative Risk Management Strategy," *Journal of Healthcare Risk Management* 30 (2011): 8–14.

21. Agency for Healthcare Research and Quality, "AHRQ Seeks to Help Patients Report Adverse Medical Events," September 24, 2012, accessed May 11, 2014, http://www.ihealthbeat.org/articles/2012/9/24/ahrq-seeks-to-help-patients-report-adverse-medical-events.

22. "Statement by The American Congress of Obstetricians on North Dakota Abortion Laws," American College of Obstetricians and Gynecologists, accessed April 11, 2014, http://www.acog.org/About_ACOG/News   Room/News-Releases/2013/North   -Dakota-Abortion-Laws.

11. MEDICAL IMAGING: DOES IT HELP?

1. C. J. Garvey and R. Hanlon, "Computed Tomography in Clinical Practice," *BMJ* 324 (2002): 1077–1088.

2. G. Liney, "Magnetic Resonance Imaging in Clinical Practice," Springer 2006, ISBN 184628161x.

3. J. Gruettner, "Clinical Assessment of Chest Pain and Guidelines for Imaging," *European Journal of Radiology* 81 (2012): 3663–3668.

4. A. Bleyer and G. Welch, "Effects of Three Decades of Screening Mammography in Breast Cancer," *New England Journal of Medicine* 367 (2012): 1998–2005.

5. C. O'Donoghue, M. Eklund, E. M. Ozanne, et al., "Aggregate Cost of Mammography Screening in the United States: Comparison of Current Practice and Advocated Guidelines," *Annals of Internal Medicine* 160 (2014): 145–153.

6. E. J. Emmanuel, "What Are the Health Care Cost Savings?" *JAMA* 307 (2012): 39–40.

7. S. V. Srinivas, R. A. Deyo, and Z. D. Berger, "Application of Less Is More," *Archives of Internal Medicine* 172 (2012):1016–1020.

8. A. Slomski, "Screening Women for Ovarian Cancer Still Does More Harm than Good," *JAMA* 307 (2012): 2474–2475.

9. T. S. Carey and C. G. Sheps, "Review: Routine Spinal Imaging Does Not Improve Clinical Outcomes in Low Back Pain," *Annals of Internal Medicine* 150 (2009): 6–7.

10. A. Martini, "What Patients Should Know about Imaging," The Hastings Center Report over 65 (online blog), 2013, 17.

11. M. Moss, "Mammography Team Learns from Its Errors," *New York Times,* June 28, 2002.

12. R. Smith-Bindman, P. Chu, D. L. Miglioretti, et al., "Physician Predictors of Mammographic Accuracy," *Journal of the National Cancer Institute* 97 (2005): 358–367.

13. E. Thompson, K. Mirocha, and K. B. Sagar, "Effect of Physician Training on Interpretation of Echocardiography," *Journal of the American Society of Echocardiography* 24 (2009): 54.

14. General Accounting Office, accessed April 15, 2015, http://tinyurl.com/mpwus6h.

15. V. M. Rao and D. C. Levin, "The Overuse of Diagnostic Imaging and the Choosing Wisely Initiative," *Annals of Internal Medicine* 157 (2012): 574–576.

16. S. Begley, "Some Medical Procedures Do More Harm Than Good," *Newsweek*, September 18, 2011 (front page).

17. O. Wegwarth and G. Gigerenzer, "Overdiagnosis and Overtreatment: Evaluation of What Physicians Tell Their Patients about Screening Harms," *JAMA Internal Medicine* 173 (2013): 2086–2088.

18. M. Bassett, "Shaming Doctors to Reduce Inappropriate Imaging? It's Worth a Try," *New York Times*, July 28, 2013.

Bibliography

42 USC 11101, *et seq*. Accessed April 28, 2014,http://www.npdb.hrsa.gov/resources/titleIv.jsp. For the secrecy provision, see 42 USC 11137(b).

42 USC 11111. Accessed April 28, 2014, http://www.law.cornell.edu/uscode/text/42/11111.

42 USC 11135. Accessed April 28, 2014, http://www.law.cornell.edu/uscode/text/42/11135.

ABIM. "Why Maintenance of Certification Matters." Accessed March 12, 2014, http://www.abim.org/pdf/publications/why-MOC-matters.pdf.

"About Dr. Roberts." Perlmutter Health Center.

"About FDA: What Does FDA Do?" US Food and Drug Administration. http://www.fda.gov/aboutfda/transparency/basics/ucm194877.htm .

"Accountable Care Organizations." Centers for Medicare and Medicaid Services, US Department of Health and Human Services. Accessed April 10, 2014, http://www.cms.gov/Medicare/Medicare-Fee-for-Service-Payment/ACO/.

Aceto v. Dougherty, 415 Mass. 654 (1993).

Adisa, A. O., Lawal, O. O., and Adejuyigbe, O. "Evaluation of Two Methods of Preoperative Hair Removal and Their Relationship to Postoperative Wound Infection." *Journal of Infection in Developing Countries* 5, no. 10 (2011): 717–722.

"Adverse Events in Skilled Nursing Facilities: National Incidence among Medicare Beneficiaries." Office of Inspector General. Accessed April 13, 2013, https://oig.hhs.gov/oei/reports/oei-06-11-00370.pdf .

Agency for Healthcare Research and Quality. "AHRQ Seeks to Help Patients Report Adverse Medical Events." September 24, 2012. Accessed May 11, 2014, http://www.ihealthbeat.org/articles/2012/9/24/ahrq-seeks-to-help-patients-report-adverse-medical-events .

———. "Questions to Ask Your Doctor." http://www.ahrq.gov/patients-consumers/patient-involvement/ask-your-doctor/index.html .

Ahmad. A., Nijpels, G., Dekker, J. M., et al. "Effect of a Pharmacist Medication Review in Elderly Patients Discharged From the Hospital." *Archives of Internal Medicine* 172 (2012): 1346–1347.

Albert, T. "Preventing Lawsuits: Coalition Pushes Apologies and Cash Up-Front." *American Medical Association News*, February 7, 2005. Accessed October 20, 2013, http://www.amednews.com/article/20050207/profession/302079966/2/.

Allen, L. A., Ambardekar, A. V., Devaraj, K. M., et al. "Clinical Problem-Solving: Missing Elements of the History." *New England Journal of Medicine* 370 (2014): 5595–5566.

American Academy of Orthopaedic Surgeons. "Current Concerns with Metal-on-Metal Hip Arthroplasty." December 2012. Accessed February 27, 2014, http://www.aaos.org/about/papers/advistmt/1035.asp.

American Board of Internal Medicine Foundation. Choosing Wisely. Accessed March 24, 2014,http://www.choosingwisely.org/doctor-patient-lists/american-geriatrics-society.

American College of Obstetricians and Gynecologists. "Statement by the American Congress of Obstetricians on North Dakota Abortion Laws." 2013. Accessed April 11, 2014, http://www.acog.org/About_ACOG/News-Room/News-Releases/2013/North-Dakota-Abortion-Laws.

American Medical Association. "Continuing Medical Education for Licensure Reregistration." Accessed March 14, 2014, http://www.ama-assn.org/resources/doc/med-ed-products/continuing-medical-education-licensure.pdf.

———. "Opinion 8.08—Informed Consent." 2014. Accessed April 26, 2014, www.ama-assn.org//ama/pub/physician-resources/medical ethics/code-medical-ethics/opinion808.page.

———. "Reporting Impaired, Incompetent or Unethical Colleagues." Accessed March 14, 2014, http://www.ama-assn.org//ama/pub/physician-resources/medical-ethics/code-medical-ethics/opinion9031.page.

American Recovery and Reinvestment Act of 2009, Public Law 111-5, Sec. 3001. Hospital Value-Based Purchasing Program.

American Social History Productions, Inc. "Upton Sinclair Hits His Readers in the Stomach." *History Matters: The US Survey Course on the Web.* http://historymatters.gmu.edu/d/572/.

Ameringer, C. F. *State Medical Boards and the Politics of Public Protection.* Baltimore, MD: John Hopkins University Press, 1999.

———. "State Medical Boards and the Problem of Unnecessary Care and Treatment." *Journal of Medical Regulation* 99 (2013): 25–32.

"An Accountable Care Organization." Kelsey-Seybold Clinic. Accessed April 10, 2014, http://www.kelsey-seybold.com/kelseycare/pages/what-is-an-accountable-care-organization.aspx.

Angell, M. *The Truth About the Drug Companies—How They Deceive Us and What to Do About It.* New York: Random House, 2004.

Anonymous. "A Randomized Trial of Propranolol in Patients with Acute Myocardial Infarction. I. Mortality Results." *JAMA* 247 (1982): 1707–1714. Accessed April 24, 2014, http://www.ncbi.nlm.nih.gov/pubmed/7038157.

Arfanis, K., Shillito, J., and Smith, A. F. "Risking Safety or Safely Risking? Healthcare Professionals' Understanding of Risk-Taking in Everyday Work." *Psychology, Health and Medicine* 16, no. 1 (2011): 66–73. doi:10.1080/13548506.2010.521566.

Arora, N., Patel, K., Engell, C. A., and Larosa, J. A. "The Effect of Interdisciplinary Team Rounds on Urinary Catheter and Central Venous Catheter Days and Rates of Infection." *American Journal of Medical Quality* (2013). Accessed April 30, 2014.

Ask. "How Many Hospitals Are in the USA? Most Current Hospital Data According to the U.S. Census Bureau." Accessed April 24, 2014, http://answers.ask.com/Education/Schools/how_many_hospitals_are_there_in_the_usa?ad=semD&an=google_s&am=broad&o=2731.

Associated Press. "Governor Signs Web Privacy, DNA Collection, Medical Apology Bills." *Channel3000,* April 8, 2014. Accessed April 15, 2014, http://www.channel3000.com/news/politics/governor-signs-web-privacy-dna-collection-medical-apology-bills/25383378?item=1.

Association for Professionals in Infection Control and Epidemiology, Infectious Diseases Society of America, and the Society for Healthcare Epidemiology of America. "Model Legislation on Public Reporting of Healthcare-Associated Infections." January 17, 2006.

Association of American Medical Colleges. Accessed April 24, 2014, https://www.aamc.org/newsroom/newsreleases/358410/20131024.html.

Atwood, D. "Impact of Medical Apology Statutes and Policies." *Journal of Nursing Law* 12 (2008): 43–53.

Audet, A-M. J., Doty, M. M., Shamasdin, J., and Schoenbaum, S. C. "Measure, Learn, and Improve: Physicians' Involvement in Quality Improvement." *Health Affairs* 24 (2005): 843–853. doi: 10.1377/hlthaff.24.3.843.

Bach, P. B. "Reforming the Payment System for Medical Oncology," *JAMA* 310 (2013): 261–262.

Banja, J. "The Normalization of Deviance in Healthcare Delivery." *Business Horizons* 53 (2010): 139. doi:10.1016/j.bushor.2009.10.006.

Basch, E. "Toward Patient-Centered Drug Development in Oncology," *New England Journal of Medicine* 369 (2013): 397–400.

Bassett, M. "Shaming Docs to Reduce Inappropriate Imaging? It's Worth a Try." *Fierce Medical Imaging,* July 28, 2013. Accessed April 29, 2014, http://www.fiercemedicalimaging. com/story/shaming-docs-reduce-inappropriate-imaging-its-worth-try/2013-07-28.

Battard-Menendez, J. "The Impetus for Legislation Revoking the Joint Commission's Deemed Status as a Medicare Accrediting Agency." *JONA'S Healthcare Law, Ethics, and Regulation* 12 (2010): 69–76. Accessed April 28, 2010, http://www.ncbi.nlm.nih.gov/pubmed/ 20733410.

Beck, M. "U.S. News: More Doctors Steer Clear of Medicare." *Wall Street Journal,* July 29, 2013. http://online.wsj.com/news/articles/.

Begley, S. "Some Medical Tests, Procedures Do More Harm Than Good." *Newsweek,* September 8, 2011. Accessed April 29, 2014, http://www.newsweek.com/some-medical-tests-procedures-do-more-harm-good-67291.

Bekelman, J. E., Kim, M., and Emanuel, E. J. "Toward Accountable Cancer Care." *JAMA Internal Medicine* 173 (2013): 958–959.

Beletsky, L., Rich, J. D., and Walley, A. Y. "Prevention of Fatal Opioid Overdose." *JAMA* 308 (2012): 1863–1864.

Bell, C. M., Brener, S. S., Gunraj, N., et al. "Association of ICU or Hospital Admission with Unintentional Discontinuation of Medications for Chronic Diseases." *JAMA* 306 (2011): 840–847.

Belsky, A. J. "PA Medical Apology Law Soon to Take Effect, JHU Study Shows Lack of Courtesy among Young Doctors." Maryland Malpractice Lawyer (blog). Accessed December 6, 2013, http://www.marylandmalpracticelawyers.com/2013/12/pa-medical-apology-law-soon-to-take-effect-jhu-study-shows-lack-of-courtesy-among-young-doctors.html.

Bennett, M. *My Father: An American Story of Courage, Shattered Dreams, and Enduring Love,* 2011.

Berens, M. J. "Investigation: Unhealthy Hospitals—Infection Epidemic Carves Deadly Path." *Chicago Tribune,* July 21, 2002.

Berge, K. H., Seppala, M. D., and Schipper, A. M. "Chemical Dependency and the Physician." *Mayo Clinic Proceedings* 84 (2009): 625–631.

Berwick, D. M. "A Transatlantic Review of the NHS at 60." *Physicians for a National Health Program,* July 1, 2008. http://www.pnhp.org/news/2010/may/a-transatlantic-review-of-the-nhs-at-60.

Bishop, T. "Cardiologist's License Revoked over Accusations of Placing Unneeded Stents." *Baltimore Sun.* Accessed April 28, 2014, http://articles.baltimoresun.com/2011-07-13/ health/ms-md-midei-license-revoked-20110713_1_midei-unneeded-stents-stent-business.

Blackmond, B. "Hospital Accreditation—Alternatives to the Joint Commission." Accessed April 28, 2014, http://www.healthlawyers.org/Events/Programs/Materials/Documents/ HHS09/blackmond.pdf.

Bleyer, A., and Welch, H. G. "Effect of Three Decades of Screening Mammography on Breast-Cancer Incidence." *New England Journal of Medicine* 367, no. 21 (November 22, 2012): 1998–2005. Accessed April 29, 2014, http://www.ncbi.nlm.nih.gov/pubmed/23171096. doi: 10.1056/NEJMoa1206809.

Boodman, S. "Rarely Mentioned Medical Mistake: Patients Harmed by High Rates of Misdiagnosis." *The California Report, State of Health.* Accessed April 16, 2014, http://blogs.kqed. org/stateofhealth/2013/05/07/doctors-mistakes-in-diagnosis-rarely-mentioned-harm-patients/.

Borden, W. B., Redberg, R. F., Mushlin, A. I., et al. "Patterns and Intensity of Medical Therapy in Patients Undergoing Percutaneous Coronary Intervention." *JAMA* 305 (2011): 1882–1889.

Bosk, C. L., Dixon-Woods, M., Goeschel, C. A., and Pronovost, P. J. "Reality Check for Checklists." *Lancet* 374, no. 9688 (2009): 444–445.

Boucher, H. W., Talbot, G. H., Benjamin, D. K., et al. "10 × '20 Progress—Development of New Drugs Active against Gram-Negative Bacilli: An Update from the Infectious Diseases Society of America." *Clinical Infectious Diseases* (2013).

Bowman, M. A., and Pearle, D. L. "Changes in Drug Prescribing Patterns Related to Commercial Company Funding of Continuing Medical Education." *Journal of Continuing Education Health Professions* 8 (1988):13–20. doi: 10.1002/chp.4750080104.

Brawley, O. W. *How We Do Harm—A Doctor Breaks Ranks about Being Sick in America* . New York: St. Martin's Press, 2012.

Brennan, N., Mattick, K., and Ellis, T. "The Map of Medicine: A Review of Evidence for Its Impact on Healthcare." *Health Information and Libraries Journal* 28, no. 2 (June 2011): 93–100. doi:10.1111/j.1471-1842.2011.00940.x.

Brennan, T. A., Horwitz, R. I., Duffy, D., et al. "The Role of Physician Specialty Board Certification Status in the Quality Movement." *JAMA* 292 (2004): 1038–1043. doi:10.1001/jama.292.9.1038.

Briesacher, B. A., Tjia, J., Field, T., et al. "Antipsychotic Use among Nursing Home Residents." *JAMA* 309 (2013): 440–442.

Brilli, R. J., McClead Jr., R. E., Crandall, W. V., et al. "A Comprehensive Patient Safety Program Can Significantly Reduce Preventable Harm, Associated Costs, and Hospital Mortality." *Journal of Pediatrics* 163, no. 6 (2013): 1638–1645.

Brown, E. G., Attorney General of the State of California, Case Number 02-2002-139527. Accessed April 28, 2014, http://www2.mbc.ca.gov/BreezePDL/document.aspx?path=%5cDIDOCS%5c20070508%5cDMRAAABI16%5c&did=AAABI070508224526093. DID&licenseType=A&licenseNumber=32120#page=1.

Brunton, L., Lazo, J., and Parker, K. *Goodman and Gilman's The Pharmacological Basis of Therapeutics*. 11th ed. New York: McGraw-Hill, 2005.

Bunting, R. "Healthcare Innovation Barriers: Results of a Survey of Certified Professional Healthcare Risk Managers." *Journal of Healthcare Risk Management* 31, no. 4 (2012): 3–16. doi:10.1002/jhrm.20099.

California Department of Public Health. Accessed April 28, 2014, http://www.cdph.ca.gov/programs/LnC/Pages/lnc.aspx.

California Healthline. "Judge Upholds Requirements on Reporting of Hospital Infections." June 23, 2011, http://www.californiahealthline.org/articles/2011/6/23/judge-upholds-requirements-on-reporting-of-hospital-infections.

Caplan, A. Interviewed by Robin Young. *Here and Now*. "Penn Joins States with I'm Sorry Law." 90.9 WBUR FM. October 25, 2013. Accessed November 13, 2013, http://hereandnow.wbur.org/2013/10/25/im-sorry-law.

Carey, J. "Medical Guesswork." *Business Week* , May 28, 2006. Accessed April 1, 2014, http://www.businessweek.com/stories/2006-05-28/medical-guesswork.

Carey, T. S., and Sheps, C. G. "Review: Immediate Routine Lumbar-Spine Imaging Does Not Improve Clinical Outcomes in Low-Back Pain." *Annals of Internal Medicine* 150, no. 12 (2009): JC6–7. Accessed http://annals.org/article.aspx?articleid=744411. doi:10.7326/0003-4819-150-12-200906160-02007.

Carroll, A. "Too Few Generalist Physicians Doesn't Necessarily Mean Too Many Specialists." June 26, 2013. Accessed April 24, 2014, http://newsatjama.jama.com/2013/06/26/too-few-generalist-physicians-doesnt-necessarily-mean-too-many-specialists/.

Carroll, R., and Nakamura, P. L. B., eds., 2011. *Risk Management Handbook for Healthcare Organizations: Volume 1: The Essentials*. San Francisco, CA: John Wiley and Sons, Inc.

Carpenter, P. "Benevolent Gesture Law Means Medical People Can Display Human Impulses." *Morning Call,* October 30, 2013. Accessed November 5, 2013, http://articles.mcall.com/2013-10-30/news/mc-pc-benevolent-gesture-legislation-20131029.

Caverly, T. J., Combs, B. P., Moriates, C., et al. "Too Much Medicine Happens Too Often." *JAMA Internal Medicine* 174 (2014): 8–9.

Centers for Disease Control and Prevention. "Media Statement, CDC statement: Public Reporting of Healthcare Associated Infections," media statement, February 2, 2010. Accessed April 15, 2014, http://www.cdc.gov/media/pressrel/2010/s100202.htm.

———. "Clostridium Difficile Infection." Accessed January 16, 2014, http://www.cdc.gov/HAI/organisms/cdiff/Cdiff_infect.html.

———. "Healthcare Facility HAI Reporting Requirements to CMS Via NHSN—Current Requirements" (2013).

————. "Making Health Care Safer: Stop Infections from Lethal CRE Germs." *CDC Vital Signs*, March 2013.

————. Accessed March 24, 2014, http://www.cdc.gov/hai/outbreaks/meningitis-map-large.html.

Centers for Medicare and Medicaid Services. Press Release. Accessed March 24, 2014, http://www.cms.gov/Newsroom/MediaReleaseDatabase/Press-Releases/2013-Press-Releases-Items/2013-08-27.html.

————. "Hospital-Acquired Conditions." Accessed April 15, 2014, http://www.cms.gov/Medicare/Medicare-Fee-for-Service-Payment/HospitalAcqCond/Hospital-Acquired_Conditions.html.

————. "Hospital Value Based Purchasing." Accessed April 15, 2014, http://www.cms.gov/Medicare/Quality-Initiatives-Patient-Assessment-Instruments/hospital-value-based-purchasing/index.html?redirect=/hospital-value-based-purchasing/.

————. Accessed April 28, 2014,http://www.gpo.gov/fdsys/pkg/CFR-2011-title42-vol5/pdf/CFR-2011-title42-vol5-sec482-21.pdf.

"CertiFacts Online Frequently Asked Questions." *American Board of Medical Specialties.* http://www.certifacts.org/faq.html#14.

Chen, D. T., Wynia, M. K., Moloney, R. M., and Alexander, G. C. "U.S. Physician Knowledge of the FDA-Approved Indications and Evidence Base for Commonly Prescribed Drugs: Results of a National Survey." *Pharmacoepidemiology Drug Safety* 18 (2009): 1094–1100. doi: 10.1002/pds.1825.

Chen, S. L., and Morgan, T. R. "The Natural History of Hepatitis C Virus (HCV) Infection." *International Journal of Medical Sciences* 3, no. 2 (2006): 47–52.

"Choosing a Patient Safety Organization: Tips for Hospitals and Health Care Providers." *Agency for Healthcare Research and Quality.* http://www.pso.ahrq.gov/sites/default/files/Choosing%20a%20PSO.pdf.

"Clinic Outcry Grows." *Las Vegas Review Journal,* February 29, 2008. http://www.reviewjournal.com/news/clinic-outcry-grows.

"Clinical Laboratory Improvement Amendments (CLIA)." *Centers for Medicare and Medicaid Services.* http://www.cms.gov/Regulations-and-Guidance/Legislation/CLIA/index.html?redirect=/clia/.

Cohn, J. N., Kowey, P. R., Whelton, P. K., and Prisant, L. M. "New Guidelines for Potassium Replacement in Clinical Practice." *Archives of Internal Medicine* 160 (2000): 2425–2429.

Colorado Department of Regulatory Agencies, Division of Registrations. "What Happens When You File a Complaint." Accessed April 16, 2014, http://www.dora.state.co.us/reg_investigations/file_complaint.htm.

Combs, V. "Activist Group Targets J&J and its Transvaginal Mesh Lawsuits with Social Media Attack." Medcity News. Accessed April 14, 2014, http://medcitynews.com/2014/04/activist-group-targets-jj-transvaginal-mesh-social-media-attack/?utm_source=MedCity+News+Subscribers&utm_campaign=2c710c8608-RSS_EMAIL_CAMPAIGN&utm_medium=email&utm_term=0_c05cce483a-2c710c8608-67014761.

Consumer Reports Best Buy Drugs. Accessed March 24, 2014, http://www.consumerreports.org/health/best-buy-drugs/index.htm.

Consumer Reports. "Hospitals Will Have to Pay for Their Mistakes." September 2008. Accessed May 8, 2014, http://www.consumerreports.org/cro/aboutus/mission/viewpoint/hospitals-will-have-to-pay-for-their-mistakes/overview/hospitals-paying-for-their-mistakes-ov.htm.

————. "Coming Clean on Hospital Infections." March 2010.

Consumers Union Safe Patient Project. "CU Testifies at Senate Hearing about California's Lax Enforcement of Patient Safety Laws." October 20, 2010. Accessed April 15, 2014, http://safepatientproject.org/document/cu_testifies_at_senate_hearing_about_californias_lax_enforcement_of_patient_safety_laws.

————. "Model Hospital Infection Disclosure Act." Accessed April 20, 2014, http://safepatientproject.org/document/model_hospital_infections_disclosure_act.

————. "Preventable Harm, California Fails to Follow through with Patient Safety Laws." March 2010. http://safepatientproject.org/CAPatientSafetyReportFinal_2.pdf.

————. "Testimony of Advocate Carole Moss before CA Senate Health Committee." October 20, 2010. Accessed April 15, 2014, http://safepatientproject.org/document/testimony_of_ advocate_carole_moss_before_ca_senate_health_committee.

Crowley, C. "Medical Board Soft on Doctors." *Times Union*, August 20, 2012. Accessed March 12, 2014, http://www.timesunion.com/local/article/Medical-board-softer-on-doctors-3798607.php.

Cullen, B. "Commission Case Reports." *Washington State Medical Quality Assurance Commission Update* 3. Winter 2013. Accessed April 16, 2014, http://www.doh.wa.gov/Portals/1/Documents/3000/658-002%28December2013%29.pdf.

Dahms, K., Sharkova, Y., Heitland, P., et al. "Cobalt Intoxication Diagnosed with the Help of Dr. House." *Lancet* 383 (2014): 573–574.

Davidson, K. "How Much is an Apology Worth?" *Marketplace Economy*, November 12, 2013. Accessed January 3, 2014, http://www.marketplace.org.

Davis, D. A., Mazmanian, P. E., Fordis, M., et al. "Accuracy of Physician Self-Assessment Compared with Observed Measures of Competence: A Systematic Review." *JAMA* 296 (2006):1094–1102. doi:10.1001/jama.296.9.1094.

Davis, J. M., Connor, E. M., and Wood, A. J. J. "The Need for Rigorous Evidence on Medication Use in Preterm Infants—Is It Time for a Neonatal Rule?" *JAMA* 308 (2012): 1435–1436.

Day, M. "Doctors Are Told to Ditch 'Disease Spreading' Neckties." *BMJ* 332, no. 7539 (2006): 442.

Deeny, S. R., Cooper, B. S., Cookson, B., et al. "Targeted Versus Universal Screening and Decolonization to Reduce Healthcare-Associated Mehicillin-Resistant Staphylococcus Aureus Infection." *Journal of Hospital Infection* 85, no. 1 (2013): 33–44.

Department of Health and Human Services. "National Action Plan to Prevent Health Care-Associated Infections: Road Map to Elimination." Accessed April 15, 2014, http://www.health.gov/hai/prevent_hai.asp#hai_plan.

Derbyshire, R. C. "How Effective is Medical Self-Regulation?" *Law and Human Behavior* 7 (1983): 193–202.

DesRoches, C. M., Rao, S. R., Fromson, J. A., et al. "Physicians' Perceptions, Preparedness for Reporting, and Experiences Related to Impaired and Incompetent Colleagues." *JAMA* 304 (2010): 187–193. doi: 10.1001/jama.2010.921.

DHHS. Office of Inspector General. "Federal Initiatives to Improve State Medical Boards' Performance," oei-01-93-00020, February 1993.

————. Office of Disability, Aging and Long-Term Care Policy, Office of the Assistant Secretary for Planning and Evaluation. *State Discipline of Physicians: Assessing State Medical Boards through Case Studies*, by Randall R. Bovbjerg, Pablo Aliaga, and Josephine Gittler. Contract #HHS-100-03-0011. Washington, DC, 2006. http://aspe.hhs.gov/daltcp/reports/2006/stdiscp.htm.

————. Office of Inspector General, Office of Analysis and Inspections. *Medical Licensure and Discipline: An Overview*. Control Number: P-01-86-00064, Boston, MA: 1986.

————. Office of Inspector General. *State Medical Boards and Medical Discipline*. oei-01-89-00560, August 1990.

————. *Performance Indicators, Annual Reports, and State Medical Discipline: A State-by-State Review*. oei-01-89-00563, July 1991.

————. *Federal Initiatives to Improve State Medical Boards' Performance*. oei-01-93-00020, February 1993.

Daneman, N., Gruneir, A., Bronskill, S. E., et al. "Prolonged Antibiotic Treatment in Long-Term Care." *JAMA Internal Medicine* 173 (2013): 673–682.

Dmyterko, K. "ASE: More Training Needed to Avoid Echo Discrepancies, High Costs." *Health Imaging*, June 14, 2010. Accessed April 29, 2014, http://www.healthimaging.com/topics/cardiovascular/ase-more-training-needed-avoid-echo-discrepancies-high-costs.

Donnon, T., Al Ansari, A., Al Alawi, S., and Violato, C. "The Reliability, Validity, and Feasibility of Multisource Feedback Physician Assessment: A Systematic Review." *Academic Medicine* 89 (2014): 1–6.

Douglas County Health Department. "Rating List Information." http://www. douglascountyhealth.com/food-a-drink/food-facility-ratings/rating-list-information.

Drake, D. "How Being a Doctor Became the Most Miserable Profession." Daily Beast. Accessed April 24, 2014, http://www.thedailybeast.com/articles/2014/04/14/how-being-a-doctor-became-the-most-miserable-profession.html.

Dubinsky, I., Jennings, K., Greengarten, M., and Brans, A. "360-Degree Physician Performance Assessment." *Healthcare Quarterly* 13 (2009): 71–76.

"Earn CME Credits on Your Own Time, Take the Vacation You Want and Get the Education You Need." Travel Medical Seminars.com. Accessed March 25, 2014, http://www. travelmedicalseminars.com/index.php.

Eddy, D. M. "Evidence-Based Medicine: A Unified Approach." *Health Affairs* 24 (2005): 9–17. doi: 10.1377/hlthaff.24.1.9.

Eisler, P., and Hansen, B. "Thousands of Doctors Practicing Despite Error, Misconduct." *USA Today*, August 20, 2013. Accessed March 20, 2014, http://www.usatoday.com/story/news/ nation/2013/08/20/doctors-licenses-medical-boards/2655513/.

Elbein, S. "Anatomy of a Tragedy." *Texas Observer*, August 28, 2013. Accessed March 20, 2014, http://www.texasobserver.org/anatomy-tragedy/.

Emanuel, E. J. "What Are the Health Care Cost Savings?" *JAMA* 307, no. 1 (2012): 39–40. doi:10.1001/jama.2011.1927. Accessed April 29, 2014, http://jama.jamanetwork.com/ article.aspx?articleid=1104822.

"Enhancing Patient Safety by Reducing Healthcare-Associated Infections: The Role of Discovery and Dissemination." *Infection Control and Hospital Epidemiology* 31, no. 2 (2010): 118–123.

Epstein, R. M., Alper, B. S., and Quill T. E. "Communicating Evidence for Participatory Decision Making." *Journal of the American Medical Association* 291, no. 19 (2004): 2359–2366. doi:10.1001/jama.291.19.2359.

Estey, M. P., Diamandis, E. P., Van Der Straeten, C., et al. "Cobalt and Chromium Measurement in Patients with Metal Hip Prostheses." *Clinical Chemistry* 59 (2013): 880–886.

Fábregas, L. "New PA Law Allows Doctors to Be Human." *TribLive*, December 7, 2013. Accessed December 10, 2013, http://triblive.com/opinion/luisfabregas/4614305-74.

Fain, K., Daubresse, M., and Alexander, C. G. "The Food and Drug Administration Amendments Act and Postmarketing Commitments," *JAMA* 310 (2013): 202–204.

"Fast Facts on US Hospitals." *American Hospital Association.* http://www.aha.org/research/rc/ stat-studies/fast-facts.shtml.

Federation of State Medical Boards. "The Exchange, vol. 1. Licensing Boards, Structure and Disciplinary Functions" (Euless, TX: FSMB, loose-leaf compilation), 2003.

———. "2009 State of States Physician Regulation." Accessed March 6, 2014, http://www. fsmb.org/pdf/2009_state_of_states.pdf.

———."Summary of 2010 Board Actions." Accessed April 16, 2014, http://www.fsmb.org/ pdf/2010-summary-of-board-actions.pdf.

———. "What Is a State Medical Board? Answers to Your Questions about the Role of State Medical Boards in Health Care." Accessed March 6, 2014, http://www.fsmb.org/what_is_a_ smb.html.

———. "Physician Profile Information—Board-by-Board Overview." Accessed March 22, 2014, http://www.fsmb.org/pdf/GRPOL_Physician_Profiling.pdf.

———. "U.S. Medical Regulatory Trends and Actions." March 2014.

Feudner, C., Dai, D., Hexem, K. R., et al. "Prevalence of Polypharmacy Exposure among Hospitalized Children in the United States." *Archives of Pediatrics and Adolescent Medicine* 166 (2012): 9–16.

"Fourth Decennial International Conference on Nosocomial and Healthcare-Associated Infections." *MMWR Weekly*, February 25, 2000. Accessed April 15, 2014, http://www.cdc.gov/ mmwr/preview/mmwrhtml/mm4907a4.htm.

Food and Drug Administration (2013), http://www.fda.gov/Drugs/ResourcesForYou/ Consumers/default.htm. Accessed March 24, 2014.

———. (2010). Accessed March 24, 2014, http://www.fda.gov/drugs/newsevents/ucm219716. htm.

————. "Information for Patients Who Have Metal-on-Metal Hip Implants." January 17, 2013. Accessed February 27, 2014, http://www.fda.gov/MedicalDevices/ ProductsandMedicalProcedures/ImplantsandProsthetics/MetalonMetalHipImplants/ ucm241766.htm.

————. "Information for Patients Considering a Metal-on-Metal Hip Implant System." January 17, 2013. Accessed February 27, 2014, http://www.fda.gov/MedicalDevices/ ProductsandMedicalProcedures/ImplantsandProsthetics/MetalonMetalHipImplants/ ucm241767.htm.

Freixas, N., Bella, F., Limon, E., et al. "Impact of a Multimodal Intervention to Reduce Bloodstream Infections Related to Vascular Catheters in Non-ICU Wards: A Multicentre Study." *Clinical Microbiology and Infection* 19, no. 9 (2013): 838–844.

Fuchs, V. R. "Major Trends in the US Health Economy Since 1950." *New England Journal of Medicine* 366 (2012): 973–977.

Gandhi, T., and Lee, T. "Patient Safety beyond the Hospital." *New England Journal of Medicine* 363 (2010): 1003.

Garfinkel, D., and Mangin, D. "Feasibility Study of a Systematic Approach for Discontinuation of Multiple Medications in Older Adults." *Archives of Internal Medicine* 170 (2010): 1648–1654.

Garman, A., and Scribner, L. "Leading for Quality in Healthcare: Development and Validation of a Competency Model." *Journal of Healthcare Management*, November 1, 2011. Accessed July 7, 2013, http://www.biomedsearch.com/article/Leading-quality-in-healthcare-development/274519826.html.

Garvey, C. J., and Hanlon, R. "Computed Tomography in Clinical Practice." *BMJ* 324, no. 7345 (May 4, 2002): 1077–1080. Accessed April 29, 2014, http://www.ncbi.nlm.nih.gov/ pmc/articles/PMC1123029/.

Gawande, A. "Big Med: Restaurant Chains Have Managed to Combine Quality Control, Cost Control, and Innovation. Can Health Care?" *New Yorker*, August 13, 2012. Accessed April 10, 2014,http://www.newyorker.com/reporting/2012/08/13/120813fa_fact_gawande? currentPage=all .

————. "The Disturbing Truth about Doctors and Your Medical Safety." truthout. Accessed January 15, 2014, http://www.truth-out.org/archive/item/70678:atul-gawande--the-disturbing-truth-about-doctors-and-your-medical-safety.

General Accounting Office. "Medicare Imaging Accreditation: Establishing Minimum National Standards and an Oversight Framework Would Help Ensure Quality and Safety of Advanced Diagnostic Imaging Services." Accessed April 15, 2015.

Gentry, C. "Alternative-Medicine Doctor Reprimanded, Fined in Hepatitis C Outbreak." *WUSF News*, October 12, 2014.http://wusfnews.wusf.usf.edu/post/alternative-medicine-doctor-reprimanded-fined-hepatitis-c-outbreak.

Gheorghaide, M., Gattis, W. A., and O'Conner, C. M. "Treatment Gaps in the Pharmacologic Management of Heart Failure." *Reviews in Cardiovascular Medicine* 3 (2002): S11–S19.

Glabman, M. "Lobbyists That the Founders Just Never Dreamed Of." *Managed Care Magazine*, August 2002. http://www.managedcaremag.com/archives/0208/0208.lobbying.html.

Goldacre, B. *Bad Pharma—How Drug Companies Mislead Doctors and Harm Patients.* New York: Faber and Faber, 2012.

Good Morning America. "Doctor Sued for Inserting Screwdriver into Patient's Back." February 17, 2006. http://abcnews.go.com/GMA/story?id=1630844.

Gorwitz, R. J., Kruszon-Moran, D., McAllister, S. K., et al. "Changes in the Prevalence of Nasal Colonization with Staphylococcus Aureus in the United States, 2001-2004." *Journal of Infectious Diseases* 197, no. 9 (2008): 1226–1234.

Gotzsche, P. *Deadly Medicines and Organised Crime—How Big Pharma has Corrupted Healthcare.* London: Ratcliffe Publishing, 2013.

Gould, D. "Survey Reveals Growing Consumer Demand for Antibiotic-Free Meat." *Forbes.* Accessed March 2, 2014, http://www.forbes.com/sites/daniellegould/2012/06/26/survey-reveals-growing-consumer-demand-for-antibiotic-free-meat/.

Government Accountability Office. VA Healthcare, December 2013. Accessed April 28, 2014, http://www.gao.gov/assets/660/659378.pdf.

———. "Health-Care-Associated Infections In Hospitals: Leadership Needed from HHS to Prioritize Prevention Practices and Improve Data on These Infections," Testimony before the Committee on Oversight and Government Reform, House of Representatives (April 16, 2008).

———. "Report to the Chairman, Committee on Oversight and Government Reform, House of Representatives: An Overview of State Reporting Programs and Individual Hospital Initiatives to Reduce Certain Infections" (September 2008).

———. "FDA Should Take Steps to Ensure That High-Risk Device Types Are Approved through the Most Stringent Pre-market Review Processes." GAO-09-190 (January 2009). Accessed February 26, 2014, http://gao.gov/new.items/d09190.pdf.

Goyal, A., and Bornstein, W. A. "Health System-Wide Quality Programs to Improve Blood Pressure Control." *JAMA* 310 (2013): 695–696.

Graber, M. L. "Diagnostic Errors in Medicine: A Case of Neglect." *Joint Commission Journal on Quality and Patient Safety* 31 (2005): 106–113.

———. "The Incidence of Diagnostic Error in Medicine." *BMJ Quality and Safety* 22 (2013): ii21–ii27. doi:10.1136/bmjqs-2012-001615.

Grant, D., and Alfred, K. C. "Sanctions and Recidivism: An Evaluation of Physician Discipline by State Medical Boards." *Journal of Health Politics, Policy and Law* 32 (2007): 867–885.

Graves, S. E. "What Is Happening with Hip Replacement?" *Medical Journal of Australia* 194 (2011): 620–621.

Graves, S. E., Rothwell, A., Tucker, K., et al. "A Multinational Assessment of Metal-on-metal Bearings in Hip Replacement." *Journal of Bone and Joint Surgery American Volume* 93 Suppl 3 (2011): 43–47.

Groskerry, P. "From Mindless to Mindful Practice—Cognitive Bias and Clinical Decision Making." *New England Journal of Medicine* 368 (2013): 2445–2448. doi:10.1056/NEJMp1303712.

Gruettner, J., Henzler, T., Sueselbeck, T., Fink, C., Borggrefe M., and Walter, T. "Clinical Assessment of Chest Pain and Guidelines for Imaging. http://www.ncbi.nlm.nih.gov/pubmed/21396792 (December 2012): 3663–3668. Accessed April 29, 2014, doi: 10.1016/j.ejrad.2011.01.063.

Guillermo, M. "Dipak Desai Gets Life in Prison in Hep C Outbreak Case." KVVU Broadcasting Corporation, January 2, 2014. http://www.fox5vegas.com/story/23780441/dipak-desai-gets-life-in-prison-in-hep-c-outbreak-case.

Guy, A. Y., Thompson, N. D., Schaefer, M. K., et al. "Patient Notification for Bloodborne Pathogen Testing Due to Unsafe Injection Practices in the US Health Care Settings, 2001-2011." *Medical Care* 50 (2012): 786.

Hacek, D. M., Paule, S. M., Thomson Jr., R. B., et al. "Implementation of a Universal Admission Surveillance and Decolonization Program for Methicillin-Resistant Staphylococcus Aureus (MRSA) Reduces the Number of MRSA and Total Number of S. Aureus Isolates Reported by the Clinical Laboratory." *Journal of Clinical Microbiology* 47, no. 11 (2009): 3749–3752.

Hahn, A. "Would You Go under Anesthesia If Your Doctor's Only Backup Plan Was to Call 911?" *Online Metroland*, October 21, 2004. http://metroland.net/back_issues/vol_27_no43/features.html.

Hall, W., Violato, C., Lewkonia, R., et al. "Assessment of Physicians' Performance in Alberta: The Physician Achievement Review." *Canadian Medical Association Journal* 161 (1999): 52–57.

Halloran, J. "The Overuse of Antibiotics in Food Animals Threatens Public Health." Consumers Union. Accessed March 2, 2014, http://consumersunion.org/news/the-overuse-of-antibiotics-in-food-animals-threatens-public-health-2.

Hamilton, H., Gallagher, P., Ryan, C., et al. "Potentially Inappropriate Medications Defined by STOPP Criteria and the Risk of Adverse Drug Events in Older Hospitalized Patients." *Archives of Internal Medicine* 171 (2011): 1013–1019.

Hartocollis, A. "With Money at Risk, Hospitals Push Staff to Wash Hands." *New York Times.* Accessed January 18, 2014, http://www.nytimes.com/2013/05/29/nyregion/hospitals-struggle-to-get-workers-to-wash-their-hands.html?_r=0.

Haskell, H. "Many Medical Errors Don't Happen in the Hospital But in Doctors' Offices." *TEDMED Great Challenges 2012* (unpublished).

Hazlewood, K. A., Brouse, S. D., Pitcher, W. D., and Hall, R. G. "Vancomycin-Associated Nephrotoxicity: Grave Concern or Death by Character Assassination?" *American Journal of Medicine* 123, no. 2 (2010): 182 e1-7.

"Health Information Privacy." US Department of Health and Human Services. http://www.hhs.gov/ocr/privacy/.

Healy, D. *Pharmageddon*. Berkeley and Los Angeles: University of California Press, 2012.

Healy, R. "(Non) Profit Hospitals: Charity Pays." 100 Reporters—New Journalism for a New Age. Accessed April 14, 2014, http://100r.org/2014/04/nonprofit-hospitals-charity-pays/.

"Healthcare Associated Infections." Data.Medicare.Gov. (2012). https://data.medicare.gov/Hospital-Compare/Healthcare-Associated-Infections/ihvx-zkyp.

"HEDIS and Quality Compass." *National Committee for Quality Accreditation*. http://www.ncqa.org/HEDISQualityMeasurement/WhatisHEDIS.aspx.

Heisel, W. "State Medical Boards Leave Patients in Danger and in Dark." *Reporting on Health*, December 29, 2010. Accessed March 21, 2014, http://www.reportingonhealth.org/node/10331.

———. "Off the Record: Legislators Try to Put Doctor Discipline behind the Curtain." *Reporting on Health*. Accessed March 10, 2014, http://www.reportingonhealth.org/2014/02/28/record-legislators-try-put-doctor-discipline-behind-curtain.

"HHS Has Taken Steps to Address Unsafe Injection Practices, But More Action Is Needed." US Government Accountability Office, July 2012. GAO-12-712.

Hicks, L. A., Taylor, T. H., and Hunkler, R. J. "U.S. Outpatient Antibiotic Prescribing, 2010." *New England Journal of Medicine* 368, no. 15 (2013): 1461–1462.

Hines, L. "Retail Clinics Challenging Pediatricians for Business." *Houston Chronicle*, April 13, 2014: D5.

Ho, B., and Liu, E. "Does Sorry Work? The Impact of Apology Laws on Medical Malpractice." Job Market Paper, Cornell University and University of Houston (October 2010). Accessed September 14, 2013, http://irving.vassar.edu/faculty/bh/Ho-Liu-Apologies-and-Malpractice-nov15.pdf.

Ho, K., Jarvis-Selinger, S., Norman, C. D., Li, L., Olatunbosun, T., Cressman, C., and Nguyen, A. "Electronic Communities of Practice Guidelines from a Project." *Journal of Continuing Education in the Health Professions* 30, no. 2 (2010): 139–143. doi:10.1002/chp.20071.

Hollings, R. L., and Pike-Nase, C. *Professional and Occupational Licensure in the United States*. Westport, CT: Greenwood Press, 1997.

Horowitz, R. *In the Public Interest: Medical Licensing and the Disciplinary Process*. New Brunswick, NJ: Rutgers University Press, 2013.

House of Representatives, 99th Congress, 2d. Session, Rpt 99-903. Report to Accompany HR 5540 [by the Committee on Energy and Commerce], p. 2.

"How Safe Is Your Hospital?" *Consumer Reports*, January 2003, 16.

"How to Choose a Doctor." ConsumerReports.org, March 2013. http://www.consumerreports.org/cro/2012/12/how-to-choose-a-doctor/index.htm.

Hughes, C. M., and Tunney, M. M. "Improving Prescribing of Antibiotics in Long-Term Care." *JAMA Internal Medicine* 173 (2013): 682–683.

Illinois General Assembly. Senate Bill 59. 93rd General Assembly, August 20, 2003. Accessed April 15, 2014, http://www.ilga.gov/legislation/BillStatus.asp?GA=93&DocTypeID=SB&DocNum=59&GAID=3&SessionID=3&LegID=49.

Institute for Healthcare Improvement. "Overview of the 100,000 Lives Campaign." Accessed April 15, 2014, http://www.ihi.org/Engage/Initiatives/Completed/5MillionLivesCampaign/Documents/Overview%20of%20the%20100K%20Campaign.pdf.

Institute of Medicine. *To Err Is Human: Building a Safer Health System*. Washington, DC: National Academies Press, 2000. Accessed March 30, 2014, http://www.nap.edu/openbook.php?record_id=9728.

———. *Conflict of Interest in Medical Research, Education, and Practice*. Washington, DC: National Academies Press, 2009. Accessed March 20, 2014, http://www.ncbi.nlm.nih.gov/books/NBK22942/.

———. *Preventing Medication Errors* (Washington: National Academies Press, 2007), 4.

———. *Ethical and Scientific Issues in Studying the Safety of Approved Drugs* (Washington, DC: National Academies Press, 2012). Accessed March 24, 2014. http://tinyurl.com/cxovshm.

———. *Medical Devices and the Public's Health: The FDA 501(k) Clearance Process at 35 Years* (Washington: National Academies Press, 2011), 1–12.

———. *Toward Quality Measures for Population Health and the Leading Health Indicators* (Washington, DC, National Academies Press, 2013). Accessed April 29, 2014, http://www.iom.edu/Reports/2013/Toward-Quality-Measures-for-Population-Health-and-the-Leading-Health-Indicators.aspx.

———. "Clinical Practice Guidelines We Can Trust" (2011). Accessed April 11, 2014, https://tinyurl.com3t9hj8t.

Jacobs, J. J. "Commentary on an Article by Stephen S. Tower, MD: 'Arthroprosthetic Cobalt-ism: Neurological and Cardiac Manifestations in Two Patients with Metal-on-metal Arthro-plasty. A Case Report.'" *Journal of Bone and Joint Surgery American Volume* 92 (2010): e35.

James, J. T. *A Sea of Broken Hearts, Patient Rights in a Dangerous, Profit-Driven Health Care System*. Bloomington, IN: AuthorHouse, 2007.

———. "A New, Evidence-Based Estimate of Patient Harms Associated with Hospital Care." *Journal of Patient Safety* 9 (2013): 122–128. doi: 10.1097/PTS.0b013e3182948a69.

Jena, A. B., Seabury, S., Lakdawalla, D., et al. "Malpractice Risk According to Physician Specialty." *New England Journal of Medicine* 365 (2011): 629–636.

Jewell, K., McGiffert, L. "To Err Is Human, To Delay Is Deadly." May 2009, 4. Accessed May 12, 2014, http://safepatientproject.org/safepatientproject.org/pdf/safepatientproject.org-ToDelayIsDeadly.pdf.

Johnson, D., and Talmage, L. "The Evolution of Medical Discipline in 20th Century America." Federation of State Medical Boards. Accessed March 15, 2014, http://www.iamra.com/pdf/IAMRA%20Conference%20%20October%203/Workshops/Evolution%20of%20Medical%20Discipline%20in%2020th%20Century%20America.pdf.

Johnson, D. C., and Kazemi, H. "Disorders of Ventilatory Control." *UpToDate* (2007): 1–11.

Johnson, K. "Denver Woman Sentenced in Hepatitis Infection Case." *New York Times*, February 24, 2010. http://www.nytimes.com/2010/02/25/us/25hepatitis.html?_r=0.

Jones, P., and Greenstone, M. "Carbonic Anhydrase Inhibitors for Hypercapnic Ventilatory Failure in Chronic Obstructive Pulmonary Disease." *Cochrane Database of Systematic Reviews* 1 (2001). Art. No. CD002881. doi:10.1002/14651858.CD002881.

Joseph, B. "Flaws Found in State Consumer Protection Enforcement." *Orange County Register*, October 26, 2012. http://www.ocregister.com/articles/boards-375814-board-cases.html.

Joynt, K. E., Orav, E. J., and Jha, A. K. "Mortality Rates for Medicare Beneficiaries Admitted to Critical Access and Non-Critical Access Hospitals, 2002-2010." *JAMA* 309 (2013): 1379–1387.

Kachalia, A., and Mello, M. M. "New Directions in Medical Liability Reform." *New England Journal of Medicine* 364, no. 16 (2011): 1564–1572. Accessed January 11, 2014. doi/full/10.1056/NEJMhpr1012821.

Kahn, J. M., and Angus, D. C. "Going Home on the Right Medications—Prescription Errors and Transitions of Care." *JAMA* 306 (2011): 878–879.

Kelly, T., Bauer, S., and Tower, S. "Power, Credibility and Expertise in a Colonized Medical Discourse." PhilSci Archive, 3rd Annual Values in Medicine, Science, and Technology Conference, Dallas, TX, May 22–24, 2013. Accessed May 29, 2014, http://philsci-archive.pitt.edu/9777/.

Kenniston, E. "The Joint Commission and Patient Safety Outcomes: Have Accreditor Policies Improved Patient Safety?" 2011. Accessed April 28, 2014,http://hlaw.ucsd.edu/prospectivestudents/documents/Kenniston_HavePoliciesImprovedPatientSafety.pdf.

Khanna R. R., Victor, R. G., Bibbins-Domingo, K., et al. "Missed Opportunities for Treatment of Uncontrolled Hypertension at Physician Office Visits in the United States, 2005 through 2009," *Archives of Internal Medicine* 172 (2012): 1344–1345.

Kirsch, M. "How Should a Physician Apologize after a Medical Error?" *KevinMD.* December 18, 2013. http://www.kevinmd.com/blog/2013/12/physician-apologize-medical-error.html.

Klaidman, S. *Coronary: A True Story of Medical Care Gone Awry.* New York: Scribner, 2008.

Klevens, R. M., Edwards, J. R., Richards Jr., C. L., et al. "Estimating Health Care-Associated Infections and Deaths in U.S. Hospitals, 2002." *Public Health Reports* 122, no. 2 (2007): 160–166.

Kliff, S. "How Much Does an Appendectomy Cost? Somewhere between $1,529 and $186,955." *Washington Post,* April 24, 2012. Accessed April 25, 2014, http://www.washingtonpost.com/blogs/wonkblog/post/how-much-does-an-appendectomy-cost-somewhere-between-1529-and-186955/2012/04/24/gIQAMeKMeT_blog.html.

Knight, S. R., Aujla, R., and Biswas, S. P. "Total Hip Arthroplasty—Over 100 Years of Operative History." *Orthopedic Reviews 2011.* Accessed February 27, 2014, http://www.pagepress.org/journals/index.php/or/article/view/or.2011.e16/3190.

Kohler, J. "Missouri Secretive, Lax on Doctor Discipline." *St. Louis Post-Dispatch,* December 12, 2010. Accessed March 21, 2014, http://www.stltoday.com/lifestyles/health-med-fit/fitness/article_5cc342ba-dd6c-5428-b25e-99f8faeca638.html.

———. "Sole Layman on Healing Arts Board Is Attorney for Doctors." *St. Louis Post-Dispatch,* December 14, 2010. http://www.stltoday.com/lifestyles/health-med-fit/fitness/sole-layman-on-healing-arts-board-is-attorney-for-doctors/article_f64e5713-5f13-509e-9364-eb59402a09b3.html.

Kruger, J., and Dunning, D. "Unskilled and Unaware of It: How Difficulties in Recognizing One's Own Incompetence Lead to Inflated Self-Assessments." *Journal of Personality and Social Psychology* 77 (1999): 1121–1134. doi: 10.1037/0022-3514.77.6.1121.

Kuehnert, M. J., Kruszon-Moran, D., Hill, H. A., et al. "Prevalence of Staphylococcus Aureus Nasal Colonization in the United States, 2001-2002." *Journal of Infectious Diseases* 193, no. 2 (2006): 172–179.

Kwon, Y-M, Lombardi, A. V., Jacobs, J. J., et al. "Risk Stratification for Management of Patients with Metal-on-Metal Hip Arthroplasty." *Journal of Bone and Joint Surgery American Volume* 96 (2014): e4.

Landro, L. "Taming the Wild West of Outpatient Surgery—Doctors' Offices." *Wall Street Journal,* October 26, 2010. http://blogs.wsj.com/health.

———. "Why Hospitals Want Patients to Ask Doctors, 'Have You Washed Your Hands?'" *Wall Street Journal.* Accessed October 1, 2013, http://online.wsj.com/news/articles/SB10001424052702303918804579107202360565642.

Lee, T. H. "Eulogy for a Quality Measure." *New England Journal of Medicine* 357 (2007): 1175–1177.

Legal Info. 2014. "Gross Negligence and Lack of Informed Consent." Accessed April 26, 2014, www.legalinfo.com/content/medical-malpractice/gross-neglignece-and-lack-of-informed-consent.html.

"Legislative Reference." American Association for Accreditation of Ambulatory Surgery Facilities, Inc. http://www.aaaasf.org/pub/OPT_Legislative_Reference.pdf.

Levine, A., Oshel, R., and Wolfe, S. "State Medical Boards Fail to Discipline Doctors with Hospital Actions against Them." Accessed March 20, 2014, http://www.citizen.org/hrg1937.

Levinson, D. R. "Prescribers with Questionable Patterns in Medicare Part D." Office of the Inspector General, Department of Health and Human Services, June 2013, OEI-02-09-00603.

Levitt, P. "Still Unsafe: Why the American Medical Establishment Cannot Reduce Medical Errors." *Skeptic Magazine* 18 (2013): 44–48.

Lexi-Corp. *Acetazolamide: Drug Onformation.* In *UpToDate ,* 1978–2006.

Lieber, R. "Your Money: The Web Is Awash in Reviews, but Not for Doctors. Here's Why." *New York Times,* March 9, 2012.http://www.nytimes.com/2012/03/10/your-money/why-the-web-lacks-authoritative-reviews-of-doctors.html?pagewanted=all.

Liebman, C. B., and Hyman, C. S. "A Mediation Skills Model to Manage Disclosure of Errors and Adverse Events to Patients." *Health Affairs* 23 (2004): 22–32. Accessed August 23, 2013, doi: 10.1377/hlthaff.23.4.22.

Light, D. W., Lexchin, J., and Darrow, J. J. "Institutional Corruption of Pharmaceuticals and the Myth of Safe and Effective Drugs." *Journal of Law, Medicine and Ethics* 14 (2013): 590–600.

Lindberg, C., Downham, G., Buscell, P., et al. "Embracing Collaboration: A Novel Strategy for Reducing Bloodstream Infections in Outpatient Hemodialysis Centers." *American Journal of Infection Control* 41, no. 6 (2013): 513–519.

Liney, G. *MRI from A to Z: A Definitive Guide for Medical Professionals.* Springer, second edition, 2006. ISBN 978-1-84996-134-9. Accessed April 29, 2014, http://www.slideshare.net/LETUONG_XQ/mri-from-a-toz-adefinitiveguideformedicalprofessionals-secondedition-2010.

Linsky, A., and Simon, S. R. "Reversing Gears—Discontinuing Medication Therapy to Prevent Adverse Events." *JAMA Internal Medicine* 173 (2013): 524–525.

Little, M. "Engaging Bioethics: A Field without Apology." *The Hoya, Georgetown University's Newspaper*, September 24, 2013. Accessed December 5, 2013, http://www.thehoya.com/engaging-bioethics-an-approach-to-ethics-rooted-in-architecture.html.

Localio, A. R., Lawthers, A. G., Brennan, T. A., et al. "Relation between Malpractice Claims and Adverse Events Due to Negligence. Results of the Harvard Medical Practice Study III." *New England Journal of Medicine* 325 (1991): 245–251.

Logan, A. C., Yank, V., and Stafford, R. S. "Off-Label Use of Recombinant Factor VIIa in U.S. Hospitals: Analysis of Hospital Records." *Annals of Internal Medicine* 154 (2011): 516–522.

Longtin, Y., Sax, H., Allegranz, B., et al. "Patients' Beliefs and Perceptions of Their Participation to Increase Healthcare Worker Compliance with Hand Hygiene." *Infection Control and Hospital Epidemiology* 30, no. 9 (2009): 830–839.

Luks, A. M., and Swenson, E. R. "Medication and Dosage Considerations in the Prophylaxis and Treatment of High-Altitude Illness." *Chest* 133 (2008): 744–755.

MacCourt, D., and Bernstein, J. "Medical Error Reduction and Tort Reform Through Private, Contractually Based Quality Medicine Societies." *American Journal of Law and Medicine*, 35 (2009): 505–561.

MacDonald, O. W. "Physician Perspectives on Preventing Diagnostic Errors." *QuantiaMD*, September 2011. Accessed March 16, 2014, http://www.quantiamd.com/q-qcp/QuantiaMD_PreventingDiagnosticErrors_Whitepaper_1.pdf.

Macedo de Oliveira, A., White, K. L., and D. P. Leschinsky, et al. "An Outbreak of Hepatitis C Virus Infections among Outpatients at a Hematology/Oncology Clinic." *Annals of Internal Medicine* 142 (2005): 901.

Machado, C., Appelbe, A., and Wood, R. "Arthroprosthetic Cobaltism and Cardiomyopathy." *Heart, Lung and Circulation* 21 (2012): 759–760.

Magill, S. S., Edwards, J. R., Bamberg, W., et al. "Multistate Point-Prevalence Survey of Health Care–Associated Infections." *New England Journal of Medicine*, March 27, 2014: 1198–1208.

Makary, M. *Unaccountable: What Hospitals Won't Tell You and How Transparency Can Revolutionize Health Care.* New York: Bloomsbury Press, 2012, 74, 147.

———. Video trailer promoting book *Unaccountable* (at 1:56). Accessed November 21, 2012, http://www.youtube.com/watch?v=d9Pi8F-lWuA&feature=em-share_video_use.

Mäkelä, K. T., Visuri, T., Pulkkinen, P., et al. "Risk of Cancer with Metal-on-Metal Hip Replacements: Population Based Study." *BMJ* 345 (2012): e4646. Accessed February 27, 2014, http://www.bmj.com/content/345/bmj.e4646.

Mansour, M., Mela, T., Ruskin, J., and Keane, D. "Successful Release of Entrapped Circumferential Mapping Catheters in Patients Undergoing Pulmonary Vein Isolation for Atrial Fibrillation." *Heart Rhythm* 1 (2004): 558–561.

Mao, X., Wong, A. A., and Crawford, R. W. "Cobalt Toxicity—An Emerging Clinical Problem in Patients with Metal-on-Metal Hip Prostheses?" *Medical Journal of Australia* 194 (2011): 649–651.

Marigliano, A., Barbadoro, P., Pennacchietti, L., et al. "Active Training and Surveillance: 2 Good Friends to Reduce Urinary Catheterization Rate." *American Journal of Infection Control* 40, no. 8 (2012): 692–695.

Martin Luther King, Jr. Hospital History. Accessed April 28, 2014, http://www. mlkcommunityhospital.org/our-story .

Martini, A. "What Patients Should Know about Imaging." The Hastings Center Report over 65 (online blog), 2013, 17. Blog site: http://www.over65.thehastingscenter.org/what-patients-should-know-about-medical-testing/.

Maryland Hospital Association Council on Legislative and Regulatory Policy. Minutes. January 14, 2005.

Mason, R. J., Broaddus, V. C., Martin, T., et al. *Murray and Nadel's Textbook of Respiratory Medicine.* 4th ed. Philadelphia, PA: Elsevier Saunders, 2005.

Mayo Clinic. Accessed March 24, 2014, http://www.mayoclinic.com/health/breast-cancer-prevention/WO00091.

McGuckin, M., Stor, J., Longtin, Y., et al. "Patient Empowerment and Multimodal Hand Hygiene Promotion: A Win-Win Strategy." *American Journal of Medical Quality* 26, no. 1 (2011): 10–17.

McIntyre, F. J., and McCloy, R. "Shaving Patients before Operation: A Dangerous Myth?" *Annals of the Royal College of Surgeons of England* 76, no. 1 (1994): 3–4.

McKibben, L., Horan, T., Tokars, J. I., et al. "Guidance on Public Reporting of Healthcare-Associated Infections: Recommendations of the Healthcare Infection Control Practices Advisory Committee." *American Journal of Infection Control* (May 2005): 217–226.

McKnight, E. V., and Bennington T. T. *A Never Event: Exposing the Largest Outbreak of Hepatitis C in American Healthcare History.* History Examined, 2010.

McKnight, E. V., and Lollini, L. "Service above Self—Johnny Robertson's Story." *Hepatitis Outbreaks National Organization for Reform* (October 28, 2013). http://www.honoreform. org/blog/?p=141#more-141.

———. "There Isn't Anything I Can't Do—Melisa French's Story." *HONOReform.org*, March 17, 2014. http://www.honoreform.org/blog/?cat=2.

"Medicaid Fraud Control Units—MFCUs Office of Inspector General." Office of Inspector General US Department of Health and Human Services. https://www.oig.hhs.gov/fraud/ medicaid-fraud-control-units-mfcu/index.asp.

Medicare Hospital Compare. Accessed April 28, 2014, http://www.medicare.gov/ hospitalcompare/search.html?AspxAutoDetectCookieSupport=1.

MEDICINEWISE N. "Monitoring for Potential Toxicity in Patients with Metal-on-Metal Hip Prostheses: Advice for Health Professionals." 2013.

Meeker, D., Knight, T. K., Friedberg, M. W., et al. "Nudging Guideline-Concordant Antibiotic Prescribing—A Randomized Clinical Trial." *JAMA Internal Medicine* 174 (2014): 425–431.

Mehlman, M. J. "Medical Practice Guidelines as Malpractice Safe Harbors: Illusion or Deceit?" *Journal of Law, Medicine and Ethics* 40, no. 2 (Summer 2012): 286–300.

———. "Professional Power and the Standard of Care in Medicine." *Arizona State Law Journal* 44 (2012): 1165–1235.

Meier, B. "Johnson & Johnson in Deal to Settle Hip Implant Lawsuits." November 19, 2013. Accessed February 27, 2014, http://www.nytimes.com/2013/11/20/business/johnson-johnson-to-offer-2-5-billion-hip-device-settlement.html?_r=0.

Meldi, D., Rhoades, F., and Gippe, A. "The Big Three: A Side by Side Matrix Comparing Hospital Accrediting Agencies." January/February 2009. Accessed April 28, 2014, http:// cms.ipressroom.com.s3.amazonaws.com/107/files/20125/Comparing_Accreditation_ Programs_Synergy_pdf.

Meryhew, R., and Howatt, G. "Minimum Standards Mean Less Discipline." *Star Tribune.* February 6, 2012. Accessed March 12, 2014, http://www.startribune.com/local/138692919. html?page=all&prepage=1&c=y#continue.

Miller, S. H. "American Board of Medical Specialties and Repositioning for Excellence in Lifelong Learning: Maintenance of Certification." *Journal of Continuing Education in the Health Professions* 25 (2005): 151–156.

Mitka, M. "Drug for Severe Sepsis Is Withdrawn from Market, Fails to Reduce Mortality." *JAMA* 306 (2011): 2439–2440.

———. "Nursing Home Antipsychotics." *JAMA* 307 (2012): 134.

Morbidity and Mortality Weekly Report (MMWR). "Monitoring Hospital-Acquired Infections to Promote Patient Safety—United States, 1990-1999." March 3, 2000, 149–153.

Morden, N. E., Schwartz, L. M., Fisher, E. S., and Woloshin, S. "Accountable Prescribing." *New England Journal of Medicine* 369 (2013): 299–302.

Morris, L., and Taitsman, J. K. "The Agenda for Continuing Medical Education—Limiting Industry's Influence." *New England Journal of Medicine* 361 (2009): 2478–2482.

Moss, M. "Mammography Team Learns from Its Errors." *New York Times*, June 28, 2002. Accessed April 29, 2014, http://www.nytimes.com/2002/06/28/health/28MAMM.html.

Muto, C. A., Jernigan, J. A., Ostrowsky, B. E., et al. "SHEA Guideline for Preventing Nosocomial Transmission of Multidrug-Resistant Strains of Staphylococcus aureus and Enterococcus." *Infection Control and Hospital Epidemiology* (May 2003): 362–386.

National Conference of Insurance Legislators. "Lawmakers Unanimously Adopt Patient Safety Model Law, Support Medical Error Reporting." *NCOILetter* 3, December 2005. Accessed April 24, 2014, http://www.ncoil.org/news/2005_NewsLetters/December2005.pdf.

National Conference of State Legislatures. "Ensuring Public the Trust 2012, Program Policy Evaluation's Role in Serving State Legislatures." Accessed March 11, 2014, http://www.ncsl.org/legislators-staff/legislative-staff/program-evaluation/survey-ensuring-the-public-trust.aspx.

National Practitioner Data Bank. http://www.npdb-hipdb.hrsa.gov/hcorg/register.jsp.

———. 2010 Annual Report. Available at http://www.npdb-hipdb.hrsa.gov/resources/reports/2010NPDBAnnualReport.pdf, Table 6. The 2010 Annual Report is the latest report available as of November 10, 2012.

———. Accessed April 28, 2014, http://www.npdb-hipdb.hrsa.gov/hcorg/billingAndFees.jsp. Users may also enroll practitioners in the Data Bank's continuous query service, which provides immediate copies of all new reports on enrolled practitioners. This service costs $3.25 per year per name enrolled.

———. 2002 Annual Report, page 11. http://www.npdb-hipdb.hrsa.gov/resources/reports/2002NPDBAnnualReport.pdf.

———. Accessed April 28, 2014, http://www.npdb.hrsa.gov/.

Nelson, H. D., Smith, B., Griffin, J. C., and Fu, R. "Use of Medications to Reduce Risk for Primary Breast Cancer: A Systematic Review for the U.S. Preventive Services Task Force." *Annals of Internal Medicine* 158 (2013): 604–614.

Nicolau, D. P. "Carbapenems: A Potent Class of Antibiotics." *Expert Opinion on Pharmacotherapy* 9, no. 1 (2008): 23–37.

Norcini, J. J., Boulet, J. R., Dauphinee, W. D., et al. "Evaluating the Quality of Care Provided by Graduates of International Medical Schools." *Health Affairs* 8 (2010): 1461–1468.

Nyquist, A. C., Gonzales, R., Steiner, J. F., and Sande, M. A. "Antibiotic Prescribing for Children with Colds, Upper Respiratory Tract Infections, and Bronchitis." *JAMA* 279, no. 11 (1998): 875–877.

O'Connell, K. "Two Arms, Two Choices: If Only I'd Known Then What I Know Now." *Health Affairs*, August 2012, 1895–1899.

O'Donoghue, C., Eklund, M., Ozanne, E. M., and Esserman, L. J. "Aggregate Cost of Mammography Screening in the United States: Comparison of Current Practice and Advocated Guidelines." *Annals of Internal Medicine* 160, no. 3 (February 4, 2014): 145–153. doi:10.7326/M13-1217. Accessed April 29, 2014, http://annals.org/article.aspx?articleID=1819118.

"Office-Based Surgery (OBS) Frequently Asked Questions (FAQ's) for Practitioners." New York State Department of Health. http://www.health.ny.gov/professionals/office-based_surgery/obs_faq.htm.

Office of Inspector General, Department of Health and Human Services. "Adverse Events in Hospitals: National Incidence among Medicare Beneficiaries." November 2010. OEI-06-09-00090. Page ii. http://oig.hhs.gov/oei/reports/oei-06-09-00090.pdf.

"Office-Related Antibiotic Prescribing for Persons Aged </= 14 Years—United States, 1993-1994 to 2007-2008." *MMWR Morbidity and Mortality Weekly Report* 60, no. 34 (2011): 1153–1156.

OIG News. December 11, 2003. Accessed April 28, 2014, https://oig.hhs.gov/publications/docs/press/2003/121103release.pdf.

Open Notes. http://www.myopennotes.org/. Accessed March 24, 2014.

Oregon State Medical Board. "Anatomy of a Complaint." Accessed April 16, 2014, http://www.oregon.gov/omb/Investigations/Documents/anatomy-of-complaint.pdf.

"OSHA Fact Sheet: OSHA Inspections." *Occupational Safety and Health Administration.* https://www.osha.gov/OshDoc/data_General_Facts/factsheet-inspections.pdf.

Ostrom, C. M. "Legislative Measure Seeks Medical-Board Transparency." *Seattle Times,* March 16, 2011. Accessed March 22, 2014, http://seattletimes.com/html/localnews/2014517578_doctorcomplaints17m.html.

Ottum, A., Sethi, A. K., Jacobs, E. A., et al. "Do Patients Feel Comfortable Asking Healthcare Workers to Wash Their Hands?" *Infection Control and Hospital Epidemiology* 33, no. 12 (2012): 1282–1284.

Outterson, K. "Regulating Compounding Pharmacies after NECC." *New England Journal of Medicine* 367 (2012): 1969–1972.

———. "Punishing Health Care Fraud—Is the GSK Settlement Sufficient?" *New England Journal of Medicine* 367 (2012): 1082–1085.

———. "The Drug Quality and Security Act—Mind the Gaps." *New England Journal of Medicine* 370 (2014): 97–99.

Overeem, K., Wollersheim, H. C., Arah, O. A., et al. "Evaluation of Physicians' Professional Performance: An Iterative Development and Validation Study of Multisource Feedback Instruments." *BMC Health Services Research* 12 (2012): 8. Accessed April 24, 2014, http://www.biomedcentral.com/1472-6963/12/80.

Patel, G., Huprikar, S., Factor, S. H., et al. "Outcomes of Carbapenem-Resistant Klebsiella Pneumoniae Infection and the Impact of Antimicrobial and Adjunctive Therapies." *Infection Control and Hospital Epidemiology* 29, no. 12 (2008): 1099–1106.

Patient Centered Outcome Research Institute. Accessed April 14, 2014, http://www.pcori.org/.

Pittet, D., Hugonnet, S., Harbarth, S., et al. "Effectiveness of a Hospital-Wide Programme to Improve Compliance with Hand Hygiene. Infection Control Programme." *Lancet* 356, no. 9238 (2000): 1307–1312.

Prasad, V., Rho, J., and Cifu, A. "The Inferior Vena Cava Filter." *JAMA Internal Medicine* 173 (2013): 493–495.

President Clinton: Patient Bill of Rights, February 20, 1998. Accessed April 14, 2014, http://archive.ahrq.gov/hcqual/press/pbor.html .

"Problems Paying Medical Bills: Early Release of Estimates from the National Health Interview Survey, January 2011–June 2012." Centers for Disease Control and Prevention. Accessed April 14, 2014, http://tinyurl.com/ky27w8q.

Pronovost, P., Needham, D., Berenholtz, S., et al. "An Intervention to Decrease Catheter-Related Bloodstream Infections in the ICU." *New England Journal of Medicine* 355, no. 26 (2006): 2725–2732.

Pronovost, P. J. "Enhancing Physicians' Use of Clinical Practice Guidelines." *Journal of the American Medical Association* 30, no. 23 (2013): 2501–2502. doi:10:1001/jama.2013/281334.

ProPublica. http://projects.propublica.org/checkup/. Accessed March 24, 2014.

Public Citizen. Accessed February 11, 2014, http://www.worstpills.org/includes/page.cfm?op_id=552.

———. "State Medical Boards Fail to Discipline Doctors with Hospital Actions against Them." March 2011. http://www.citizen.org/documents/1937.pdf.

Raju, T. N. "Ignac Semmelweis and the Etiology of Fetal and Neonatal Sepsis." *Journal of Perinatology* 19, no. 4 (1999): 307–310.

Rao, V. M., and Levin, D. C. "The Overuse of Diagnostic Imaging and the Choosing Wisely Initiative." *Annals of Internal Medicine* 157, no. 8 (2012): 574–576. Accessed April 29, 2014, http://annals.org/article.aspx?articleID=1355170. doi:10.7326/0003-4819-157-8-201210160-00535.

Ray, W. A., Murray, K. T., Hall, K., et al. "Azithromycin and the Risk of Cardiovascular Death." *New England Journal of Medicine* 366 (2012): 1881–1890.

"Recovery Audit Program." *Centers for Medicare and Medicaid Services.* http://www.cms. gov/Research-Statistics-Data-and-Systems/Monitoring-Programs/Medicare-FFS-Compliance-Programs/Recovery-Audit-Program/?redirect=/recovery-audit-program/.

Regehr, G., and Eva, K. "Self-Assessment, Self-Direction, and the Self-Regulating Professional." *Clinical Orthopaedics and Related Research* 449 (2006): 34–38.

Reid, T. R. *The Healing of America—A Global Quest for Better, Cheaper, and Fairer Health Care* (New York: Penguin Press, 2009), 171.

"Restaurant Inspections in Your Area." *Food Safety News.* http://www.foodsafetynews.com/restaurant-inspections-in-your-area/#.UlRyKRbAXfg.

Rhode Island General Assembly. "An Act Related to Courts and Civil Procedure: Admissibility of Heatlh Care Providers Reports' of Medical and Health Care Errors." January 2014. Accessed February 28, 2014, http://lawprofessors.typepad.com/tortsprof/2014/01/ri-medical-apology-bill-introduced.html and http://lawprofessors.typepad.com/tortsprof/2014/01/ri-medical-apology-bill-introduced.html.

Rich, K. L., Reese, S. M., Bol, K. A., et al. "Assessment of the Quality of Publicly Reported Central Line-Associated Bloodstream Infection Data in Colorado, 2010." *American Journal of Infection Control* 41, no. 10 (2013): 874–879.

Roddy, D., Malloy, D. "Rep. John Murtha Dies at 77." *Pittsburgh Post-Gazette.* Accessed March 1, 2014, http://www.post-gazette.com/nation/2010/02/08/Rep-John-Murtha-dies-at-77/stories/201002080195.

Rodwin, M. A. "Drug Advertising, Continuing Medical Education, and Physician Prescribing: A Historical Review and Reform Proposal." *Journal of Law, Medicine and Ethics* 38 (2010): 807–815. doi: 10.1111/j.1748-720X.2010.00534.x.

Rogan, G. N., Sebat, F., and Grady, I. *How Peer Review Failed at Redding Medical Center, Why It Is Failing across the Country and What Can Be Done about It.* June 1, 2008. Accessed April 28, 2014, http://www.allianceforpatientsafety.org/redding-failure.pdf.

Roman, B. R., and Asch, D. A. "Faded Promises: The Challenge of Deadopting Low-Value Care." *Annals of Internal Medicine,* April 29, 2014. http://www.ncbi.nlm.nih.gov/pubmed/24781317.

Rosoff, A. J. "Evidence-Based Medicine and the Law." *AHRQ: Research Findings and Reports.* Accessed May 10, 2014, http://www.ahrq.gov/research/findings/evidence-based-reports.

Rundle, R. "Some Push to Make Hospitals Disclose Rates of Infection." *Wall Street Journal,* February 1, 2005.

Saman, D. M., and Kavanagh, K. T. "A Tale of Two Cows: Why We Have a Cow Map and Not a Healthcare Acquired Infection Map." 2013. http://www.cddep.org/blog/posts/tale_two_cows_why_we_have_cow_map_and_not_healthcare_acquired_infection_map .

Saman, D. M., Kavanagh, K. T., and Abusalem, S. K. "Redefining the Standardized Infection Ratio to Aid in Consumer Value Purchasing." *Journal of Patient Safety* 9, no. 2 (2013): 55–58.

Saman, D. M., Kavanagh, K. T., Johnson, B., and Lutfiyya, M. N. "Can Inpatient Hospital Experiences Predict Central Line-Associated Bloodstream Infections?" *Plos One* 8, no. 4 (2013): e61097.

Sanderson, R. "Outbreak of Hepatitis C in an Outpatient Alternative Medicine Clinic." Association of Professionals in Infection Control, 2010 Annual Conference and Educational Meeting, July 11-15, New Orleans, LA.

Sarosiek, S., Crowther, M., and Sloan, J. M. "Indications, Complications, and Management of Inferior Vena Cava Filters." *JAMA Internal Medicine* 173 (2013): 513–517.

Sawicki, N. "Character, Competence, and the Principles of Medical Discipline." *Journal of Health Care Law and Policy* 13 (2010): 285–323.

Schiff, G. D., Hasan, O., Kim, S., et al. "Diagnostic Error in Medicine, Analysis of 583 Physician-Reported Errors." *Archives of Internal Medicine* 169 (2009): 1881–1887.

Schwartz, J. 2012. "A Dose of Reality for Medical Malpractice Reform." *New York University Law Review* advance online publication. http://ssrn.com/abstract=2104964.

Scott, R. D. "The Direct Medical Costs of Healthcare Associated Infections in US Hospitals and the Benefits of Prevention." March 2009.

Seattle Times. "License to Harm." April 25, 2006. Accessed March 20, 2014, http://seattletimes.com/news/local/licensetoharm/index.html.

Shapiro, D. "Beyond the Blame: A No-Fault Approach to Malpractice." *New York Times*, September 23, 2003. Accessed November 17, 2013, http://www.nytimes.com/2003/09/23/health/essay-beyond-the-blame-a-no-fault-approach-to-malpractice.html.

Sharma, G., Awashi, S., Dixit, A., and Sharma, G. "Patient Safety Risk Assessment and Risk Management: A Review on Indian Hospitals." *Chronicles of Young Scientists* 2, no. 4 (October–December 2011): 186–191.

Shebi, N., Franklin, B., and Barber, N. 2012. "Failure Mode and Effects Analysis Outputs: Are They Valid?" *BMC Health Services Research* 12, no. 1: 150–159. doi:10.1186/1472-6963-12-150.

Shoemaker, L. K., Kazley, A., and White, A. 2010. "Making the Case for Evidence Based Design in Healthcare: A Descriptive Case Study of Organisational Decision Making." *Health Environments Research and Design* 4, no. 1: 50–99.

Sievert, D. M., Ricks, P., Edwards, J. R., et al. "Antimicrobial-Resistant Pathogens Associated with Healthcare-Associated Infections: Summary of Data Reported to the National Healthcare Safety Network at the Centers for Disease Control and Prevention, 2009-2010." *Infection Control and Hospital Epidemiology* 34, no. 1 (2013): 1–14.

Similowski, T., Whitelaw, W., and Derenne, J-P, eds. *Clinical Management of Chronic Obstructive Pulmonary Disease, Lung Biology in Health and Disease, Volume 165*. New York: Marcel Dekker, 2002.

Singh, H., Mayer, A. N. D., and Thomas, E. J. "The Frequency of Diagnostic Errors in Outpatient Care: Estimations from Three Large Observational Studies Involving US Adult Populations." *BMJ Quality and Safety* (2014). doi:10.1136/bmjqs-2013-002627.

Singleton, M. M. "I'm Sorry for Your Loss." *AAPS A Voice for Private Physicians*. November 11, 2013. Accessed February 8, 2014, http://www.aapsonline.org/index.php/site/article/im_sorry_for_your_loss/.

Skipor, A. K., Campbell, P. A., Patterson, L. M., et al. "Serum and Urine Metal Levels in Patients with Metal-on-Metal Surface Arthroplasty." *Journal of Materials Science: Materials in Medicine* 13 (2002): 1227–1234.

Slomski, A. "Screening Women for Ovarian Cancer Still Does More Harm Than Good." *JAMA* 307, no. 23 (2012): 2474–2475. doi:10.1001/jama.2012.5646. Accessed April 29, 2014, http://jama.jamanetwork.com/article.aspx?articleid=1187925.

———. "Falls from Taking Multiple Medications May be a Risk for Both Young and Old." *JAMA* 307 (2012): 1127–1128.

Smith-Bindman, R., Chu, P., Miglioretti, D. L., Quale, C., Rosenberg, R. D., Cutter, G., Geller, B., Bacchetti, P., Sickles, E. A., and Kerlikowske, K. "Physician Predictors of Mammographic Accuracy." *Journal of the National Cancer Institute* 97, no. 5 (March 2, 2005): 358–367. Accessed April 29, 2014, http://www.ncbi.nlm.nih.gov/pubmed/15741572.

Smith, T. J., and Hillner, B. E. "Bending the Cost Curve in Cancer Care." *New England Journal of Medicine* 364 (2011): 2060–2065.

Snowbeck, C. "Compromise Approved on Reporting Infections; Focuses on Those Acquired in Hospitals." *Pittsburgh Post-Gazette*, March 5, 2004.

Society for Healthcare Epidemiology of America, Infectious Diseases Society of America and Pediatric Infectious Diseases Society. "Policy Statement on Antimicrobial Stewardship by the Society for Healthcare Epidemiology of America (SHEA), the Infectious Diseases Society of America (IDSA), and the Pediatric Infectious Diseases Society (PIDS)." *Infection Control and Hospital Epidemiology* 33, no. 4 (2012): 322–327.

Sorrell, J. "Ethics: Ethics in Healthcare Organisations: Struggling with New Questions." *Online Journal of Issues in Nursing* 13, no. 3 (2008): 1–4. doi:103912/OJIN.Vol13No03EthCol01.

Sotos, J. G., and Tower, S. S. "Systemic Disease after Hip Replacement: Aeromedical Implications of Arthroprosthetic Cobaltism." *Aviation, Space, and Environmental Medicine* 84 (2013): 242–245.

Srinivas, S. V., Deyo, R. A., and Berger, Z. D. "Application of 'Less Is More' to Low Back Pain." *Archives of Internal Medicine* 172, no. 13 (July 9, 2012): 1016–1020. Accessed April

29, 2014, http://www.ncbi.nlm.nih.gov/pubmed/22664775. doi: 10.1001/archintern-med.2012.1838.

Srinivasan, A., Craig, M., and Cardo, D. "The Power of Policy Change, Federal Collaboration, and State Coordination in Healthcare-Associated Infection Prevention." *Clinical Infectious Diseases* 55, no. 3 (2012): 426–431.

Staff Report on Cardiac Stent Usage at St. Joseph Medical Center. December 2010. Accessed April 29, 2014, http://www.finance.senate.gov/newsroom.

Stafford, R. S. "Regulating Off-Label Drug Use—Rethinking the Role of the FDA." *New England Journal of Medicine* 358 (2008): 1427–1429.

Starfield, B. "Is US Health Really the Best in the World?" *JAMA* 284 (2000): 483–485.

"State Medical Boards' Disciplinary Actions." *Public Citizen.* Accessed March 20, 2014, http://www.citizen.org/statemedicalboardsdisciplinaryactions.

"Statement by the American Congress of Obstetricians on North Dakota Abortion Laws." American College of Obstetricians and Gynecologists. Accessed April 11, 2014, http://www.acog.org/About_ACOG/NewsRoom/News-Releases/2013/North -Dakota-Abortion-Laws.

State of California. Accessed April 28, 2014, https://www.breeze.ca.gov/datamart/detailsCADCA.do?selector=false&selectorType=&selectorReturnUrl=&anchor=b727bcb.0.0.

State of Maryland license sanctions, July 2011. Accessed April 28, 2014, http://www.mbp.state.md.us/forms/jul11sanctions.pdf.

Stein, A. "Doctors Who Get Away with Killing and Maiming Must Be Stopped." February 2, 1986. Accessed April 16, 2014, http://www.nytimes.com/1986/02/02/opinion/doctors-who-get-away-with-killing-and-maiming-must-be-stopped.html.

Stramer, A. J. "Rates of Medical Errors and Preventable Adverse Events among Hospitalized Children Following Implementation of a Resident Handoff Bundle." *JAMA* 310, no. 21 (2013): 2262–2270. doi:10.1001/jama.2013.281961.

Strand, R. D. *Death by Prescription—The Shocking Truth Behind an Overmedicated Nation.* Nashville, TN: Thomas Nelson Publishers, 2003.

Straus, S., Tetroe, J., and Graham, I. "Defining Knowledge Translation." *Canadian Medical Association Journal* 181, no. 3–4 (2009): 165–168.

Sutton, R., Fisher, J. D., Linde, C., and Benditt, D. G. "History of Electrical Therapy for the Heart." *European Heart Journal* 9 (Suppl 1) (2007): 13–20.

Swenson, B. R., Hedrick, T. L., Metzger, R., et al. "Effects of Preoperative Skin Preparation on Postoperative Wound Infection Rates: A Prospective Study of 3 Skin Preparation Protocols." *Infection Control and Hospital Epidemiology* 30, no. 10 (2009): 964–971.

Taft, L. "Disclosing Unanticipated Outcomes: A Challenge to Providers and Their Lawyers." *Health Lawyers News* 12, no. 5 (2008): 13–18.

Tamkins, T. "Medical Bills Prompt More Than 60 Percent of U.S. Bankruptcies." CNN Health. Accessed April 14, 2014, http://www.cnn.com/2009/HEALTH/06/05/bankruptcy.medical.bills/.

Testimony of Ed Lawton, House Committee on Oversight and Government Reform. April 16, 2008. Accessed April 15, 2014, http://oversight-archive.waxman.house.gov/documents/20080416112456.pdf.

Texas Department of State Health Services. "Recommendations and Key Findings Advisory Panel on Health Care-Associated Infections Submitted to Meet the Reporting Requirements of SB 872, 79th Legislature, Regular Session." 2006, 3.

The Joint Commission. "The Joint Commission Sentinel Event Alert: Issue 51." 2013. Accessed April 26, 2014, http://www.jointcommission.org/sea_issue_51.

———. "Surgical Care Improvement Project." August 15, 2012. Accessed April 14, 2014, http://www.jointcommission.org/surgical_care_improvement_project/.

Thompson, D. L., Makvandi, M., and Baumbach, J. "Validation of Central Line-Associated Bloodstream Infection Data in a Voluntary Reporting State: New Mexico." *American Journal of Infection Control* 41, no. 2 (2013): 122–125.

Thompson, E., Mirocha, K., and Sagar, K. B. "Effect of Physician Training on Interpretation of Echocardiography." *Journal of the American Society of Echocardiography* 24 (2009): 54

Tonsing, B. *Stand in the Way—Patient Advocates Speak Out*. Lulu Publishing Services, Lulu.com, 2014, xi–xiii.

Torrey, T. "How to Find a Doctor's Medical Malpractice Track Record." About.com. http:// patients.about.com/od/doctorinformationwebsites/a/malpracticeinfo.htm.

Tower, S. S. "Arthroprosthetic Cobaltism Associated with Metal on Metal Hip Implants." *BMJ* 344 (2012): e430.

———. "Arthroprosthetic Cobaltism: Identification of the At-risk Patient." *Alaska Medicine* 52 (2010): 28–32.

———. "Arthroprosthetic Cobaltism: Neurological and Cardiac Manifestations in Two Patients with Metal-on-Metal Arthroplasty: A Case Report." *Journal of Bone and Joint Surgery American Volume* 92 (2010): 2847–2851.

Twohey, M. "Dr. Ricardo Arze and Sex Abuse Cases Shows Disconnect between Law Enforcement, State Regulators of Doctors." *Chicago Tribune*, July 29, 2010. Accessed March 21, 2014, http://www.chicagotribune.com/health/ct-met-doctor-sex-charges-20100729,0,5520049.story.

Urman, R., and Shapiro, F. "Improving Patient Safety in the Office: The Institute for Safety in Office-Based Surgery." Spring-Summer 2011. http://www.apsf.org/newsletters/html/2011/ spring/02_officesafety.htm.

Valaitis, R. K., Akhtar-Danesh, N., Brooks, F., Binks, S., and Semogas, D. "Online Communities of Practice as a Communication Resource for Community Health Nurses Working with Homeless Persons." *Journal of Advanced Nursing* 67, no. 6 (2011): 1273–1284. doi:10.1111/j.1365 2648.2010.05582.x.

Van Zee, A. "The Promotion of OxyContin: Commercial Triumph, Public Health Tragedy." *American Journal of Public Health* 99 (2009): 221–227.

Vila Jr., H., Soto, R., Cantor, A. B., et al. "Comparative Outcomes Analysis of Procedures Performed in Physician Offices and Ambulatory Surgery Centers." *Archives of Surgery* 138 (2003): 994.

"Viral Hepatitis Outbreaks: Viral Hepatitis Statistics and Surveillance, Healthcare-Associated Hepatitis B and C Outbreaks Reported to the Centers for Disease Control and Prevention (CDC) in 2008-2012." Centers for Disease Control and Prevention. http://www.cdc.gov/ hepatitis/Outbreaks/HealthcareHepOutbreakTable.htm.

Vincent, C. "Understanding and Responding to Adverse Events." *New England Journal of Medicine* 348, no. 11 (2003): 1051–1055.

Wahlberg, D. "Wisconsin Doctors Who Make Mistakes Often Don't Face Serious Consequences." *Wisconsin State Journal*, January 26, 2013. Accessed March 20, 2014, http://host. madison.com/news/local/health_med_fit/wisconsin-doctors-who-make-mistakes-often-dont-face-serious/article_3c6f0602-673d-11e2-a66c-001a4bcf887a.html.

Wald, H., Richard, A., Dickson, V. V., and Capezuti, E. "Chief Nursing Officers' Perspectives on Medicare's Hospital-Acquired Conditions Non-Payment Policy: Implications for Policy Design and Implementation." *Implementation Science*, August 28, 2012. Accessed April 14, 2014, http://www.implementationscience.com/content/7/1/78.

Walter, D. *Collateral Damage—A Patient, a New Procedure and the Learning Curve* (privately published in Charleston, SC, 2011), 1–182.

Weeks, J. C., Catalano, P. J., Cronin, A., et al. "Patients' Expectations about Effects of Chemotherapy for Advanced Cancer." *New England Journal of Medicine* 367 (2012): 1616–1625.

Wegwarth, O., and Gigerenzer, G. "Overdiagnosis and Overtreatment: Evaluation of What Physicians tell their Patients about Screening Harms." *JAMA Internal Medicine* 173 (2013): 2086–2087.

Weissman, J. S., Schneider, E. C., Weingart, S. N., et al. "Comparing Patient-Reported Hospital Adverse Events with Medical Record Review: Do Patients Know Something That Hospitals Do Not?" *Annals of Internal Medicine* 149 (2008): 100–108. doi:10.7326/0003-4819-149-2-200807150-00006.

"WFP Health Talk: The Benefits of Integrative Medicine with Dr. Carol Roberts, MD." *Wiseman Family Practice*. http://www.wisemanfamilypractice.com/wfp-healthtalk-the-benefits-of-integrative-medicine-with-dr-carol-roberts-m/.

Whalen, J. "Glaxo in $3 Billion Settlement." *Wall Street Journal*, July 3, 2012. Accessed October 7, 2013.

"What to Ask Healthcare Providers." *One and Only Campaign.* http://oneandonlycampaign. org/content/what-ask-healthcare-providers.

White, C. M., Statile, A. M., Conway, P. H., et al. "Utilizing Improvement Science Methods to Improve Physician Compliance with Proper Hand Hygiene." *Pediatrics* 129, no. 4 (2012): e1042–1050.

"Why Intuitive Issued a Recall for da Vinci Surgical System." Accessed April 14, 2014, http:// www.advisory.com/daily-briefing/2013/12/06/intuitive-says-da-vinci-surgical-system-can-stall-issues-recall.

*WHO Guidelines on Hand Hygiene in Health Care: First Global Patient Safety Challenge Clean Care Is Safer Car*e. Geneva: World Health Organization, 2009.

Williams, J. R., Mechler, K. M., Akins, R. B., et al. "The Rural Physician Peer Review Model©: A Virtual Solution." http://www.ahrq.gov/downloads/pub/advances2/vol2/Advances-Williams_115.pdf.

Wilson, D. "Mistakes Chronicled on Medicare Patients." *New York Times*, November 15, 2010. http://www.nytimes.com/2010/11/16/business/16medicare.html?_r=0.

Winters, B., Custer, J., Galvagno Jr., S. M., et al. "Diagnostic Errors in the Intensive Care Unit: A Systematic Review of Autopsy Studies." *BMJ Quality and Safety* 21 (2012): 894–902. doi:10.1136/bmjqs-2012-000803.

Wojcieszak, D., Saxton, J. W., and Finkelstein, M. M. *Sorry Works! Disclosure, Apology, and Relationships Prevent Medical Malpractice Claims*. Indiana: AuthorHouse, 2010. Accessed July 17, 2013, http://books.google.com/books.

Wolf, S. Sidney Wolf to Secretary Kathleen Sebelius, Department of Health and Human Services. March 15, 2011. Accessed March 1, 2014, http://www.citizen.org/documents/1937A.pdf.

Wolfe, S. M., Williams, C., and Zaslow, A. "Public Citizen's Health Research Group Ranking of the Rate of State Medical Boards' Serious Disciplinary Actions, 2009-2011." May 17, 2012. http://www.citizen.org/documents/2034.pdf.

Wu, A. W., Cavanaugh, T. A., McPhee, S. J., et al. "To Tell the Truth: Ethical and Practical Issues in Disclosing Medical Mistakes to Patients." *Journal of General Internal Medicine* 12, no. 12 (1997). Accessed August 20, 2013, doi:10.1046/j.1525-1497.1997.07163.

Yessian, M. R., and Kvaal, M. B. "Quality Assurance Activities of Medical Licensure Authorities in the United States and Canada." *US Department of Health and Human Services Office of Inspector General*. http://oig.hhs.gov/oei/reports/oei-01-89-00561.pdf.

Young, A., Chaudhry, A. J., Rhyne, M. D., and Dugan, M. "A Census of Actively Licensed Physicians in the United States, 2010." *Journal of Medical Regulation* 96, no. 4. (2011): Table 1.

Zhao, J., and Pablos, P. "Regional Knowledge Management: The Perspective of Management Theory." *Behaviour and Information Technology* 30, no. 1 (2011): 39–49. doi:10.1080/044929X2010.492240.

Zimmerman, R. "Delicate Doctoring Moments: A Medical Error by Another Physician." *Common Health Reform and Reality*, November 1, 2013. Accessed February 20, 2014, http://commonhealth.wbur.org .

Zipperer, L., and Amori, G. "Knowledge Management: An Innovative Risk Management Strategy." *Journal of Healthcare Risk Management* 30, no. 4 (2011): 8–14. Retrieved from wileyonlinelibrary.com. doi: 10.1002/jhrm.20064.

Zrelak, P., Utter, G., Banafseh, S., Sadeghi, B., Cuny, J., Baron, R., and Romano, P. "Using the Agency for Healthcare Research and Quality Patient Safety Indicators for Targeting Nursing." *Journal of Nursing Care Quality*, 27, no. 2 (2012): 99–108. doi:10.1097/NCQ0b013e318237e0e3.

Zuckerman, D. M., Brown, P., and Nissen, S. E. "Medical Device Recalls and the FDA Approval Process." *Archives of Internal Medicine* 171 (2011): 1006–1011.

Index

Contributors

Cheryl Brown, DBA, RN, U.S. Army Nurse retired, serves as an Army Medical Command Patient Safety Nurse Consultant for patient safety managers assisting with Sentinel Event root cause analysis and providing feedback for process improvement. She served as Commander of a Combat Support Hospital and is a trauma nurse veteran of the Persian Gulf War. She contributed clinical expertise for a ground nurse character in the book *Centerline*. She completed research on Automated Dispensing Cabinet Improvements Implemented in Army Hospitals to Decrease Medication Errors and is a co-author for "Overcoming Benchmarking Reluctance: A Literature Review" (*Benchmarking: An International Journal*, 2012).

John T. James, PhD, is the former chief toxicologist at a federal agency where he received numerous meritorious awards and wrote many book chapters and monographs dealing with spaceflight safety. As a result of the loss of his oldest son to medical errors in 2002, he has become a patient safety activist, having published a book in 2007 about his son's care (*A Sea of Broken Hearts*) and proposing a national patient bill of rights to empower and protect patients. He publishes a monthly electronic newsletter on patient safety issues and has been appointed to the State of Texas Healthcare Acquired Infection and Preventable Adverse Event Advisory Panel. He just published an evidence-based, peer-reviewed study in a medical journal in which he estimated that more than 400,000 Americans have their lives shortened by medical errors in hospitals. He founded Patient Safety America whose website is http://PatientSafetyAmerica.com.

Rosemary Gibson is a national authority on US health care. At the Robert Wood Johnson Foundation, she designed and led national initiatives to improve health care quality and safety. She was vice president of the Economic and Social Research Institute and served as senior associate at the

American Enterprise Institute. She is principal author of *Wall of Silence*, *The Treatment Trap*, and *The Battle over Health Care*. She serves as an editor for the *Archives of Internal Medicine* series Less Is More.

Dr. Denise S. Lasater, DBA, RN, US Army nurse retired, serves as the US Army Medical Command risk manager with thirty-eight years of experience as a professional nurse in military, government, and civilian health care delivery systems. Her role includes development, implementation, and evaluation of the risk management in a Joint Service environment promoting risk reduction in health care outcomes.

Lisa McGiffert, BA, directs Consumers Union's Safe Patient Project. Consumers Union is the advocacy arm of *Consumer Reports*. The campaign works on state and national levels to make information available to consumers about medical harm, focusing on health care–acquired infections, medical errors, physician safety, and medical device safety.

Evelyn V. McKnight, AuD, is president of the HONOReform Foundation. She is one of ninety-nine cancer survivors who contracted hepatitis C through substandard medical care in 2002. She helped found Hepatitis Outbreaks' National Organization for Reform (www.HONOReform.org) and co-authored *A Never Event: Exposing the Largest Outbreak of Hepatitis C in American Healthcare History*.

Robert E. Oshel, PhD, retired as associate director for research and disputes of the National Practitioner Data Bank in 2008. He led the US Department of Health and Human Services's research into malpractice and medical discipline issues and also headed the department's Secretarial Review process for disputed Data Bank reports.

Gerald Rogan, MD (University of Michigan,'72), of Rogan Consulting, practiced emergency medicine and general medicine for twenty-five years, then served as medical director of a Medicare and Medicaid contractor in California. He is the lead author of a disaster analysis of the Redding Medical Center debacle (1997–2002) during which more than seven hundred patients were damaged by two physicians in conspiracy with the hospital's leadership.

Kiran B. Sagar, MD, FAHA, FACC, is an adult cardiologist with keen interest in accurate imaging interpretation. She held positions of professor (tenured) and interim chief of cardiology and director of noninvasive cardiology at the Medical College of Wisconsin. She has written several scientific manuscripts and book chapters and presented at national meetings.

Daniel M. Saman, DrPH, MPH, CPH, serves as chief epidemiologist at Health Watch USA, where he has championed the implementation of standards and protocols for MRSA surveillance. His focus as associate research scientist at Essentia Institute of Rural Health is on reducing health disparities among rural Americans.

Stephen S. Tower, MD, received his medical degree from the University of Washington (Seattle) and completed internships/residencies at the Oregon Health Sciences University (Portland), Shriners Hospital for Children (Portland), and Dartmouth Hitchcock Medical Center (Lebanon, New Hampshire). He is a member of the American Academy of Orthopaedic Surgeons and the clinical faculty of the University of Washington and has served as president of the Anchorage Orthopedics Society for many years. He has practiced orthopedic medicine in Anchorage since 1992.

Yanling Yu, PhD, is a research scientist at the University of Washington, Washington State. She improves medical regulatory systems and advocates for patient safety. She is cofounder of a Washington State patient safety organization promoting accountability, quality, safety, and responsibility in patient care. She and her husband were instrumental in enacting a Washington State law improving medical board transparency.